THE
BREAST CANCER
COMPANION

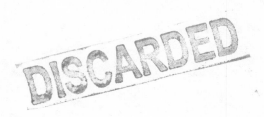

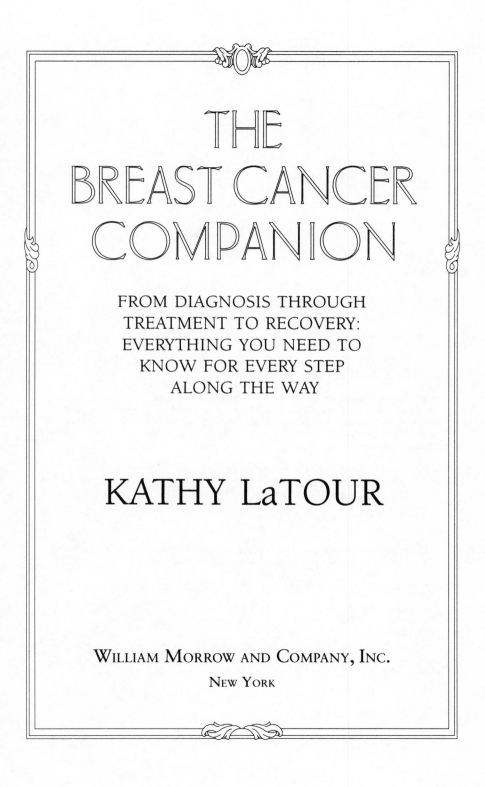

THE BREAST CANCER COMPANION

FROM DIAGNOSIS THROUGH
TREATMENT TO RECOVERY:
EVERYTHING YOU NEED TO
KNOW FOR EVERY STEP
ALONG THE WAY

KATHY LaTOUR

WILLIAM MORROW AND COMPANY, INC.

NEW YORK

Library of Congress Cataloging-in-Publication Data

LaTour, Kathy.
    The breast cancer companion : from diagnosis through treatment to recovery : everything you need to know for every step along the way / Kathy LaTour.
        p.   cm.
    Includes bibliographical references and index.
    ISBN 0-688-11931-X
    1. Breast—Cancer—Popular works.   I. Title.
    RC280.B8L29   1993
    616.99'449—dc20   93-7473
                                                                                    CIP

Printed in the United States of America

First Edition

1   2   3   4   5   6   7   8   9   10

BOOK DESIGN BY MM DESIGN 2000, INC./MICHAEL MENDELSOHN

Dedicated to my husband, Tom Perkins, without whose love and support I would have survived neither breast cancer nor the writing of this book.

To my mother, Mary Josette Stevenson LaTour, who taught me how to ask questions and who died of breast cancer on May 22, 1992.

To my agent, Judy Semler, who kept telling me how important this book was and who began her own battle with breast cancer in May 1992.

And
to my precious daughter, Kirtley, for whom I demand a cure to this insane disease.

CONTENTS

PART II
EMOTIONAL ISSUES AND HEALING:
THE BODY AND THE SPIRIT

PART III
LIFE AFTER BREAST CANCER:
EMOTIONAL AND PHYSICAL ISSUES

ACKNOWLEDGMENTS

This is a book of voices—mine but one—and without the willingness of those closest to this disease to talk about it, it would have been a very short book. I want to thank:

The women whose experiences are the heart and soul of this book. I found them and they found me through flyers I distributed at doctors' offices, through friends, and friends of friends across the country. If anything distinguishes these women it is their diversity: They represent a cross section of American life and experience. The youngest was twenty-three at diagnosis; the oldest was seventy-three, but they shared many of the same feelings. They were black, white, gay, straight, married, single, divorced, mothers, and women without children. Their personalities were as diverse as their backgrounds. Some laughed through the interview and others cried. They represent all levels of education and socio-economic standing. In some instances, I spoke with the men and children in their lives, whose insights into what this disease does to a family were poignant. I felt strongly for these "strong" men, brought to their knees by a threat to the fabric of their family that they could neither kill nor fix with all the resources they possessed.

My special thanks to the twenty professionals from across the country who took time out from their daily struggle with this disease to share their expertise. Dr. Sally Knox, in addition to being my surgeon, is associated with Baylor University Medical Center, which is seeing numbers of breast cancer patients as is Memorial Sloan-Kettering Cancer Center in New York City, which is home to breast specialist Dr. Jeanne Petrek, who gave of her time to comment on the mastectomy vs. lumpectomy issue.

In Dallas we are also fortunate to have a plastic surgeon who has been named by his colleagues as one of the best in the country. Dr. Fritz Barton, Jr., former head of the Division of Plastic Surgery at Southwestern Medical School and pioneer of many reconstruction techniques, brings years of experience in discussing reconstruction options.

Medical oncologist Dr. Robert Mennel and oncologic gynecologist Dr. Allen Stringer offer a combined wealth of information as part of Texas Oncology, one of the largest medical oncology groups in the country.

Dr. Michael Lagios, at California Pacific Medical Center, has seen the birth of modern mammography in his tenure as a pathologist and offers expertise about the in situ diagnosis, while his West Coast colleague radiation oncologist Dr. John Gebert of West Coast Radiology and Western Medical Center comments on the newest advances in radiation therapy.

Dr. Joseph Fay, who established one of the country's first bone marrow transplant programs at Duke University Medical School, and is now the director of the Bone Marrow Transplant Unit at Baylor University Medical Center in Dallas, offers the perspective of one who has seen the procedure move from experimental to one that can save the lives of high-risk women.

And Dr. Amanullah Khan, Ph.D., an oncologist, hematologist, and immunologist at St. Paul Medical Center in Dallas, combines immunology and oncology to treat his breast cancer patients while also spending a significant amount of time researching ways to unlock the body's own ability to fight cancer naturally.

While these excellent physicians struggle daily with the physical manifestations of this disease, an entire cadre of professionals assist with the equally important healing of the spirit.

My love and thanks go to Jan Pettigrew, R.N., Ph.D., now in Little Rock, Arkansas, whom I met when she began a support group through my surgeon's office in 1989. At that time, only a few physicians in the country were conceding that there was more to healing than scars and hair growing back. Since then I have seen an explosion in the acceptance of the need for our soul healers. People such as Jan, and Charles Kluge, Ph.D., a Dallas clinical psychologist whose practice includes many cancer patients. Dr. Michael Fitzpatrick, a psychiatrist and professor at University of Texas Southwestern Medical School at Dallas, began the first support group in the country only for the men whose significant other had been diagnosed with breast cancer. He is in the process of creating videos to help couples talk during this crisis. And Julie Steele, R.N., brings her years of dealing with children's developmental needs in the midst of cancer in the family to help sort out children's issues during this time.

Also in Dallas we are fortunate to have one of only a few risk analysis experts in the country. Barbara Blumberg, Sc.M., Director of Education at Komen Alliance Clinical Breast Center, counsels women from across the country about their true medical risk.

And who could be more qualified to talk about sex after breast cancer than nurse counselor Lois Green, R.N., a breast cancer survivor who was a single at the time of her diagnosis, and a former head of the Nashville, Tennessee, Council on Human Sexuality. Just as George Liepa, Ph.D., nutritionist, and college professor at Texas Woman's University, brings a special poignancy to his discussion of nutrition since his wife is a four-year survivor.

And for those whose mission is to help us die a healthy death when the reality and inevitability descend, I want to thank Family Hospice counselor Joanne Pryor-Carter and grief counselor the Reverend Judy Kane-Smith, whose gifts transcend what most of us can comprehend.

And to my support group. For so many things. For being willing to offer their stories for this book. For listening to me talk about "the book" endlessly, offering solace when I was crazy, coming up with the *Mam-O-Gram* to remind us that we can still laugh at life when we have had cancer; that it is in fact essential that we do. But most of all for teaching me how to live until I die.

To Jane Albritton, Diana Rowden, and Elaine Liner, my friends and, very handily, excellent editors, who suggested, cajoled, inspired, and read endless rewrites.

To the Southern Methodist University Center for Communication Arts, particularly chairman John Gartley, who invited me back to teach while I was still undergoing chemotherapy and helped with time and support for this project so that I could continue teaching college sophomores where to put commas and how to spell *accommodate* while writing this book. And my fine friend David McHam, my first ever writing professor and mentor and now my colleague, without whose early encouragement I would have given up writing altogether.

And finally, to two wonderful editors: Liza Dawson at William Morrow for her faith, trust, and enthusiasm.

And Marjorie Braman at Avon Books for being in her office the day my agent dropped by, and for surviving her own breast cancer experience so that she might be the perfect midwife to this child of mine.

INTRODUCTION

HOW TO USE THIS BOOK

"Your mammogram came back highly suspicious," said the voice on the phone.

"What does that mean?" I asked.

"It means you probably have breast cancer," she said.

Now I understood the cliché "gripped by fear." Seven little words, but they cut through my life very cleanly, dividing it neatly into a *before* and *after*.

When I learned in October 1986, at the age of thirty-seven, that I had breast cancer, friends immediately asked if I was keeping good notes for the book that they were sure would follow. Being a writer, I too expected that I would be drawn to the word processor, where words would work their usual magic in my life.

But I didn't write about my cancer. In fact, I couldn't. Anytime I began thinking about writing the word *cancer,* panic struck. Indeed, not until the fall of 1989, three years after my diagnosis, did I begin to feel the urge to write of my experiences. All of a sudden I felt safe.

I understand now that in order to write about breast cancer, I had to feel that I would live through it.

When, all of a sudden, I wanted to write about breast cancer, it became an obsession. There were so many things that I knew now that I wish I had known then—the day I got the call. I became determined that other women would have that information in as much detail and range of experience as I could manage from the real experts in this disease, the women who had been there.

Indeed, as soon as I hung up the phone that fateful Friday, my journalist persona took over as I walked into the bedroom and calmly told my husband, Tom, what had transpired and explained that I wanted to go to the bookstore *now*. I didn't understand then why he kept reminding me to breathe. My sense of control in life has always come from information. I was out of control. It was as if there were two people functioning simultaneously in my body: the thinking "me" and the panic-stricken "other."

My trip to the bookstore didn't help. I expected to find many books on the subject—books that would tell me I wasn't going to die, books that would speak to the fear consuming me, books that would tell me how to be a wife and mother (to an infant and four stepchildren in their teens) and to continue with my writing career while *doing cancer*.

I was going to have to make medical decisions very soon in a language that I didn't speak, and my emotional state made absorbing information difficult. I desperately needed to talk to other women who had been through this—but where were they? I think I might have been afraid to look. Were they all dead?

No, we aren't dead. We are here for you in the pages that follow—many of us who either are experiencing or have experienced what you or a loved one is facing.

The women and men who were interviewed for this book are very real people. They could be your neighbors or your family, and their individual stories can be found at the back of the book. They represent the entire spectrum of diagnosis and prognosis. I have tried to offer you a wide range of experience, because, as I am sure you are learning quickly, breast cancer is far from a black-and-white issue.

As you begin reading, you may begin to see yourself in one woman's voice—or in a combination of women. Look for them in the back alphabetically and begin to look for their perspective. You may find you have made a new friend. The women in this book range in age from twenty-three to seventy-three when they were diagnosed, and all chose what would be called an orthodox medical approach to their cancer, although many combined medicine with "complementary" healing, such as nutrition and psychological methods that include visualization, positive thinking, and relaxation.

If you have just learned you have breast cancer, start at page 1 and know that the next few months will be difficult. For you this book becomes a "How to" manual. The movement will be chronological. The medical procedures may result in dramatic changes to your body as you battle the physical aspects of the disease. In these pages you will also hear directly from the health-care professionals who specialize in treating both the physical and emotional aspects of the disease. I tried to ask the questions you would have asked had you been there with me. The medical professionals address the latest in treatment options, while those who care for our spiritual healing look at the possible emotional reactions.

The emotional battle, which is much less clearly defined, will be one of inches and feet before it is miles. Your enemy here is not a mass of nasty cells but fear, guilt, anger, uncertainty, and depression. Just as you overcome one, another will emerge.

If you found this book in the midst of treatment, don't concern yourself with what you should have done that you didn't. Go to Part II and understand where you are emotionally with all its confusion and ambiguity—that every feeling is normal.

This book recognizes that breast cancer is a battle that must be fought on two fronts—physical and emotional. The physical battle, with variations, becomes primarily a battle of endurance. The emotional battle is unique to each woman and varies greatly with her history, her personal power, her sense of self, her support system, and her determination.

Know that this is not a book just for the first few months of breast cancer. Resolution of this disease is a process that takes years—and for some of us it has become a mission. I hope that you will find yourself referring to it over and over again and then lending it to friends and family so that they will understand how you are and where you are.

If you are reading and the first comment doesn't fit where you are, continue on. For you must understand is that this is a unique process. For example: Women vary in their feelings about their physical selves. Some have found their definition and self-worth in their physical attributes. For these women the removal of a breast cuts much deeper than through tissue and skin. You will hear the voices of those who feel this loss keenly, while you may not. But even those of us whose self-esteem exists in spite of our physical selves must grieve the loss of a body part.

While some women felt the loss of a body part was the most traumatic issue of this disease, others felt it was insignificant compared to the thought of confronting one's mortality, which is frightening and life-changing. And for those of us with children remains the chilling, gut-wrenching thought that we may not live to rear them.

But no matter where you are in this disease, you share with each of us the sense that the future has been irrevocably altered. Gone is the innocent faith that it would be for us always as it has been, ready to be shaped and planned for. Plans, dreams, and hopes are put on hold at worst and tainted with constant uncertainty at best. Our lives have become a maybe.

My sincerest hope is that you will never personally need the chapter that addresses dying. I do know that if you are remotely involved in the breast cancer community, you will be faced with this issue head on—46,000 of us will die this year, as we did last year. Yet coming to an understanding of death is life-affirming work, and when you are ready, it will be the work that takes you to depths of this disease—a place where true healing can begin. I personally have come to believe that in order to live with this disease, we must struggle with the fact that we could die from it.

And this will all take place in relation to the family you have now or hope to have one day. Yours is not an isolated struggle but one that involves lovers, husbands and husbands to come, children and children wished for, families and future families.

Your present now revolves around being sick, getting well, staying well, and living with (and making peace with) the fear that such a struggle dictates. And we're here to help.

Also know that you are not alone in your search for information. The American Cancer Society estimates that 182,000 women will be diagnosed with invasive breast cancer in 1993. Thousands more women will undergo surgery and treatment for an intraductal/in situ diagnosis. This year's figures are higher, as each year's figures have been for the past decade. While the numbers increase, the ages of the women decrease. What used to be a disease primarily of women over sixty has in the past two decades begun to appear with increasing frequency in women in their twenties, thirties, and forties. Why? To a degree the increasing numbers of young women can be attributed to better screening and earlier detection, but that's only part of the answer. The other factors of this epidemic remain a mystery.

While the incidence of breast cancer has risen significantly in the past decade, early detection and improved treatment have kept the death rate basically unchanged since 1930. *So while many more women than ever before are getting breast cancer, many more women than ever before are surviving breast cancer.*

Today, no matter where you are in the breast cancer process, you are a survivor. You have joined the 1.5 million of us who go on in the wake of this epidemic. How you will do that presents many options, some of which are spoken by women who have crossed that chasm.

In this book you will find both the unique aspects that each woman brings to the disease and the collective experience—those issues with which we all struggle. Although I thought I had no expectations when beginning this book, I soon found that I could be surprised again and again in interviews. Indeed, the outline for this book was a creation with a life of its own as women addressed issues and questioned me about issues relating to breast cancer. *They wanted to know if I knew why they had gotten breast cancer.* It is the question for which we all seek an answer. We have heard the list of high-risk factors, some of which we can own as ours. But there is also the compelling statistic that around 70 percent of the women being diagnosed today have *none* of the high-risk factors.

As I talked to women who were physically fit, bore their children young, and had no family history, it became clear that there is no simple answer to the question Why?

As these women shared their experiences, there were commonalties such as doctors and treatment options. But the reactions and feelings about these common areas varied greatly.

We shared panic attacks and a fear of dying. But our personal reactions to the emotional recovery from breast cancer were unique. If there is a truism about breast cancer, it is that it does not discriminate. Some of the women in this book began the breast cancer experience as passive, disengaged women to whom life happened. They came out of it with a new sense of identity and purpose, having chosen through the experience to finally engage in life. Other women sank deeper into life's pain. Others made dramatic life-style changes. Some sought help in groups or with an individual counselor to explore not only how to cope with cancer but how to cope with life. Some sought no help, but now wish they had. Some found their interpersonal relationships dramatically restructured, requiring a new level of communication with husbands and loved ones.

They know now that a woman shouldn't do this without support. It is one of the clearest messages they have for you, and one that has added emphasis by the medical and psychological information now being released on the importance of reducing stress and its impact on the immune system.

Never before have cancer patients faced such a barrage of information about their mental well-being and its impact on disease. It is now well documented that those cancer patients who do the best are those who are active in their treatment options and feel empowered in their choices for a cure. It seems logical that in order to live, one has to *want to.*

Then there are those who blame cancer patients for their illness and admonish them to discover the secret in their past or the unresolved issue in their life that is causing cancer. If this were so, I know at least two dozen people who should have died years ago, so beset are they by dysfunctional families and unresolved issues.

Some of the women accepted responsibility for their cancer, citing divorce, illness, or other catastrophic events in the eighteen months prior to their cancer. Others said the time preceding their cancer was the best of their lives.

Much remains unknown and unclear about the mind/body connection in disease and healing. The psychological variables when combined with physical variables result in countless combinations for each individual, some of which may have contributed to cancer. Such combinations make the scientific study of such links all but impossible. Medical science for the most part tends to discount anything it cannot study, and the human spirit remains one of those intangibles that defies control-group analysis.

The women in this book took many paths in their treatment options—with varied outcomes. Some had a positive prognosis and followed all suggested treatment and did well. They are considered cured. Others with the same prognosis followed the same path and suffered recurrence. During and since breast cancer many have married, divorced, dated, given birth to children, and reared children. Many continued professional careers—few could "take time off" for cancer.

It's a unique sorority and one to which you now hold a lifetime membership.

MY STORY

When the call came that October evening in 1986, the voice on the other end of the phone was my obstetrician, who was also my friend.

One year earlier, she had held my hand through a very difficult pregnancy and the premature birth of my daughter, Kirtley. In fact, it was at my one-year visit just the week before that I had pointed out a small lump in my right breast that I had discovered the previous week as the result of a strange, painful itching. Neither of us was concerned. At thirty-seven I was too young for breast cancer, and everyone knows that cancer has no feeling (two myths debunked!). But she suggested a mammogram. I sensed that it was not something to delay and went the next day.

She called on Friday night with the results. I recall her explaining that the lump would have to be taken out and biopsied and that I would have to find a surgeon. Someplace in my gut I was screaming, "I can't find a surgeon, I can't do anything; I have cancer. I am going to die. I have a one-year-old daughter, and she won't even remember me." It was a thought too crushing to sustain for more than an instant.

I moved through the house like an image from a carnival fun house. My head went first, followed by a body that seemed to undulate from the shoulders down. My body had turned on me. It was trying to kill me.

What followed for me was five months that included surgery and chemotherapy and seven years that have included an indescribable journey into myself and out again.

Like all breast cancer patients, I'll never know the critical moment when some aberrant cell in my body decided to go haywire and begin multiplying. What I do choose to acknowledge are factors that I believe led to my cancer. They are unique to my history and not meant to be a guideline for any other women.

But like most other women I have talked to, I needed to decide why I got breast cancer in order to better cope with it and to accept that these factors could affect my daughter's risk of breast cancer.

At thirty-six I became a first-time mother to a 3 lb. 14 oz. premature infant who didn't sleep for six hours straight until she was three months old. My diet after Kirtley's birth became more erratic at a time when I should have been building my immune system. I was emotionally and physically spent. My estrogen level had been up and down, and I was already at high risk by having had my first child after age thirty-five.

In October 1991, almost five years to the day after my diagnosis, my mother was diagnosed, and I learned I had another high-risk factor—family history.

In addition, while information concerning birth control pills and breast cancer is contradictory at best, new studies point to those of us who took the pill in the late sixties, when the dosage was four to five times what women take today. We took them early in our childbearing years for extended periods, and new studies (some of which are refuted by other studies) indicate that that combination could result in a risk five times greater than normal for developing breast cancer.

I consider myself an open person, but the possibility that unexpressed anger was causing stress has prompted me to be much more open about my feelings (my husband, Tom, says I am succeeding).

Lest I sound like one of those who has bought entirely the idea that I caused my cancer, I also blame our environment and the endless combinations of carcinogens to which we have been exposed growing up in the twentieth century. I remember clearly my pesticide-covered neighborhood—free of mosquitoes, but covered with a fine mist of chemicals twice a week. What effect, I wonder, did the twice-weekly DDT spraying have on my health? How many other carcinogens played a part in my cancer, I will never know, but in spring 1992 studies showed that the breast tissue of women who had had breast cancer showed much higher levels of PCBs found in pesticides! How I can protect my daughter from the possibility of breast cancer in light of all the questions for which there are no answers is another set of issues.

Physically, I have recovered well from breast cancer. After undergoing a modified radical mastectomy in October 1986, I underwent six rounds of chemotherapy, due to one malignant lymph node.

The chemotherapy experience can only be described as the most difficult thing I have ever experienced. For two years following chemo, I became nauseated just driving in the general direction of my oncologist's office. During chemo I threw up until I thought I would die; I lost every hair on my head; I had a mouth full of ulcers for two months. It took months for my energy to return and to begin to feel human.

I also know I would do it again in a minute after researching this issue for more than two years (and the introduction in 1990 of the antinausea drug Zofran, which has eliminated nausea for a significant percent of women). I have also talked to women who lost only a part of their hair and bounced back well. It isn't easy watching your hair accumulate in the drain, but it is easier than watching your baby toddle toward you and to know you aren't doing everything possible to ensure you will be around to rear her.

In 1988 I had a back-flap breast reconstruction, in which my back muscle was moved to my chest wall, along with a wedge of skin, underneath which a silicone implant was placed. The nipple was formed with skin from my upper thigh and then tattooed to match the existing nipple. The left breast was lifted to match the newly constructed breast. No, I don't look the same. I have a long scar down my back, and the scars on my reconstructed breast are still a little pink. But I can move my new breast, and I am gradually regaining feeling in the armpit and surrounding areas. And with the changes on the left breast, my chest looks like it did when I was eighteen: firm and straight ahead.

While I am constantly amazed at the physical result of reconstruction, I was totally unprepared for the enormous emotional change that occurred after reconstruction. In a way, I am whole again physically. When I'm dressed in bathing suits and nightgowns, no one would know I had ever had breast cancer.

I wish my soul and psyche were so easily restored. Emotionally, I remain on the roller-coaster ride that is life after breast cancer. On my good days, I praise medical science for the speed and efficiency with which they removed the cancer. I think of myself as a cancer survivor and even find myself grateful for chemotherapy. I can even have a sense of humor about breast cancer from time to time, and on my good days I list the positive changes cancer has wrought in my life. My panic attacks seem farther apart now, and I no longer lie in bed and cry quietly as I wonder how my daughter will cope with adolescence after I have died.

On my bad days I have a pain that quickly becomes chronic. Sure that I am dying, I call my oncologist. I scan reports of those who have died of cancer, comparing and contrasting my pathology. I know deep in my heart that this insidious disease can lurk for years before being triggered to attack. I have planned my own funeral and made my husband promise I could die at home if that time ever comes.

But the bad days are fewer now than last year, which was better than the year before that. I just read one statistic that says it takes us three years to (choose one) get over, assimilate, cope with, recover from, deal with breast cancer. No, I don't think "get back to normal" is a choice in that sentence. How your life will change as a result of breast cancer is up to you.

I have learned a number of things about myself since discovering I had breast cancer. Before being diagnosed, I was in the middle of the postpartum blues as I tried to decide personal directions. I was irritated with little things. My prayer life consisted of questions such as, Where am I going? What do you want from me? Help me see what is important in life.

Now I know what is important. And while I am not to the point that I can call my cancer a gift, it certainly clarified my life for me and provided a few truths:

I can live without a breast.

Relationships are not based on breasts.

I have a high pain tolerance.

I don't like to vomit.

Hair grows back.

Children grow up no matter what.

On the more introspective level, I have come to accept that I have had cancer, but that fact does not have to ruin or rule my life. I have a lot to live for, and I intend to live for it. I know now that fear can be more painful than surgery. But most of all I know I now have the personal power to make my own decisions.

This last truth is perhaps my greatest wish for you in the pages of this book: That from the women who have been there you find the personal power to live with and through breast cancer to whatever outcome there is. And that by hearing from those who travel the path with you will come a better understanding of your ability to make choices for your life and find the most effective tools to live with peace, love, dignity—and cancer.

Kathy LaTour
Dallas, Texas
July 1993

GLOSSARY

In the last section of the book you will read the short biography of each woman interviewed for this book. What you do not know about these women is the individual pathology analysis of their particular cancer cells. DNA testing has resulted in the identification of many variations of breast cancer cells. This information now determines treatment and prognosis with greater certainty than ever before, but each one is a highly individual case.

In this book you will be introduced to a new vocabulary. Begin to listen for the new words, and always ask your doctors for their definitions. Here is the basic dictionary for breast cancer.

Adjuvant treatment: Preventive treatment when the tumor has been removed and, while there is no evidence of disease, the surgeon and oncologist feel that there might be microscopic cells lurking. Chemotherapy, hormone therapy, and radiation therapy are all adjuvant.

Aspirate: Many lumps are fluid-filled cysts. A surgeon will first try to remove the fluid with a needle, which is called aspirating. Performed by a **surgeon.**

Axillary dissection: The name of the procedure to remove the lymph nodes. Every woman has a different number clustered like grapes under her arms. In some instances, when it appears the cancer is contained, a surgeon may remove just a few. In other instances, where the surgeon feels that the cancer may have moved into the lymph nodes, all may be removed for examination.

Benign: Not cancerous.

Biopsy: Removal of some cells or the entire tumor from the body by either a needle or through surgery to be studied by a **pathologist** to determine if the tumor is malignant or benign and to determine a number of other factors about the cells in the tumor.

Calcifications: Areas in the breast where the cells have died and calcium salts from the blood have calcified are common and do not necessarily indicate malignant cells, but certain patterns of calcifications are more likely to indicate malignancy.

Chemotherapy: Cancer-killing chemicals administered to the entire body through the bloodstream to kill any cancer cells in the blood that may have traveled from the primary tumor site.

Ducts: The hollow tubes in the breast that carry the milk to the nipples.

Intraductal carcinoma (also called noninvasive carcinoma and ductal carcinoma in situ): The cancer has remained inside the ducts. It may mean there is a tumor within the ducts or it may mean there are masses of cells.

Invasive (also called infiltrating) ductal carcinoma: The cancer has broken through the duct walls into the surrounding tissue.

Lobular carcinoma in situ: A precancerous condition in the lobules that may or may not develop into invasive cancer. Women with lobular carcinoma are at greater risk of developing it in the other breast also.

Lobules: The part of the breast tissue that makes milk.

Localized breast cancer: Only the breast tissue is involved.

Lymph nodes: Clustered like grapes under each arm (and in many other places in the body), these nodes move the lymph fluid throughout the body while fighting infection and diseases. The lymph nodes act as a barrier, and the number of nodes invaded by the cancer indicate to what degree cells have moved into the body. The more **positive** (malignant) nodes involved, the greater the chance that the cancer has spread to other parts of the body, or will in the future. The number of positive nodes will have a direct impact on treatment and prognosis.

Malignant (cancerous): The cell is not normal and divides at a much more rapid rate than normal cells, taking over healthy tissue.

Mammogram: The X ray of the breast that shows variations in tissue. There are degrees of sensitivity on mammograms that can detect areas of concern. Those done at mobile units offer a general screening, while technology at certified sites can do more specific and closer inspection. Read by a **radiologist.**

Metastatic breast cancer: Either at diagnosis or after diagnosis, the breast cancer appears in another organ of the body. This is still considered breast cancer because it is a breast cancer cell that is growing elsewhere.

No Evidence of Disease: After the tumor is removed, you have no obvious signs of cancer in the body. You are NED.

Protocol: The treatment selected for your cancer. Usually prescribed by a **medical oncologist.**

Radiation: Used to kill cancer cells by radiation of the affected area. Performed by a **radiation therapist** or a **radiation oncologist.**

Recurrence: Evidence of new tumor growth in the body after a time of No Evidence of Disease. Can be local, in the area of the breast, or elsewhere in the body. Breast cancer most often recurs in the liver, lungs, or bones.

Systemic breast cancer: Lymph nodes are involved, indicating that microscopic cancer cells have made it past the body's natural defense and may end up in another part of the body.

Trial: A new treatment that has not yet been accepted as a general treatment. A drug or protocol that is being tested for effectiveness.

Tumor: Mass of cells that has formed into a hard mass.

Wire (or needle) localization: When the cancerous area is very small, as is frequently the case with calcifications, the radiologist will first guide a thin wire to the cancerous spot, using mammography, and then the surgeon will remove the wire and the suspicious area.

PART I

DOCTORS, DIAGNOSIS, SURGERY, and RECONSTRUCTION

THE MEDICAL AND EMOTIONAL ISSUES

Chapter 1

---◆---

IT BEGINS

WELCOME TO SHOCK

"Breast cancer is one big title for tumors that vary greatly. I have seen tumors the size of an orange with no spread to the lymph nodes. I have also seen cases when the tumor is the size of a pen eraser and there are already nodes involved."

—Dr. Sally Knox, breast surgeon

The diagnosis of cancer catapults us into the senseless world of shock and denial. Our listening is impaired, and at a time when we need information to make critical decisions, we can barely concentrate on the daily paper.

A couple of months after my mastectomy, I remember wondering out loud about something relating to my surgery. My husband, Tom, responded, "Don't you remember, the doctor said . . ."

No, I didn't remember. I really didn't, and I had paid careful attention—or so I thought. I am a journalist; listening is my profession. Yet it became increasingly clear to me that Tom had heard many things that somehow escaped my consciousness. Some call it "selective hearing," born of a desperate need to hear the right answers. After the first few interviews for this book, I found that I was not alone in having missed some critical information. Almost every woman I talked to described herself as in some form of shock or denial during the time surrounding the diagnosis.

Betty was four months pregnant with a very wished for child when she learned she had breast cancer. She recalls the surgeon saying immediate surgery was necessary due to the size of the tumor. When they returned home, she asked her husband to tell their six-year-old son.

"He said he would tell him that we found out today that your mom has cancer and that means she's going to be sick for a while and she's going to have to have chemo, and it'll make her sick and her hair's going to fall out. I said, 'Oh, honey, those are just wives' tales. Things like that don't happen anymore.' And he started crying because the oncologist had told us all of that and I had no memory of it. I just lost it. I truly did not hear a word."—Betty

Tip—It is estimated that patients hear 10 percent of what is said to them during an initial diagnosis of cancer.

"We had gone back to the surgeon several times before it dawned on me that we were going to see a doctor in a building for cancer patients and the doctor was a cancer doctor. My mind just had a very difficult time accepting that. Dot is the healthiest person I have ever known in my entire life, and I have never seen her sick. To suddenly be confronted with accepting the ultimate sickness is something I still have a hard time with."—Dot's husband, Jack

One woman said that being diagnosed with breast cancer was like being caught in a tornado: *"I was being whipped around by this tremendous force that left me totally out of control."*

So take a deep breath. If you are reading this, you are probably caught in that tornado. The situation dictates that you act quickly, but the relationships you form and decisions you make in the next few weeks have long-term implications.

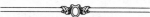

Tip—Get as much information as you can and demand to be a participant in your care. As one woman said, "Make speed, not haste."

At a time when you feel least able, you must make choices about who will care for you, what kind of care you want, and where you will receive that care. Family decisions must also be made about your care and who will care for the children during your recovery. If you are alone, you must rally friends or family to be close. Your employer needs basic information about your condition—information you may not yet know.

This time is hard. One woman called it "free fall." Even if you are good at crisis management and function well under stress, this is different. This is about mortality.

This chapter focuses on those issues facing you immediately in a simple, clear fashion. In order to be an active participant in the decision-making process, you need basic information. I remember feeling left out during the early months of my cancer diagnosis and treatment. It was like being in the room but not being present. I felt talked about. My surgeon, Sally Knox, would ask if I had any questions, but I couldn't think of any—I know now that I was overwhelmed.

This chapter also addresses your immediate needs: understanding your diagnosis, choosing doctors, understanding your surgical options, and getting information. You will also hear directly from two **breast specialists** and a **pathologist** on diagnosing breast cancer, finding a surgeon, and making the choice for lumpectomy or mastectomy.

Read as much as you can. If you can't handle all the information now, read the tips and save the rest for later.

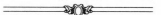

Tip—Buy a notebook with pockets and a calendar. Make dividers with blank paper for each topic: doctors, surgery, insurance, etc. Begin keeping a jour-

nal of dates and people talked to. The pockets are
great for storing copies of your letters, notes, and
reports from doctors. Keep a file at home to transfer
all paperwork for insurance claims. Keep everything.

TAKING CHARGE

*"If you think something is wrong, don't let a doctor tell you there's not.
Don't let him say you're just a tired housewife or whatever, because if
your body is telling you something, you need to listen even if it takes
going to ten doctors in a row. I knew something was wrong, and everybody kept telling me, 'You're fine, you're fine,' and eventually I let them
convince me."*—Leanne

I used to think *doctor* was a generic term. A doctor is a doctor is a
doctor. And they are always right because they went to medical school,
and they are all caring and have our best interests at heart because that's
why they became doctors.

Wrong on all counts. Doctors, like all other professionals, are people
with varied pasts, interests, personalities, and skill levels. They are not
gods; they are people with quirks and limitations—just like the rest of
us there are excellent doctors, good doctors, and bad doctors. It's up
to *you* to find the one who's right for you.

Yet, most of us have been taught to trust them all equally. From the
pediatrician we had as a child, to the ob/gyn we saw when we became
women, we have handed over our lives. Unfortunately for young
women, many of our well-care physicians, whether general practitioners
or gynecologists, are still unaware that this disease can strike young and
very young women and therefore do not act aggressively when women
explain that they have found a lump.

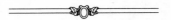

Tip—Trust your body and your instincts about
what your body is telling you. Don't let anyone talk

**you out of your instincts. There is *no way* of know-
ing absolutely whether a lump is benign or malignant unless those cells are examined under a
microscope.**

---

*"The doctor is a human and humans make errors, but there's some-
thing instinctive inside you that tells you. I went back twice, saying this
isn't right. You saw something in the mammogram that's abnormal.
They allayed my fears, yet there was something inside me saying, 'Do
something,' and I didn't act on it soon enough."*—Sylvia

*"She did an examination, and the very first thing she said to me
was, 'I'm sure it's benign, because women your age do not get breast
cancer. But just in case, I'm scheduling a mammogram this afternoon.'
A lot of doctors would have sent me home, but she said, 'You're too
young, but we are going to do this anyway.' "*—Theresa

Newspapers reported an advisory by the Physician Insurers Association of America in June 1990 that cautioned doctors not to ignore
young women who had found lumps, citing an increase in the number
of malpractice claims being paid due to delayed diagnosis of breast
cancer.

"Self-discovery often may be ignored, especially in younger
women, where the incidence of malignancy is thought to be less
than in older women, and is more difficult to detect," said the report. The study also said that the most common reason for delay in
the diagnosis was that *"the physical findings at the examination failed
to impress the physician."*

"Failure to impress" was reported in 55 percent of the women for
whom diagnosis was delayed. The second most common reason was
that the mammogram reports were negative. Indeed, 35 percent of
the women who ultimately were paid claims for delayed diagnosis
had negative mammograms, and in 14 percent of the cases, the
mammogram was inconclusive.

The study concluded that doctors should not depend entirely on
mammograms and should follow any suspicious findings with a biopsy.

Leanne found the lump herself at age twenty-eight in 1987 and her ob/gyn assured her it was a blocked milk duct since she had just breast-fed her second child. But he also suggested a mammogram. When it came back negative, Leanne was reassured. *"About six months later I started feeling bad. I started to lose weight and was really run-down and had a low-grade fever. I went to my internist. He ran a blood test and urine test and said I was fine, and then he said, 'You've got two little kids at your house and you're tired. It's normal.' I didn't feel right, and everyone was telling me it was normal. So I went to a surgeon and he took one look at my breast and you could see the color drain from his face. He said 'Why didn't you come in before?' I said, 'I have been to two doctors.' "*

Angela was twenty-two when she found a lump, which her regular doctor said should be watched. A year later he finally did a biopsy on what he was still sure was a benign lump. Angela recalls him attempting to waken her enough from the anesthesia to sign the release for an immediate mastectomy. She refused, found an oncologist who began chemotherapy, and never had the remainder of the tumor removed. *"I had too much trust in my doctor and not enough education. I basically laid my life in his hands and that was a dumb move on my part. It's something I'll never do again. But you're brought up to trust your doctors. That's what your mom says: 'Do what the doctor tells you to do.' "*

Joanne had been watching a small lump for two and a half years while her doctor reassured her that it was nothing. *"I ate properly and jogged four miles a day. I thought I was taking good care of myself. I was seeing a doctor and he said the lump was a fatty tumor because nothing showed on the mammogram. I was thinking the whole time, There's something wrong. This is not right. I walked around with that for two years, believing everybody. They couldn't stop me from getting cancer, but I didn't have to have lymph node involvement."*

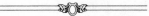

Tip—If you are a very young woman with a lump, it is probably not breast cancer, but be aware that the younger you are, the less effective the mammogram, and if it is cancer, the delay in diagnosis could result in death. Demand a biopsy.

THE PROFESSIONALS

Our primary-care physicians are well-care doctors. You are now looking for a veritable troop of urgent-care doctors and health care professionals who may be your lifelong partners in a life and death struggle.

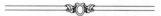

> **Tip—You have some time to find a surgeon. With few exceptions, a few weeks is not going to make a difference in your situation. The immediacy of your individual case will become apparent if you will listen. There is a difference in "You need to have that biopsied," and "You need to have that biopsied today."**

"My internist found the lump, but he didn't think it was suspicious. The mammogram didn't show anything. I really didn't trust that and wanted a surgeon to look at it. I had had a friend the year before whose doctor said not to worry, but it was malignant, and by the time she took it out, it had spread."—Karen

In your cancer care, you will be dealing with more than one doctor, including: a **radiologist,** who reads the mammogram; a **surgeon,** who removes the cancer from your body; a **pathologist,** who studies the cancer cells and reports to the surgeon; and possibly a **medical oncologist,** whose specialty is treating cancer with drugs and the systemic treatment of the disease; and a **radiation oncologist,** who specializes in the external use of radiation to kill cancer cells locally. I would add to this list a **psychiatrist, psychologist,** or **oncology R.N.,** whose specific expertise is your mental well being.

"I was raised in the era when doctors were gods and they were God's helpers. And they are, big-time. In this life that's what they're here for and that's who sent them, the good ones. But they're not gods. They need to work with you as part of your team. Most of them, if they're

good, want your input, because they understand that's how these people heal. That's how they get well."—Joyce

Each doctor and nurse is a specialist. The oncologist and radiation therapist are recommended by the surgeon, who will be the primary contact. Usually, the surgeon will remove the tumor and discuss the pathology report with you before recommending an oncologist. But in some instances, **chemotherapy** may be needed before surgery to shrink the tumor. In that case, you will be seeing the oncologist first. A good, caring surgeon will also be able to put you in contact with a psychologist. If he or she can't, you will be best served by obtaining recommendations from other women who have been there.

I want to stress the word *recommend*. The choice of doctors is up to you. While your primary-care physician may recommend someone, it is up to you to choose that person. Just because you like your surgeon, you don't have to use any other doctor that he or she recommends.

After telling me that my mammogram probably meant that I had breast cancer, my obstetrician said she could recommend a good general surgeon. I remember thinking, "Why can't you do this? I'm afraid; I don't want a stranger doing this and I know you."

Like most young women, my experience with an ongoing relationship with doctors was limited to my ob/gyn. My C-section the year before was my first hospitalization ever. As I contemplated cancer, the idea of a strange doctor didn't help.

I took the name of the general surgeon my ob offered while at the same time thinking that I wanted to find someone at the medical center on my side of town. I remember thinking, after traveling across town twice a day while Kirtley was in the preemie nursery, this cancer stuff will be easier if I am close to home.

My reasoning at that moment had to do with distance and time in the car and convenience for my family. What I would soon learn was that distance would become secondary to finding a doctor who specialized in breast cancer.

I am now glad that the fateful call came on a Friday night. Initially, I was angry. There was nothing I could do until Monday, so I had two whole days to phase in and out of terror. But I also had those days to assimilate as much information as possible about finding a doctor.

I made a hasty trip to the bookstore, where I secured a copy of Rose

Kushner's *Alternatives*. Only a few pages into the book, I realized that I wanted a breast specialist. Why go to a surgeon who has done ten mastectomies and seen fifty lumps in the last year when there is someone who has done one hundred mastectomies and seen five hundred lumps? And just as important, why count on a pathologist who sees fifty lumps when there are those who see thousands?

Bridie lived in Connecticut, not far from the Yale Medical School breast center. When she told her general surgeon, who was in New York City, that she had decided to go to Yale, he wasn't pleased.

> *"He said he didn't believe in these things called breast surgeons. I told him I knew a lot of people who have had this surgery who can't move their arm. Besides these people specialized in breasts. I wasn't going to be dealing with the guy who does spleens on Thursdays and tonsils on Fridays. This guy told me he hadn't done a mastectomy or even a lumpectomy in a year and a half. Gimme a break. I get my tires changed more often than that."*—Bridie

This in no way means that a competent **general surgeon** won't do an excellent job, and for many women who live in smaller towns or have an insurance plan that offers only general surgeons, they are the only choice. But even when the choice is limited, you may find that in your community there is a general surgeon who has become the "breast" surgeon. Often, general surgeons will have a special interest in one kind of surgery. If you are in a small town, find women who have had breast surgery. Does one surgeon's name continue to come up? Ask about him or her. Also look at the next larger town, where your choice may be wider.

For those on an insurance plan that covers them only for doctors involved in the plan, you can still shop around. Victoria belonged to a Health Maintenance Organization (HMO) and didn't like the first doctor she was referred to. She called around and found another in the plan who better suited her needs and who she felt was better qualified. *"I knew that the first one was not for me when he said he might have to 'chop off my breast.' I got on the phone and found a surgeon who had specialized in oncological surgery, or removing cancer. He was great."*

For those of us who are in or close to major metropolitan areas, the decision often is overwhelming because there seem to be so many doctors to choose from. I had the advantage of being only ten minutes from Baylor University Medical Center in Dallas, a designated comprehensive cancer treatment center that offered the most up-to-date treatment and was engaged in a number of studies of breast cancer.

As soon as I determined I wanted a specialist, I put out a call that rivaled the urgency of Paul Revere's midnight ride. Friends and family began calling with recommendations, and when I heard the name Dr. Sally Knox twice from trusted friends, I felt I had found a good choice. I called for an appointment the next day.

What you must decide is whether you will find the same quality of care in the smaller medical center near your home that you would find in a larger city, where cases are frequently shared by staff and the latest equipment and treatment are available. Indeed, it may be that the idea of traveling any distance from home is too frightening. If this is the case, you will probably be dealing with a general surgeon instead of a specialist, a choice that many women have made with excellent results.

But choosing a small general hospital that is not recognized as a cancer treatment center will require more knowledge on your part. Some cancer patients do not receive the most current treatment because their doctors simply are not up on the latest protocols. One woman I met while writing this book was diagnosed at the same time I was. She had a tumor of a similar size and one malignant lymph node. She received what she thought was good treatment from a small suburban hospital close to her home. But her doctor did not recommend chemotherapy as an adjuvant treatment—a protocol that was recommended at all comprehensive treatment centers at that time for women with positive nodes and one that was recommended to me. Subsequently, she experienced a recurrence and died.

On the other hand, just because a doctor serves a rural area doesn't mean he or she is not up on the latest treatment. Kit lived in a small east Texas town when she was diagnosed. She consulted her obstetrician, who asked if she wanted to go to the next larger town. She said no, so the doctor recommended a local surgeon with whom Kit was well pleased. *"The tumor was like a jelly roll and he said it looked fibrocystic. The frozen biopsy showed it was benign. But he told me he didn't like the looks of the tissue and wanted to send it to another lab for further testing. He explained that sometimes the cancer cells don't show up in the frozen state. Well, there were cancer cells in the tumor, and when they did the mastectomy the next week, I already had six lymph nodes that were positive."*

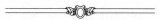

> **Tip—In considering a hospital, try to balance the need for the most up-to-date care with the need to be close to your support system of family and friends.**

Sherry and her husband, Kerry, visited a breast specialist at a cancer treatment center for a second opinion. He agreed with the diagnosis of the original general surgeon, whom she had seen at the suburban hospital near her home. *"One friend insisted we go to a specialist because he said he was the best. I said, Wait a minute—this is my decision. I want to go to Dr. X. I want to be close to home and my babies. I didn't want Kerry to have to drive forty-five minutes every day to come visit me."*

Sherry estimated that they talked with seven or eight doctors before she underwent her mastectomy. They had lived in Dallas for thirteen years and, at the time of diagnosis, had no doctor other than their pediatrician. They asked each doctor they visited about the other doctors they had seen and his or her qualifications and recommendations. *"The surgeon had done a whole bunch of mastectomies, and I also asked for a plastic surgeon to close the incision. I was demanding all these things, and I'd never asked a doctor for anything before."*

> **Tip—Find a doctor who has been well recommended and then get a second opinion. If you still feel uncertain, get a third opinion. And so on.**

At my first appointment with Dr. Knox, I told her who I would be seeing for a second opinion. She agreed that the surgeon was well qualified and encouraged me to see her.

Finding a doctor when you either don't trust your primary physician or don't have one can be more complicated. Other women who have been there are a great source of information, and there are many of us out there now. Nurses and doctors in your community are good sources. Ask friends to ask around, and soon your phone will be ringing with recommendations. There is also a list of sources at the end of this chapter.

After you get some names, make up a list of preliminary questions for the surgeon's nurse, with whom you will talk when you call. Their responses to these questions will narrow your list. Also, the nurses will give you a good introduction to the doctors.

I now listen closely to what the nurse says and her attitude about questions, having found that the nurse is usually a good reflection of the doctor. Doctors tend to hire people much like themselves. And since it's the nurse with whom you will speak when trying to get in touch with the doctor, I am particularly sensitive to how she responds.

QUESTIONS TO ASK THE NURSE

Is the doctor board-certified?

When was the last time he or she updated that certification?

Where did he or she get her training?

How long has he or she been in practice?

Is he or she a general surgeon, or has he or she specialized in either breast or oncologic surgery?

How many biopsies has he or she performed?

How many mastectomies (lumpectomies) has he or she done?

Could you give me the names of some women patients who would be willing to talk to me?

Breast Surgeon Dr. Sally Knox, Baylor University Medical Center, Talks About Finding a Surgeon

How is a breast specialist different from a general surgeon?

After five years of general surgical residency, I did one year specializing in breast oncology. There are also surgical oncologists, who spend two years or more after residency specializing in oncology surgery (removal of malignant tumors); they would also be considered specialists.

I did some extra study concerning breast cancer, but there are many general surgeons who have devoted extra time and interest to the study of breast cancer during their practice. Some of these surgeons spend 50 to 75 percent of their working time caring for women with breast cancer and are well-qualified individuals. The best guide for a patient might be to look for a surgeon who is known to see a high volume of breast patients or indicates a special interest in that field. Almost all surgical oncologists will see a high volume of breast patients.

What should a woman ask a general surgeon?

Ask how many breast cancer patients he or she has seen in the past year or what percentage of his or her patients have breast complaints. Also, it isn't out of line to ask for the name of someone they have treated for breast cancer. A doctor can only give out a name of a patient who has volunteered for this service, but it can't hurt to ask.

How can a woman get the names of surgeons in her area?

The county medical society can supply names of qualified doctors and tell you their qualifications, such as whether they are board-certified. The local chapter of the American Cancer Society

(continued)

can also be helpful, as are other physicians, nurses, or health care workers.

A woman should only go to a board-certified surgeon. In major hospitals you won't find any nonboard-certified surgeons. But in the countryside you will find a lot.

To be board-certified you have to complete a five-year residency, and for specialists, one or more additional years. Also, there is a written and oral exam. They must take an exam in their specialty and must have had training in a good setting. At any major hospital, physicians are required to have continuing medical education each year, and surgeons must recertify every ten years.

What are the red flags a woman should look for in finding a surgeon?

There needs to be a good rapport between patient and physician. Physicians realize that from time to time, regardless of surgical skill, there is just not a good rapport between patient and doctor. Even if that woman is only going to have a biopsy, that may lead to further surgery and an ongoing relationship for many years. Before she has the first biopsy done, she should be confident in her surgeon and feel good about the rapport, feel that she is being heard and that the surgeon is answering questions. If there isn't a good chemistry right then, she should go somewhere else. It doesn't hurt my feelings if a patient finds a better chemistry with another doctor. That is healthy for both parties.

What about getting a second opinion?

A qualified surgeon should not be threatened or angry at a patient's request for further information or a second opinion. My only caution is that it needs to come from another qualified physician and not "Aunt Netti," who had a mastectomy ten years ago. Well-meaning friends or relatives may offer advice or counsel that unintentionally fosters confusion or fear.

A DOZEN REASONS TO LOOK FOR ANOTHER DOCTOR

- The surgeon recommends a Halsted radical or radical mastectomy, an outdated surgery in which the woman's chest muscles were routinely removed. This is appropriate today only if there is an indication that the pectoral muscles are directly involved with the tumor.
- The surgeon says there is no need for a two-step procedure (biopsy and then discussion with patient before mastectomy). If the mammogram or other factors indicate a high probability of malignancy, you and your surgeon may agree on the one-step procedure, but the decision should be up to you.
- The surgeon is defensive about your questions and you feel bullied.
- The surgeon does not want you to get a second opinion.
- The surgeon tells you not to worry about all the details, that he/she will take care of everything.
- The surgeon says there is no time to discuss what you have asked, saying, "Just trust me."
- The surgeon will not look directly at you when addressing you.
- The surgeon balks at giving you copies of your lab work and other paperwork.
- The surgeon balks at having a tape recorder or friend present.
- You get the sense he or she is not telling you everything.
- You feel rushed, as if he or she is eager to get to the next patient.
- You just don't like him or her.

DOCTORS—THE EMOTIONAL MATCH

"I wouldn't buy a pair of shoes from a guy with that kind of attitude. I'll be damned if I let him cut into my body and pay him for the privilege. Forget it. But that's the way it is when we're forced into situations. You're terrified and you don't know the language. You thought you were a healthy person, and someone says you're dying."
—Bridie

"I can't stress enough to women to find doctors who they like and trust. I saw someone first and didn't feel comfortable with her and went to Dr. H for a second opinion and it made a tremendous difference.

The first doctor was very abrupt and cold and I wanted to talk to her before she examined me and she didn't want to do that and she stood in the room while I took my clothes off."—Amy

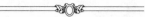

Tip—Don't say yes when your gut says no. You have the right not to like a doctor.

Personality and style are important issues in choosing a doctor. You know if you are the serious type or if you prefer someone whose bedside manner is open and casual.

Some doctors excel at treating a disease but flunk at treating a patient's *disease*. The converse is also true: a doctor may have a consoling and warm personality and not be a great clinician. Bridie met with a plastic surgeon to talk about immediate reconstruction and was unclear about her choices. When she asked a question about one possibility, he said it was stupid. *"I just left. I walked out. He called me and apologized. I told him he was very insensitive. Then he told me why he was making the suggestion he was, and was more explanatory instead of dogmatic."*

Laura Mae described her doctor as impatient with her show of emotion at the diagnosis. She liked his attitude. *"When he first told me I was going to lose my breast, I broke down and sobbed, and I could tell he didn't like it. He said, 'I can save your life. I am offering you life.'"*

At one point during interviews for this book, I interviewed two women who had used the same surgeon for the biopsy. This particular surgeon is a specialist and well known in the city. She works closely with her patients and is involved in facilitating a group at the hospital where she operates. She has excellent credentials.

One of the women interviewed chose to go to another surgeon for her subsequent mastectomy, saying she thought the surgeon was too pretty and was too restrained and unnatural in her communication style. She found the surgeon's personal style unprofessional and disliked her immediately.

The very next interview I conducted was with a woman who thought the *same* surgeon was an outstanding physician and person. She commented on how much she liked her casual nature and easy style. Both of these women were articulate and educated and knew what they wanted. They just wanted and needed different things in a doctor, which is each woman's right.

You also have a responsibility to tell the doctor what you want and expect. If you want a team approach, tell him or her. Make clear how much information you want and how you want to receive it. Keep these "I" statements, such as "I want a doctor who will tell me exactly what is happening and not keep anything from me." Or, "I want someone who is open and caring and will be honest with me, but only on the questions I am ready to ask."

Then realize what a complicated relationship this is when two personalities are brought together in a crisis situation that may or may not be resolved in wellness. You have expectations and fears that you may direct to a doctor, who may or may not be doing what you consider is his or her best, to help you in an area you know nothing about. The best you can do is to be an informed patient and then be as open and honest as possible and expect the same from your doctor.

Marsha says her doctor asked her how much she wanted to know. *"He said this was what he would do as far as the biopsy. Then he stopped and said, 'Is that all you want to know, or do you want to know your options at this point? Some women say, 'We'll just do that and maybe it will be okay and I won't have to deal with it.' I told him I wanted to hear it all right then. So he explained if it was a certain way, we could just do a lumpectomy. If not, we'd have to do the mastectomy. And he really kind of drew out a little flow chart of the decision processes and what we would be deciding on and all that."*

I find it very empowering to listen to women's reactions to doctors. What you should hear in these situations is that you have choices in deciding who will care for you.

"When he arrived, he had a coffee cup in his hand and sleep in his eyes. He did not introduce himself. He asked me to lie down on the bed in his office, and because he didn't introduce himself, I said, 'I assume you are Dr. X.' The nurse said, 'Oh yes, this is Dr. X.' I said, 'Hello, my name is Lise,' and he just said, 'Hello.' He said, 'Why are you here,' while he was getting the needle ready. I asked if he had not looked at my chart even or the mammogram. He said, 'No.' He preferred to get it personally from the patient. I told him to look at my chart before he stuck the needle in."—Lise

Marjorie B was discussing her mammogram with a surgeon when his receptionist entered the examining room twice to hurry him. *"The second time she came in I turned to her and said, 'Do you mind, because this man is telling me I should have a mastectomy.' I turned to him and said, 'You know what? Any doctor who's letting his receptionist do something like this is not somebody I want to deal with. So goodbye.' I felt so empowered by that. I felt like, You're not going to run rough-shod over me."*

Ultimately, Marjorie chose a surgeon at New York's Memorial-Sloan Kettering. *"I didn't like him. He was very abrupt, he was very brusque, and he had no bedside manner, but I traded off. This guy cuts breasts for a living. I don't need my hand held by him. I just need his expertise as a clinician."*

THE FIRST APPOINTMENT

"I took my sister to my appointment, and that weekend I was digging through books looking for information and there was this three-page typed thing and I was like, What is this? Where did it come from? And she had typed up the notes from our meeting with the doctor and it was all the information I was looking for in the books."—Anne

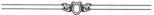

> **Tip**—Take a tape recorder to sessions with the doctor. This way you don't have to stop listening to write down notes. You can listen to the tape at home as many times as it takes for the information to sink in. If you don't have a tape recorder, take a friend who is close enough to care but distant enough to be objective. Ask this person to take notes as you talk with the doctor.

Let's slow the action now and focus on your first appointment with the surgeon you have chosen.

At this point you have a suspicious lump or area on a mammogram that your ob or your internist feels should be biopsied. You have called the surgeon's office and told the receptionist or appointment secretary what you know concerning the immediacy of the situation. Before you meet with your surgeon, he or she may ask that: (a) you have a mammogram if you haven't had one; (b) you bring your existing mammogram film with you for your appointment; or (c) you have another mammogram done at a location of his or her choice.

Remember that all mammogram technicians are not equally skilled and that the younger the woman, the less effective the procedure can be, because of the density of the breast tissue. Unfortunately, the proliferation of mammogram sites in the past few years has given women a false sense of security—the percentage of false readings increases dramatically in the hands of someone not certified to read them. A mammogram is only a tool to help your surgeon make a sound diagnosis.

Tip—Your mammogram should be performed by a center accredited by the American College of Radiology. Ask if there is a board-certified radiologist on staff and ask for a copy of your report.

The majority of breast cancers are detected because there is a suspicious spot on the mammogram or a lump under the skin that has no feeling. How it feels and how it appears on the mammogram may indicate to a certain degree the probability that it is malignant (cancerous), but it must be biopsied before you can be 100 percent sure. This can happen in a number of ways.

- The surgeon may be able to do a needle biopsy in the office. In this procedure, some cells are drawn up through a hollow needle for study.
- You may need to go into the hospital for day surgery to have the lump or suspicious area removed and studied. This procedure may result in an immediate lumpectomy or mastectomy, which is something you need to discuss with your doctor beforehand.
- If you have a small suspicious spot (not a lump) on the mammogram, you may need a needle localization before the spot is removed surgically. Your breast is placed in the mammography

equipment and then, using the projected image, the radiologist guides a thin wire to the exact suspicious spot. The wire is left in, and you are taken to surgery where the wire and the suspicious area are removed.

Of the first twenty women I surveyed, seven said their tumors did not show up on a mammogram. While my mammogram indicated a 90 percent probability of cancer, many younger women have lumps that either don't show up on the mammogram at all or show up in such a way as to make biopsy necessary. Indeed, in some instances the reluctance to see breast cancer in very young women leads some medical professionals to mislabel a tumor, calling it dense tissue.

Rula, twenty-eight, called her surgeon's office with her mammogram results, which the radiologist had just told her was clear except for an area of density. Her breast specialist, suspecting from the physical exam that all was not well, asked to see the film and assured her it was not dense tissue but a massive tumor. Rula had a 10-centimeter tumor with twelve nodes involved. *"He excused himself after we talked, explaining he was going to go downstairs and have a talk with the radiologist."*

Mammograms work by contrast. Fatty tissue in the breast is clear, while regular breast tissue is white. As a woman ages, her breast tissue tends to be replaced by fatty tissue. Since a tumor also shows up as white on a mammogram, those women with dense breasts may have a clearly palpable lump that will not show up on the mammogram, making a biopsy the only way to be certain that the lump is not cancerous.

According to statistics compiled by Baylor University Medical Center, those lumps that do show up on mammograms as round with distinct borders have a 98 percent probability of being benign. Most cancerous tumors have irregular borders or have a star-shaped appearance.

Improved mammography has also greatly increased the number of women being diagnosed when the cancer cells are still **in situ,** or contained within the ducts or the lobules of the breast. This condition often appears when **calcifications,** which show up on a mammogram like white specks, are clustered. Calcifications are frequently an indicator of **intraductal** cancer (also called **noninfiltrating** or **noninvasive,** as opposed to **invasive** or **infiltrating**), where the cells may or may not be a tumor but have remained contained inside the ducts of the breast.

Women with **lobular carcinoma in situ** (which is precancerous) have a higher risk of the same problem with the other breast.

> *"She showed me the mammogram and it was like somebody had flicked white paint where the calcifications were, and the lump was right there. She said it looked like a textbook case of intraductal cancer."*—Madeline

Therefore, the younger a woman, the more important the skill of the doctor at **palpating** (externally feeling) the lump to determine whether it should be **biopsied.**

A surgeon will generally do a physical exam and then meet with you to make his or her recommendations. Usually, the first exam is done with just the woman; her husband, partner, or friend can join her in the surgeon's office. This is the time to introduce to the surgeon the person who is in this with you and his or her relationship, whether it be spouse, family member, close friend, or significant other.

Today's complex relationships may need clarification for the doctor. A number of the women I talked with had long-term, domestic relationships, and they wanted the other person considered their spouse whether male or female. Unconventional relationships need to be made clear to the surgeon and dealt with both emotionally and legally.

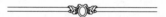

Tip—If you are not legally married, you will need to explore powers of attorney or living wills in your state in order to define who will make the decisions for you if you are unable. Otherwise, the legal party will be parents, children, or closest relative. As of December 1991, anytime you enter the hospital, you will have to address these issues as part of admission.

Before the physical exam begins, ask the surgeon if he or she will talk you through the exam, answering questions such as, "What are you feeling for?" If the surgeon says it would disrupt concentration, then ask that it be explained before the procedure is begun.

In the physical exam, the surgeon will be palpating the lump and the lymph nodes under the arm. In some instances the surgeon will be able to determine a probability of malignancy by touching the breast. If there are palpable lymph nodes under the arm, meaning enlarged nodes, this could be an indication of tumor in the nodes—or they could be swollen from an infection. But they need to be looked at.

In some cases it will be clear from the way the breast looks that there is a greater chance of malignancy. Redness, swelling, pain, and a dimpled surface referred to as *peau d'orange* (because it looks like orange peel) can indicate inflammatory cancer, a more aggressive cancer that will dictate immediate (that day) action.

After the exam, the surgeon will explain what he or she has seen and offer the next step. At this point you should be ready with questions. Here are a few suggestions:

- If the surgeon recommends removing the area or lump surgically, ask him or her to go through the specifics. Will the lump be removed and the cells examined while you are still in the operating room? Will the lymph node be removed at the same time if the lump is clearly malignant? How will you be told the results of the pathology report on the tumor—on the phone or in person? When you are at a loss, just say, "And then what happens?"
- Ask why he or she is making a specific recommendation. Is it based on studies, etc.? Is there any conflicting research? Are there any consensus papers they can give you to read?
- What would your other options be? (There is usually more than one route.)
- Ask him or her to compare procedures—lumpectomy vs. mastectomy.
- Ask how many of these procedures he or she has done. And who does he or she use for pathology; and can you take your slides to an independent pathologist?
- Ask if any of his or her former patients have indicated they would talk to new patients.
- Ask what he or she offers for your emotional recovery during this time.

- If a mastectomy is discussed as an option, ask about immediate reconstruction, done at the time of surgery, and his or her feelings on it. Ask which plastic surgeon he or she works with and whether there should be a consultation if you are interested in reconstruction at any time.
- Does he or she leave skin for reconstruction? How does he or she close the wound? What will the scar look like? Are there any pictures? Ask if he or she uses a plastic surgery stitch to close. If not, you may want to consider asking for a plastic surgeon to close the incision.
- Is there a breast specialist (if he or she is not one) that could be recommended for a second opinion?
- How does he or she feel about you? Would the two of you make a good team?

When I called Dr. Knox's office, she asked that I bring my mammogram film with me rather than get a new one done, since I had had my mammogram done at one of the few accredited locations in the city. She did the initial exam, and then my husband, Tom, and I met with her in her office. At that time she explained that because of the way the tumor looked on the mammogram, she was 85 percent sure it was malignant. She showed us the mammogram and explained that the irregular star (stellate) shape of the tumor was the primary indicator for this diagnosis.

She also said the tumor was small, about 2 centimeters, and because it was in the upper, outer quadrant of the breast, I was a good candidate for a **lumpectomy** (just removing the lump and the lymph nodes). While I ultimately had to have a mastectomy when it became clear that my little tumor had long tentacles, I began preparing for surgery thinking that I would be able to save my breast.

Because the mammogram suggested such a high probability of malignancy, Dr. Knox said the tumor would be biopsied to confirm malignancy in the operating room instead of her office, so that she could then finish the surgery and move me directly to a hospital room. She made the surgery date and an appointment with the radiation oncologist for that afternoon so Tom and I could discuss the procedure for radiation, which follows lumpectomy, to kill any remaining cells in the immediate breast tissue.

The next day I met with the second surgeon, who told me essentially the same information, except that in her estimation there was a 90 to 95 percent probability of malignancy from the look of the mammogram. I asked her opinion of Dr. Knox, and she said I was in excellent hands. I also remember asking her what she would do if I were seeing a surgeon she felt was not good for my case. She was clearly uncomfortable with the issue, but she basically said that if a patient pressed for her opinion of a surgeon, she would offer it if she had knowledge of that surgeon's abilities.

At that time, Tom and I prepared for the biopsy and what we knew would be subsequent surgery of one form or another.

THE BIOPSY

Nothing is certain in breast cancer until the suspicious cells or the lump are examined under a microscope and other sophisticated tests are performed.

Biopsy procedures vary, depending on the mammogram and physical exam. A surgeon may be able to do a fine-needle aspiration in the office, in which a few cells from a tumor are drawn up through a needle. There are also larger needle sections that can be taken with a hollow needle. But in most instances you will be set up for day surgery to have the whole lump removed.

The kind of biopsy a patient has is going to be determined by the factors that point to malignancy—both during the breast examination and on the mammogram. Once the tumor cells are removed, a number of tests will indicate the next step proposed and which combination of therapies is right for you.

In some instances, there are physical signs that indicate surgery is not the immediate answer but rather that the patient needs preliminary chemotherapy before surgery to shrink an existing tumor.

"What determines whether a woman will have preoperative chemotherapy or radiation therapy are specific findings on physical examination. Things such as swelling, redness, an orange skin appearance (dimpled), tumor that is eroding through the skin, or a very large tumor are some of the factors that may prompt a recommendation for preoperative chemotherapy.

"These findings may be associated with a rapidly progressing tumor called inflammatory cancer, so named because it looks much like an ordinary infection or 'inflammation.' Tumors that are not necessarily inflammatory cancers but have not been detected early may also show some of the same signs of swelling, redness, etc. In either of these cases, chemotherapy can usually shrink the tumor substantially and help much of the swelling to disappear, so that when a mastectomy is done, it is easier to get cleanly around the tumor with better long term results."

PATHOLOGY: TESTS ON CANCER CELLS

Dr. Sally Knox explains the procedures.

What is done with the tumor when it is removed?

We do a frozen section immediately while still in the operating room. The tumor is frozen and sliced very thin and examined under a microscope, and that will give us an answer within fifteen minutes if it is cancerous. If it is, then we send the tumor for special tests for estrogen and progesterone receptors and other tests that help us characterize the tumor.

What do the tests for estrogen and progesterone tell you?

Determining if a cancer cell is sensitive to estrogen or progesterone— in other words, has receptors to these hormones—is important for two reasons. We know that those tumors that are hormone-receptive tumors are slower-growing and have a better prognosis than tumors that aren't. It also tells us whether the tumor can be treated with some kind of hormonal therapy, such as tamoxifen.

What do DNA tests show?

The DNA test looks at the individual cells to determine if there are too many or too few pairs of chromosomes. If there are too few or too many, the cell is *aneuploid*. If there are the correct number, it is *diploid*. Diploid is a good sign because it says that the tumor cell is not as abnormal as the one that has mixed-up DNA. The other thing that the DNA analysis will measure is the S-phase, which gives us information regarding the growth rate of the tumor. The S-phase is an indirect measure of what percentage of the tumor cells are actively dividing and thus producing new tumor cells right now. If it is a high number, the tumor is growing more quickly, and a low number means it is growing slower.

There are many other tumor substances that various labs around the country are looking at to help predict which tumors will be more aggressive—i.e., the ones that give the woman a higher risk of recurrence. The more accurately physicians can determine which tumors are likely to recur, the better we can tailor a woman's treatment to her specific needs.

How can women be sure the pathology report is correct?

Ninety-five percent of breast cancer is clear-cut on the frozen section, and a trained pathologist can tell you quickly if it's cancer. Occasionally, it is a tougher call and the pathologist will wait to review the permanent sections, which are available twenty-four to forty-eight hours after surgery. A woman certainly can request that other pathologists review the slides. The normal procedure would be for one pathology department to send slides directly to another pathology lab at the patient's request. Occasionally, when seeking a second opinion, a woman may obtain the pathology slides and report herself in order to expedite matters and have the slides available for review at the time of her second-opinion appointment. A woman may want to call a reputable cancer treatment center and explain that she has a particular diagnosis and wants another opinion. They would direct her from there.

In his excellent book *Fighting Cancer,* Richard Bloch quotes Dr. Vincent DeVita, Jr., director of the National Cancer Institute: "I've been taking care of cancer patients for a long time. I have never taken care of a doctor who didn't get a second opinion. I've never taken care of a doctor who didn't have his microscopic slide read twice by more than one pathologist to make sure that he had cancer, knowing already that he had gotten into a pretty good system. And I think there is a message in that."

AFTER THE BIOPSY

Once the suspicious site or tumor has been removed and it has been determined whether it is malignant, your treatment becomes highly individualized. If there are malignant cells, the surgeon will be discussing further surgery to examine the lymph nodes and whether more of the breast will be removed.

The pathology report, the location and size of the malignant area, if it is in situ or invasive, lymph node involvement, and the size of your breast may or may not give you the option for a lumpectomy as opposed to mastectomy and will determine further treatment options.

There is a possibility that your surgeon will recommend that you consult with an oncologist *before* surgery, due either to the size of the tumor or the type of cancer. All surgeons have an oncologist they recommend, but again, you have the final say and can repeat the same search process you used to find your surgeon.

Tip—If you receive a diagnosis of malignancy; you should consult with an oncologist. Some surgeons may not be up on the latest treatment unless they specialize in the breast or are oncology surgeons.

Oncologists are the doctors who dispense chemotherapy and other systemic treatments for breast cancer. They will also follow you after surgery to assess your wellness. If your surgeon is an oncologic surgeon and you do not have any adjuvant treatment such as chemotherapy or radiation, he or she can do your follow-up tracking and blood work. Some women still prefer to be followed by an oncologist. That is your option.

"You know the surgeons think they have the silver bullet. His idea is 'I cut it out and you're well.' But I decided from having read about adjuvant therapy, that I should at least go talk to Dr. B, the oncologist. He felt strongly that I should take tamoxifen. The surgeon didn't recommend anything."—Pat H

The surgeon who performed Mary-T's biopsy suggested an immediate mastectomy for a very large tumor. He did not recommend that she see an oncologist, which she did on her own. *"He woke me up from the biopsy telling me it was bad. It was very large—over 6 centimeters, which is approximately the size of a lemon. He suggested I have a mastectomy quickly. However, in the forty-eight hours since my tumor had been removed, I had read about it and I had talked to many women that had gone through mastectomies and breast cancer treatment. I had talked to one doctor and I made a number of appointments to see other doctors. So I went back to him armed with some questions about chemotherapy, and he said, 'Probably down the road.' I said, Well, I had read that in cases such as mine that they do immediate chemotherapy and mastectomy later, he said, 'Not in your case.' But it was in my case and that's what I chose."*

Be aware that there are general oncologists just as there are general surgeons. Then there are the oncologists whose research and primary practice is one kind of cancer. Ask how much of your oncologist's practice is breast cancer. If the oncologist is in a group, you will frequently get the benefit of shared information. Ask who determines the protocols for breast cancer that he or she will use.

In choosing the oncologist, I would add another suggestion. Project yourself a year down the road. Suppose the oncologist you are considering is well qualified and you feel confident he or she is the best for the medical aspects; but how will this doctor respond to treating your fears? When you fear that every ache is cancer, will this person be supportive and caring or irritated and terse?

The oncologist is the person you will see at regular intervals for a year and then regularly at longer intervals after that for the rest of your life. It is this doctor who will monitor your body to detect if your cancer has recurred. More so than a surgeon, this person must be someone with whom you can share your fears and ask questions.

You want reality—not pessimism from this person. And there is a big difference. It will be the oncologist who will tell you statistics for *recurrence*, but he or she should be able to offer you reality—if, for example, you are high-risk—and still celebrate every visit that you are recurrence free. Oncologists know that for every statistic they quote, there are many women who have proven them wrong.

Leanne chose the oncologist her surgeon recommended. *"I asked him what he thought my chances were, and he said, 'Well, I can tell you this— the tumor was very big, it was very aggressive, and it has spread to five lymph nodes, and being in that category, your chances are about 70 to 80 percent for recurrence, and generally when it does recur, it's terminal. There's not much we can do about it.' That was how he said it. So I thought, Well, why the hell are we doing chemotherapy if I'm gonna die anyway? I don't want to lose my hair and be sick as a dog for a whole year if I'm going to die anyway."*

When I asked how she could stand visiting him every three months, she said, *"At least I don't have to talk to him. I just go through all the scans and give blood and he calls me the next day if there is a problem. He basically said there is nothing to talk about until it comes back."*

I was appalled. I have never *not* seen my oncologist during our visits. The physical exam is a crucial part of follow-up. We also talk about any fears I have and how I am feeling overall.

At the time I first talked with her, Leanne was approaching her two-year anniversary, a milestone for breast cancer patients, since 80 percent of women who have recurrence will experience it within the first two years. I, a total stranger, told her this positive statistic. I also gave her the name of a woman who had had fourteen malignant nodes and was doing fine after five years. In October 1991, I saw Leanne and her husband and children at the Susan G. Komen Race for the Cure in Dallas. *"After talking to you last year, I changed oncologists. I never knew a doctor could be warm and caring and treat me like a human being."*

And, as this book went to press, Leanne was approaching five years cancer-free!

Sonja chose to visit an oncologist after learning her lump was malignant. She decided, and the oncologist agreed, that lumpectomy should be one of her options. The surgeon disagreed. *"I asked for the medical journals, and the surgeon said I couldn't understand them. He treated me like an imbecile. I wanted information ahead of time. I think of myself as an intelligent woman and I had no idea where to look. So I was stuck. I didn't have the money to pay $50 here and there trying to find the right doctor."*

Women who are unsure about their doctor or want another decision can get a second opinion or, in most major hospitals, ask that their case be taken before the tumor board, where it would be discussed by a number of doctors. At Baylor, patients are not allowed to sit in on their case discussion. At a number of hospitals around the country there is a multidisciplinary board at which all the patient's doctors—or doctors they want invited—meet with the patient to discuss the case.

Bridie took her biopsy information and all her records to Yale Breast

Center after the biopsy. *"I sat in on the conference. There was a surgeon, pathologist, oncologist, radiologist, endocrinologist—a whole lot of 'gists.' And they presented the case and said a lumpectomy was fine. They didn't see any infiltration at that point. They warned me that if it had spread or they felt there was an invasion, they could move very fast. So they took all the nodes and they were clear. Then I had been home for a few days and the pathology came back and they had found microscopic infiltration, so I went back a month later for a mastectomy."*

SURGERY CHOICES

After discussing your biopsy results, the surgeon will begin addressing your surgery options. It is important to understand the terminology, and you might ask if your surgeon will use pictures to illustrate. Surgeons tend to tell you what will be removed using anatomical description, which few of us understand. Below is a basic description of the surgeries now being done. What is important to understand is that while surgeons may use these terms interchangeably, they may be talking about their own version. Ask him or her to be specific on how much tissue will be removed.

Lumpectomy What has come to mean the removal of the tumor and some surrounding tissue is also called **partial mastectomy, wide excision, segmental mastectomy,** and **quadrantectomy,** depending on who is doing the surgery and how they operate. The amount of tissue removed will depend on the size of the tumor, and how breast-conserving it is will depend on how much remaining tissue there is in relation to the original size of the breast.

These are generally thought of as **breast-conserving treatments** and are combined with axillary node removal either at the same time or in subsequent surgery. But the number of lymph nodes removed may be fewer than with mastectomy, depending on indicators.

Modified radical mastectomy The most performed surgery on breast cancer patients nationwide, this involves the removal of all the breast tissue, including the skin and the lymph nodes.

Simple mastectomy For some in situ diagnoses, you may be given the option of a lesser surgery that removes the breast tissue but may leave the skin, nipple, nodes, or a combination thereof. This procedure may also be referred to as **total mastectomy** or a **subcutaneous mastectomy.** Ironically, in situ diagnoses, which are very early-stage breast cancer, are often not good candidates for breast-conserving treatment such as lumpectomy, a controversy that is addressed more later in this chapter. These are not considered breast-conserving techniques because the breast tissue is removed and must be replaced with an implant.

Total glandular mastectomy A newer terminology for a surgery that goes further than a simple mastectomy. In the TGM the breast tissue is removed, leaving the skin intact. The nipple is either removed or, possibly, cored, before being replaced, but the woman can still have her own nipple. In some instances a plastic surgeon can perform a one-step surgery, removing the breast tissue and replacing it with an implant. Lymph nodes may or may not be removed, or only a few may be removed for sampling.

It is very important to understand at this point what your options are. Surgeons have strong feelings about what is the most appropriate surgery for their patients in given situations. Depending on a number of factors, you may or may not be a candidate for one of the surgeries that will conserve some or most of the breast.

LUMPECTOMY VS. MASTECTOMY

There has been much controversy in the past about the choice of lumpectomy versus mastectomy. New studies show that for those women who are good candidates, lumpectomy coupled with radiation, and in some instances chemotherapy, is as effective as mastectomy in survival rates. Some doctors argue that the studies are not old enough or thorough enough.

In the December 1990 issue of *Oncolog,* a physician's newsletter, David Hohn, M.D., professor of surgery at the University of Texas M.D. Anderson Cancer Center, gave the results of the National Institutes of Health Treatment of Early Stage Breast Cancer Conference held in the fall of 1990. At the conference, a panel of fifteen physicians and scientists drafted a consensus from studies presented from all over the world.

"We concluded that breast conservation should be considered equivalent in terms of survival to any other treatment," said Hohn in an

Oncolog interview. "If a woman wants to keep her breast and is eligible for breast conservation, she should have that option. Absolutely no data indicate that survival is reduced by opting for breast conservation instead of mastectomy."

He went on to stress, however, that the finding was not a finding against mastectomy, and such a decision must include many factors, including adequate margins of at least 1 centimeter in all directions and axillary node dissection, or removal of the lymph nodes. Women who choose conservation must also make a long-term commitment to surveillance.

Hohn said that breast conservation may not be an option for patients with very large or very small breasts, since in a small breast the cosmetic outcome may not be good while in a large breast the amount of radiation must be increased.

Yet, Hohn said, breast conservation remains a personal decision to be made by the patient, and physicians should be sensitive to patient preference.

"I still do more mastectomies than breast conservation, and I'd like to believe I'm enlightened," Hohn told *Oncolog,* explaining that his patients make their decisions based on cost and the time commitment for daily radiation for four or five weeks following surgery.

Indeed, findings of a 1992 study of Medicare patients showed distinct regional differences in how frequently lumpectomy was performed, concluding that lumpectomy was not being chosen (and perhaps offered) as often as it could be. Women in the Northeast chose lumpectomy much more frequently than those in the South, according to the study. Whether this was a question of doctors' options, women's conservative views, or women not having convenient access to radiation treatment centers was not clear.

***

Tip—While all breast-conserving treatment has been combined in the term lumpectomy **for our discussion here, there are varying philosophies on how much surrounding tissue should be removed for the best results both cosmetically and in terms of sur-**

vival and whether any lymph nodes are going to be removed. Ask your surgeon.

To be considered a good medical candidate for lumpectomy, there are a number of major considerations: the size and location of the lump and the size of the breast. A small tumor near the nipple that would require removal of the nipple in a lumpectomy will leave a misshapen breast that cannot be reconstructed easily after radiation.

A consensus published at the May 1991 American Society of Clinical Oncology annual meeting confirms the 1990 findings. The consensus paper stated: "Breast conservation treatment (lumpectomy) is an appropriate method of primary therapy for the majority of women with Stage 1 and 2 breast cancer and is preferable because it provides survival equivalent to total mastectomy with axillary dissection while preserving the breast." The report also stated that it was the consensus of the clinical trialists presenting that certain women were *not* candidates for breast conservation. They include:

1. Women with multicentric disease, meaning in multiple locations in the breast, or women whose mammogram shows microcalcifications in multiple locations in the breast.
2. Women whose tumors are large relative to the volume or shape of the breast and consequently would not gain any cosmetic advantage.

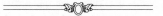

Tip—If cosmetic outcome is a major factor for you, turn to the next chapter on reconstruction now. I have seen lumpectomies that look worse than reconstructed breasts.

To be an emotional candidate for lumpectomy, which can have equal impact on the decision, a woman should be sure of her decision. This is not a choice for a "worrier," someone who will spend the remainder of her life concerned about the remaining tissue.

Breast Surgeon Dr. Jeanne Petrek, Memorial Sloan-Kettering Cancer Center, Talks About Lumpectomy vs. Mastectomy

Everybody, of course, is a candidate for mastectomy, but only certain patients are good candidates for breast conservation. A good candidate is one we feel will have the same cure rate, the same survival rate, as she would with a mastectomy. What we try to do is classify the patients into good candidates, borderline candidates, and poor candidates. We clearly have some patients who are bad candidates. We tell them directly we won't do it. Then we have a group of borderline candidates, when it's not perfect and maybe you wouldn't recommend it wholeheartedly, but the patient understands she has a slightly greater risk of recurrence—or we don't know exactly what the risk is. Those patients can still have breast preservation.

What are the factors you take into consideration?
Number one is the size of the tumor versus the size of the breast. Namely, we have some patients who have very small breasts, and even though they have very small tumors, it's just physically not possible to take out the whole tumor with all the roots and with a margin of normal tissue all the way around it without disfigurement.

Number two is that we have some women with truly large tumors. Even though they have a large breast, their cancer is 3, 4, or 5 centimeters or larger. Once a tumor gets to be—most say 4, but some say even 3 centimeters—much longer roots are present, with more invasion. The tumor is multifocal, meaning that smaller tumors could also be present in the breast even if they are not apparent by mammography or physical exam.

(continued)

Do the number of lymph nodes involved have any impact?

The lymph nodes aren't too important in determining mastectomy vs. breast preservation. They are a factor that determines if the cancer is more likely to recur in other parts of the body. But what we're considering with lumpectomy/mastectomy is the likelihood of it to recur in the breast. It is true that if you have positive lymph nodes, it's slightly more likely for the cancer to come back also in the breast, as well as in, possibly, the rest of the body.

What are the other indicators?

A lot of people are concerned about the cells' appearance. Various universities, particularly Harvard, believe that they can predict which patients will have a higher recurrence rate. If the patient has Extensive Intraductal Component—that is, in situ cancer within and around the solid tumor—if the cells' nuclei appear disordered, the cancer is more likely to recur in the breast.

Does age play a part in the decision?

Young women of course are more interested in having the breast saved. On the other hand, they sometimes have to face a much longer length of follow-up. I would not say they have more recurrence in the breast. I think it's the same percentage as middle-aged women. As a matter of fact, young women have dense, sometimes hard-to-examine breasts. The mammography is such that when the tissue is so glandular, you can't get a good radiographic image. So we are concerned that the diagnosis of any recurrence in young women could be delayed.

With the number of years young woman will live with follow-up, do you discuss the worry factor?

We point it out to some patients, and others point it out to us. Actually, some patients feel much better with a mastectomy, and some of them are the young women—because they are the ones who were told when they found the lump, "Oh it's nothing. Just

(continued)

ignore it." And then when they are biopsied eighteen months later, they are very anxious to have a mastectomy. The patients for whom everything has gone well and who have confidence in medical science are much more likely to feel optimistic about saving their breasts and about any local recurrence in the breast being diagnosed quickly. In my practice the ones who are truly Stage 1, the overwhelming percentage of them are having their breasts saved. Of the patients whose tumor is slightly larger, or perhaps they already have an enlarged lymph node, they're almost the opposite. Only a third of them are having their breasts saved.

What are the statistics for recurrence in the same breast after a lumpectomy?

Basically, over the long term, which would be five or ten years in negative node patients, it's 5 to 8 percent. And in the positive node patients, it is 10 percent or more. The women with lumpectomy treatment see the breast surgeon or their breast radiation therapist every three months for the first three years. And then every four months—or we let some go six months between visits after three years.

WOMEN TALK ABOUT THEIR SURGERY CHOICES

If you are given a choice between lumpectomy and mastectomy, it is *your* choice. It doesn't have to be a rational decision; it can be the one you want to make. Again, if you have been given the choice, it means you have the time to think and read before you make the decision. Know that if you get two or three opinions you may still hear contradictory recommendations since doctors tend to view their specialty as the best route. It is known that most surgeons in the country prefer mastectomy, while some surgeons contend that only a small percentage of women truly need mastectomy and that women with tumors 5 centimeters and under should be encouraged to choose breast conservation.

"He gave me an option of the lumpectomy or mastectomy. I really don't know why I decided for the mastectomy, and I am really an informed consumer, because of my health care background. I had a

very emotional feeling that if they took the whole breast, it would be better. I'm still not clear on it, but very happy with the decision." —Mary H

"I had huge breasts and lumpectomy was not an option I considered. She gave it to me, but it was truly not my mentality at that point. I didn't want to worry. My breasts were horribly bumpy and lumpy. All my life I had dealt with discomfort. The scarring would have made it worse. I chose a bilateral mastectomy and immediate reconstruction."—Joyce

"I was in shock, and a number of friends helped me make the decision for a mastectomy. I knew there was reconstruction, and I just didn't want to take the chance. I am very pleased with the reconstruction and know I made the right decision."—Karen

"Way back when—BC—before cancer, I always thought that if I ever got breast cancer, I would never have a lumpectomy. How stupid of those women. Just take it off. Just get it over with. Then, of course, when I was faced with it, I decided I didn't want that. I was given the option. I had read enough and felt I was educated and that if I had the option for lumpectomy, I would take it, since survival rates were the same."—Julie

"I chose lumpectomy, but I think I could have lived fairly normally with a mastectomy. The way I read the thing was, Why do more aggressive surgery than you need statistically? He gave me a lot of literature to read, and I just went on mortality rates. Dr. P told me that it was up to a 25 percent chance of local recurrence, but that statistically, he would catch it so soon that the numbers didn't show that it would increase my mortality rate."—Elizabeth T

"They had just come up with findings about lumpectomy and radiation. I was born with two breasts and decided lumpectomy was better for me. The doctor said I was stupid and that we didn't have enough statistics. The oncologist agreed with me that with lumpectomy the odds were about the same, so that was the route we went."—Sonja

"I went for a lumpectomy, hoping that it was the right decision. The day before the surgery, I saw the surgeon again and she wanted to examine me really good. She examined the breast again, and she said *if she got in there and it looked like the cancer had spread more than what we thought, she would do the mastectomy. I said yes, of course, please do what you need to do."*—Lise

Because Nancy W found her lump while breast-feeding her third child, she assumed it was a blocked milk duct. Nancy was diagnosed and had begun preoperative chemo when she decided to seek a second opinion at a university medical school in another state, where she saw a medical oncologist who knew her surgeon. Her local surgeon and the out-of-state oncologist were former colleagues and knew each other well.

"I got back home and said to my surgeon, 'Did X call you yesterday?' He said no. I said, 'Well, he said I could have a lumpectomy.' It took a minute for him to pick his jaw up off the floor. He gave me the third degree. 'Did you tell him it might be inflammatory? Did you tell him about the node under your arm?' . . . I said yes, he had all the information. So he hangs up and calls this fellow. He was shocked because he had expected the guy to agree with him. The other doctor said that I had responded well to the chemotherapy and it had shrunk the tumor and he expected I would respond well to additional chemotherapy. It's not across the board that he would recommend lumpectomy rather than mastectomy to everybody who had my initial clinical and pathological symptoms."—Nancy W

Nancy ultimately had a lumpectomy with two positive nodes. She had pre- and postoperative chemotherapy and seven weeks of radiation. At four years post-op, she is fine.

Be aware that a decision for lumpectomy may change in the operating room—as mine did—if what appeared to be a clearly defined tumor has tentacles or if the tissue around the tumor appears suspicious. A good lumpectomy procedure should allow the surgeon to get cleanly around the tumor without removing massive amounts of tissue. If there is any chance that a mastectomy will be needed instead of a lumpectomy, be sure you are clear when and why that would happen. At age seventy-one, Mary C was very body-conscious and chose a lumpectomy when given the choice. She says that the surgeon discussed the need for clear margins, and they agreed that he would do a mastectomy if needed, but she was sure that she would keep her breast.

"I remember waking up in recovery and the nurse said they had to remove the breast. My friend down the hall said she could hear me screaming. It was very traumatic. I was playing doctor, and I was so sure it was going to be a lumpectomy."—Mary C

IN SITU DIAGNOSIS

There are two kinds of in situ diagnosis: intraductal carcinoma (DCIS) also known as noninvasive duct carcinoma or duct carcinoma in situ, and lobular carcinoma in situ (LCIS). While they are both early-stage cancers, they differ in many other ways.

LCIS, which is considered a precancerous condition, is more often multicentric, or found throughout the breast, and it is more often found in both breasts, meaning that if a woman chooses mastectomy, a bilateral total glandular mastectomy is usually recommended. This surgery removes the glandular breast tissue and either the entire nipple or only the core, leaving the areola. Because it is a precancerous condition, some women choose to do nothing and monitor the situation closely. Which of the two you decide on will depend on your understanding of the risks involved, your faith in follow-up, and the fear factor.

If the choices seem complicated in the mastectomy/lumpectomy issue, they become even more complex when there is an in situ diagnosis. The ability to detect very small and even precancerous conditions with advanced mammography has resulted in a dramatic increase in the number of in situ diagnoses in the past decade—an increase that has added yet another gray area for treatment that continues to prompt disagreement from medical professionals across the country. Ironically, the argument revolves around the wisdom of breast-conserving treatment (BCT) for this very early-stage breast cancer at a time when BCT is becoming more accepted for later-stage breast cancer. This issue was further complicated by a study released in June 1993 from researchers at the University of Pittsburgh that proposed lumpectomy and radiation as an acceptable surgery choice for in situ diagnosis. The study followed 319 women who were treated with lumpectomy and radiation for an in situ diagnosis. After three years, 10 percent had had recurrence.

While specialists across the country said the findings do not mean a change in recommending mastectomy for in situ diagnosis, they called

it an important preliminary finding. Surgeons argued that the 100 percent cure rate from a mastectomy is preferable to any recurrence, since
recurrent cancer outside the breast has a very low cure rate. Other
physicians are concerned that the follow-up time is not adequate and
that more women in the study may have recurrence. The role of adjuvant treatment such as radiation, chemotherapy, and hormones for
women who chose mastectomy is yet another chapter. I offer here both
sides and the women who have faced those decisions.

*"My mammogram looked like it had the measles. I was real focused
on the one breast and they may have told me about the other one, but
I wasn't listening. When Mark and I met with the surgeon, I finally
said, 'What about my other breast?' He said it had the measles too. I
started crying. One I could see, but both? He said it was my choice. I
didn't have the clusters in the other breast, but I did have calcifications.
So I had a bilateral."*—Jo Anne

*"Probably the biggest factor in deciding for mastectomy was not
having a hundred percent assurance that we got it all. It was in the
ducts, and even though it was identified in a particular spot, that didn't
mean that there wasn't that remote possibility that some cell had broken
off and gone someplace else in the breast. I didn't want to take the
chance."*—Ann

*"After the diagnosis of lobular in situ, I thought about it, but not
that long. My mother died of endometrial cancer, and it was clear to
me that I didn't want any risk, so I chose the bilateral. But we are still
fighting with the insurance company, who said that there was no
need."*—Diana

*"I started thinking I didn't really need the surgery for the lobular
in situ diagnosis. I just found out last week one of my contacts from a
few years ago had the same breast condition that I had, and she opted
to watch it. Her friend called me last week and told me she had a
mastectomy. See, I couldn't sit on a time bomb. I don't care what it is.
I wouldn't be able to sleep at night knowing there might be a chance."*
—Kim

The concern of many doctors in discussing anything but mastectomy
for intraductal cancer is that ductal in situ cancer may be present

throughout the breast, presenting a possibility for recurrence. According to David W. Kinne, M.D., the chief of the Breast Service of Memorial Sloan-Kettering Cancer Center in an article in *Ca-A Cancer Journal for Clinicians* in March 1991: "Selection of candidates for breast preservation must be done carefully. The presence of diffuse microcalcifications throughout the breast is a contraindication; if the suspicious area can be encompassed by wide excision with clear margins (even up to quadrantectomy), breast preservation can be considered provided the patient understands the physician's concerns. Mastectomy will cure virtually 100 percent of patients with duct carcinoma in situ."

SENIOR SURGICAL PATHOLOGIST DR. MICHAEL LAGIOS, CALIFORNIA PACIFIC MEDICAL CENTER, TALKS ABOUT IN SITU DIAGNOSES

Why are in situ diagnoses increasing?

I attribute it entirely to mammography. The technological advances that made mammography reasonably reliable and cheap didn't come out until the early seventies. That's when we started to see all these tiny lesions that were represented by microcalcifications. No one can go back in time to do an experiment, but we do know that all invasive cancers originate in noninvasive disease, so it is reasonable to surmise that a good number of the lesions that we now call duct carcinoma in situ would have been neglected fifteen or twenty years ago and would not have become apparent until they became invasive.

Explain calcifications, if you would.

The calcifications don't always indicate that there's a malignancy, but one type of duct carcinoma in situ representing nearly half of all the cases is associated with a very peculiar type of linear branching calcification. The calcification is there because the tumor undergoes cell death, or what we call necrosis. As a result, the normal calcium salts that circulate in the blood leach out and

---

(continued)

get deposited in the dead tissue. You can't always tell whether calcium is really associated with malignancy or not. In fact, I would say that even when you have a very characteristic pattern of malignancy, you're only 95 percent sure. That's why we have to do a biopsy. But when you see branching linear calcifications, you know that it occurs within a duct structure of the breast, and the most common process in the breast that does that is noninvasive duct cancer.

One woman said it looked like her mammogram had the measles.

She was referring to the small microcalcifications—they look like white dots on a mammogram. And in fact, if you got a magnifying glass out, you'll see that some are actually linear and branching. You don't always see the linear branching. Sometimes they just suggest that, but sometimes they actually do form a cast of the duct and if the ducts branch, the calcification branches.

So we are not talking about an actual tumor?

Right. Noninvasive cancer can present as a palpable tumor mass if it's extensive enough because there is a reaction of the breast, of the host, so to speak, to the cancer still within the duct. But more often than not, the cancer is completely nonpalpable—certainly to the palpating hand of the surgeon or other medical worker who's examining the breast directly through the skin before the surgery.

So are we talking cancer or precancerous?

Until very recently we had no idea of what the biology of noninvasive duct cancer in particular was like. Everyone who had such a diagnosis would immediately have a mastectomy. It was like going into the hen house and seeing some eggs there; as soon as you saw an egg, you made scrambled eggs. Well, you'd never find out that those things might hatch after a while into chicks and then grow up. Or at least some of them might. That's the situation

(continued)

we have now with duct carcinoma in situ. Each individual cell might look very similar, but biologically they're very different. The ones that are inside the duct have not shown that they can move out to the outside and become invasive. Now it can be that many of them, if neglected, *will* become invasive, but it's also true that a good many will stay within the duct for a very, very long period of time or may never become invasive in the lifetime of the patient. That's one of the problems we have right now, because we're just beginning to learn about the biology of the duct carcinoma in situ. It's only in the last fifteen years that we have thought about alternative therapies for duct carcinoma in situ, and until ten years ago almost everyone treated it by total mastectomy.

What are the current controversies about treatment?

The controversies are legion. We have a situation right now where we have very little information and we're being asked to recommend therapy. When we started to do mammography in this hospital and we started to see little teeny noninvasive duct cancers, these patients were treated by standard modified radical mastectomies with node dissection and the whole works. And then after ten, fifteen, twenty such procedures in which we found no residual cancer at all in the breast, we started to rethink this procedure.

Isn't one of the concerns of ductal cancer that it may be throughout the breast?

That is one of the problems, one of the concerns of a therapist dealing with noninvasive cancer—just how extensive it is. And one of the things that we did here was to make an estimate of the extent of the disease, at least as a working hypothesis, based on how extensive the microcalcifications were in the breast. You can't treat a disease that's seen in every duct system of the breast with a limited surgical excision because the only adequate excision you can do is a total mastectomy. On the other hand, many of these mammographically detected noninvasive cancers of duct type, on

(continued)

the basis of microcalcifications, are very small and we have found that fully half of them are 25 millimeters or less in actual size. Those patients certainly have options other than total mastectomy.

What is the difference between ductal and lobular carcinoma in situ?

Well, there are a number of significant differences. The most important is that from the point of view of biology, the duct carcinoma in situ predicts risk for that breast. If you have a biopsy in the right breast and it shows duct carcinoma in situ, you have a significant chance of developing invasive cancer, but it's going to be confined to the right breast. Or at least, all of the recurrences and so on will be in the right breast. If you were to have a diagnosis of lobular carcinoma in situ, then your risk is going to be equally distributed to either breast.

A bilateral total mastectomy is often recommended for women with lobular carcinoma in situ.

We try to dissuade people from doing that here, because the level of risk is very small for lobular carcinoma in situ, approximately 1 percent a year of developing an invasive cancer in either breast. For some duct carcinomas in situ this risk is approximately 4 percent a year. We find that the alternative management is more appropriate for the level of risk in LCIS. For example, in twenty years a thirty-eight-year-old woman with a LCIS (lobular) diagnosis will have gone through about an 18 percent risk of developing invasive cancer. Not dying of cancer, but just getting the cancer. So that means that there is an 82 percent chance that she won't. We try to make sure that patients fully understand their risk and get over their initial fear reaction. So many women make a decision based on fear, which is not the way to make a decision about this kind of surgery—there is plenty of time to make a decision, particularly with lobular carcinoma in situ. Unfortunately, so much of what women perceive as risk is a reflection of

(continued)

sometimes well-meaning concern and anxiety of the surgeon, who's really programmed and directed to do surgery, and I don't think there's any way you can get around that. People who do surgery are going to have a surgical method of treating the disease. People who do radiation therapy are going to think in terms of radiation therapy, and people who are chemotherapists are going to think primarily of chemotherapy. It's always hard to see beyond ones' own nose.

RESOURCES

BOOKS:

Dr. Susan Love's Breast Book, by Susan Love, M.D. (Addison Wesley, 1991). The best book on the breast in general, from a surgeon who is at the top of the research field.

Breast Cancer: The Complete Guide, by Yashar Hirshaut, M.D., and Peter I. Pressman, M.D. (Bantam, 1992). A breast surgeon and medical oncologist offer views on all aspects of breast cancer. Good for their support of a partnership approach.

Teamwork, Talking with Your Doctor, $3, available from National Coalition for Cancer Survivorship, Fifth Floor, 1010 Wayne Avenue, Silver Spring, MD 20901. Call (301) 650-8868. Good common-sense ideas for working with your doctors. NCCS is a national advocacy group for cancer survivors. A $25 membership fee will get you quarterly newsletters about legislation and other issues pertaining to survivorship.

Spinning Straw into Gold, by Ronnie Kaye (Fireside, 1991). Good advice about emotional issues, from a survivor.

SERVICES

Cancer Information Service (a program of the National Cancer Institute) at 1-800-4-cancer

Can give you much information. Ask for a PDQ (Physician's Data

Query), a free computer printout of the most up-to-date information on breast cancer; staging information; and treatment options. Also ask for a list of publications they offer free of charge. NCI also has a list, compiled by the American College of Surgeons, of approved cancer centers around the country. It can tell you the one closest to your home.

When I called, it took about six attempts to get through, so keep trying. Eight days later I received the PDQ, a list of topics covered by other publications, and a list of approved cancer centers in my area. (My friend Diana received hers in two days.) The letterhead indicated that the information had come through the M.D. Anderson Cancer Center Public Education Office in Houston. They also sent a marvelous book called *Fighting Cancer,* by Annette and Richard Bloch. Bloch, who is the founder of H&R Block, was diagnosed with terminal lung cancer and told to go home and wait it out. Instead, he found a doctor who was willing to try surgery and extensive chemotherapy. Bloch added his own complementary therapies, and he is alive and well. The book stresses that you must call on all your resources to beat cancer and THAT IT CAN BE BEATEN. Since his cancer, Bloch has become devoted to helping people fight the disease through his Kansas City, Missouri, organization Cancer Connections, Inc. You might request this book when you call the hotline number. If they don't have it, call **Cancer Connection** at (816) 932-8453 in Kansas City, Missouri. They will send you one free of charge.

The Planetree Health Information Service, 2040 Webster Street, San Francisco, CA 94115; (415) 923-3680

Planetree is a national nonprofit consumer health organization dedicated to helping patients become active participants in their health and medical care. If you are close to San Francisco, visit this organization, which maintains a clipping file on medical issues. Otherwise, for a fee ($75 in 1993) they will send you a packet of information on any medical issue you request. When I ordered a packet on breast cancer and requested articles on alternative healing, I received a Physicians Data Query in a week and the packet in about three weeks. It contained twenty different journal articles on breast cancer. These are of value in determining diagnosis because you can read for yourself the controversies in the medical community surrounding treatment options. Planetree also has a catalog of books and other items for cancer patients.

These are good, since many bookstores may not carry books from smaller publishers.

COMPUTER SEARCH OPERATIONS

If you are in or near a city that has a major medical school, there is a good possibility that they will do a computer search of the latest in journal entries for whatever topic you want. There will probably be a fee for this service.

The Dallas public library, like many public libraries around the country, also offers searches for an hourly fee. They can give abstracts, which are short synopses, or just journal titles that you can then look up.

Also, many individuals and companies have access to one of many multiple database services through their home computer. I was able to access the NIH directly with our system and called up a current PDQ on our home computer! In addition, most of these services offer other health care databanks that can give you journal articles and articles by topic.

REFERRAL SERVICES

Your county medical society will give you names of doctors who are specialists in particular areas. When I called Dallas County Medical, they asked for my ZIP code and gave me a doctor who practiced at a small hospital near my home. They gave his name (which started with an A, indicating their list is alphabetical), where he went to school, where he did his residencies, and how long he has been in practice. Since Baylor Medical Center is not in my ZIP code, I asked if my surgeon was listed. She was.

Baylor University Medical Center has its own referral service that offers callers names of specialists on staff. Check with your local cancer center or medical center. Call the main number for the center and tell them you need a referral.

Before using one of the highly advertised phone referrals in your community, ask on what basis they take their doctors. Most just charge a fee and pay no attention to credentials.

NABCO (National Alliance of Breast Cancer Organizations)
Second Floor, 1180 Avenue of the Americas, New York, NY 10036;
(212) 719-0154

NABCO was founded to serve as a clearinghouse for information on
breast cancer. A $45 membership brings you a quarterly newsletter that
is very informative on medical issues, studies, and new drugs; in addition to a lengthy resource list.

Hot Lines Staffed by Breast Cancer Survivors

Y-ME is a national help-line in Illinois with satellite offices across the
country. Call 1-800-221-2141.
  Susan G. Komen Alliance in Dallas. Call 1-800-I'M AWARE.

IN CANADA

Cancer information line 1-800-263-6750

Canadian Breast Cancer Foundation
620 University Avenue, 9th floor
Toronto, Ontario M5G
(416) 596-6773

Canadian Breast Cancer Foundation
1917 Hosmer Avenue
Vancouver, B. C. V6J2S7
(604) 731-4723

Alberta Program for Eary Detection of Breast Cancer
(403) 262-4768

Nova Scotia Breast Screening Program
(902) 428-5960

Chapter 2

SURGERY

PLANNING AHEAD

"A qualified surgeon will not rush a patient's decision about surgery. Although a suspicious breast lump should be attended to quickly, a few days or even a week or two will not alter the likelihood of cure, and may give the patient time to think through decisions more clearly. If a woman wants to go ahead with biopsy and treatment immediately, she certainly should. But she should not feel pressured to make an on-the-spot decision if she is not ready."

—Dr. Sally Knox, breast surgeon

Don't let your surgeon rush you to surgery. Except perhaps in inflammatory or very advanced local disease, a week or two will make no difference medically, but it can make a tremendous impact emotionally. This is the time that can be spent on education and preparing emotionally to make a very stressful time easier for yourself and your family.

"The hospitalization was really great because I made it that way. I took about twenty days between biopsy and surgery. I really worked hard to get things the way I wanted them. I read Bernie Siegel's books and used a lot of his suggestions. My parents knew a nurse at the hospital, and we got a really great room with a big picture window so I could see the sky. I had tapes made of music to listen to during surgery, because there is proof you can hear while you are under. My dad helped

81

me mix all my favorite songs. I worked it out with Dr. H and we had
a tape recorder that played continually for five hours. Dr. H listened
to it and then they put the headphones on me when the plastic surgeon
came in."—Amy

MEDICAL ISSUES

You may want to visit the hospital and floor that your surgeon will
be using. If possible, talk with nurses. If for some reason you have
chosen a community hospital because there is no cancer treatment
center in the vicinity, be sure that the hospital is accredited. Accred-
itation will assure certain standards of care, safety, and quality of
practitioner care.

Most doctors have privileges at more than one hospital. Most also
have a preference where they like to operate—and where you will
get the best care. Ask if you have a choice. In one of my many hospital stays, I began talking to the nurse about her profession. She
told me she had been at a number of hospitals and this was the best
because of the nurse/patient ratio. I didn't even know such a thing
existed. She said she had quit one major cancer center because the
nurse/patient ratio was 1 to 11 and she considered that too high.
You should take such figures into consideration. Some of the more
well-known centers attract patients from all over the world and cannot help but have a lower quality of nursing care due to the number
of patients.

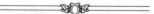

**Tip—If finances are a concern, ask your surgeon if
there is a hospital in the city that charges less and
still offers him or her operating privileges.**

If you are traveling to another city for care, extra effort will need to
go into accommodations. Call the social services office of the hospital.
Ask what is available through the hospital. Many of the larger hospitals
have a hotel on the premises.

If your surgeon has not made perfectly clear how you are to be admitted, ask for the step-by-step procedure. Becoming confused and spending the morning rushing around will add to the stress of the hospitalization.

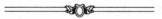

Tip—If there are strong indicators that you will have chemotherapy after your surgery, discuss veins and whether you want to explore the option of a direct line that would be inserted near your clavical at the same time the mastectomy is performed.

Hospitalization can be emotionally overwhelming. Remember that you are the client and the hospital is the provider—not the other way around.

Joyce decided she wanted to give her own blood in the event it was needed during her surgery and immediate reconstruction. *"My doctor said I didn't need to do that, but I just had a sense I should. I ended up losing four pints the night after surgery. I was a runner and my veins were like faucets. I had a bilateral and immediate reconstruction and I needed every bit of blood I had given."*

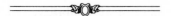

Tip—Consider giving your own blood for surgery, but this must be done no closer than seventy-two hours before surgery to allow your body to replenish.

HOSPITAL STAY

A few notes here about preparing for the hospital. Today's surgery techniques have become so advanced that women undergoing modified radicals usually spend only three or four days in the hospital. (If you are having immediate reconstruction, this may be a longer stay, depending on the procedure you chose.) Take a gown that has a loose-fitting top and a robe and slippers. If you are the kind that gets up quickly and moves around and will want to walk around the nurses' station at night, take a set of loose sweat clothes or a robe that covers you adequately.

Since my mastectomy, I have had two more hospitalizations for reconstruction and one for an infection. I now know the ropes about packing a few personal items to brighten up the room. But I thought I had heard it all until Debra told me about her husband. *"He showed up at the hospital with a lamp and picture and a rug and a jam box. I was there a week and it made a lot of difference to me. I don't know if the people at the hospital appreciated me hanging pictures, but it sure made a difference in how I felt."*

A hospital stay can bring family dynamics to the forefront. Be sure you are clear with your family about what you want. Marjorie B was in New York City when she had her first biopsy. Her mother called from out of town to ask if she wanted her to come in. *"I couldn't imagine my mother in the city. She wouldn't take a cab because it's too expensive. I can't imagine her on a bus. Forget the subway. I told her not to come and then it took me a long time to get over the fact that I was pissed off because she didn't come see me. Don't ask. Just do it or don't do it."*

Tip—To the best of your ability, tell your family where you are emotionally and what you need from them.

Diana made a list of the things she took to the hospital and the things she wishes she had taken.

WHAT TO TAKE TO THE HOSPITAL

- 2 pairs pajamas, robe, socks (the gripper kind are good because they double as slippers), slippers, underpants

- Walkman or cassette player, cassettes
- makeup mirror, travel bag of toiletries (shampoo, face cleanser, cologne, soap, feminine towelett, tampons), hair accessories (brush, ponytail holder, barrettes)
- money for machines (roll of quarters)
- list of addresses and phone numbers, stationery (thank you cards for flowers), stamps
- camera with film, to take pictures of flowers
- reading material, notepad, pencils and pens, *TV Guide*
- personal family items, such as pictures, favorite pillow, or a quilt for some color
- special food, such as fresh fruit or gum or mints

ITEMS FOR VISITING KIDS

- puzzles that fit on a small table
- a coloring book and colors or special book
- treats

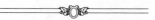

Tip—I have never tried it, but what about an answering machine? It is so frustrating not to be able to reach the phone when it rings and you are alone. Ask the hospital.

Andrea decided that to control the hospital stay, she would get up as soon as possible and put on her own clothes. There is no rule that says you can't wear loose sweats during the day and change at night. Andrea even went down to the lobby at one point. *"I just needed some fresh air. I walked outside for a few minutes and then went back up to the floor. I stopped at the nurses' station and asked for some juice. She just stared at me and said, 'Well, who are you?' I showed her my bracelet and said I was a patient. She laughed. I just refused to act sick."*

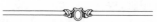

Tip—Options for hospital gifts in addition to flowers: bubble bath, nail polish, cologne, or a gift cou-
pon from one of the places that caters meals once
patients get home.

Other medical issues that you may want to explore during this time
between biopsy and surgery.

1. If you have biopsy information and have not talked to an oncol-
    ogist, this would be a good time.
2. If you are a candidate for immediate reconstruction, you probably
    already have chosen a plastic surgeon who will work in tandem
    with your surgeon. Find some women who have undergone the
    same reconstruction to get more information about how you will
    feel. The more you know, the easier the hospitalization.
3. A visit to a therapist to help with the emotional issues. Diana had
    a number of months before her surgery since her LCIS diagnosis
    was considered precancerous. She began having doubts and about
    three weeks before surgery. *"All of a sudden I was thinking, I can't
    go through with this. I started thinking I had made a mistake and I
    didn't need surgery. I was trying to find a way out. I was doing the
    physical things for surgery and decided I needed to talk to a professional
    about my anxieties. I wanted to focus my energies on healing and not
    have all these issues distracting me and interrupting my healing process.
    The therapist helped me see that my fears were legitimate, and then we
    talked about what I wanted out of life and I decided I wanted to grow
    old with my husband. I didn't want to worry about getting cancer. He
    also gave me a relaxation technique that helped me sleep more restfully
    to prepare for surgery."*

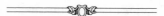

Tip—Discuss all the possibilities before surgery
with your surgeon. Ask what could happen once

you are in the operating room that would change what he or she has just told you. Be sure your husband/family have someone for support so they won't have to deal with a cancer diagnosis alone.

FAMILY ISSUES

"My husband's friends had offered to help. I wanted to take advantage of that, but my husband is the kind of person who doesn't believe in asking for help. If anybody asks you for help, you give help, you offer help. But you don't ever ask for help, and you don't accept help. And I said, 'Excuse me. We've got three little kids.' "—Nancy W

Put someone in charge of the homefront while you are away if there are children involved. This person should be someone other than your husband or partner, who will want to be with you at the hospital. The logistics of driving to and from the hospital can get tiresome.

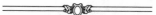

Tip—There is something incredibly exhausting about hospitals. I wonder if it isn't the tension in the atmosphere that saps our energy.

We are women of the nineties. We buy houses, have careers, are gourmet cooks. We are liberated and can do volunteer work, wash the dog, and monitor our children's TV viewing simultaneously. We should be able to handle cancer alone too, right? Wrong.

My pregnancy with Kirtley the year before I was diagnosed with breast cancer ended with six weeks of bed rest. Both my husband and I learned for the first time in our married life that it was all right to accept help. It made our friends feel useful and good, and I was neither bad nor weak for accepting it.

When Tom's mother called and offered to come help during my hospitalization, Tom said no. I told him to call her back and accept. I knew that taking care of two children, one of whom was barely walking, plus my needs, would be too much for him. She was there to cover the house to free Tom to be with me.

Remember that your husband or partner is to some degree also impaired. This diagnosis has affected him in ways that may be similar or dissimilar to yours.

> *"I went through a range of emotions—mad, scared, wondered why it happened—you name it. I went through emotions of fear for myself. Because I didn't know what I'd do without her."*
> —Cindy's fiancé, Larry

We see ourselves as "in charge" and capable of handling anything. For many of us it is a significant part of our identity. But there is a time to let go and rally the troops. The time is now. Think of it as part of your treatment. The need for emotional support is as pressing right now as are the medical decisions. For it is the emotional support that will help you cope with and make the very difficult medical decisions.

> *"It is very hard for me to ask people to do things for me. I tell everybody that I don't need help. I had friends who wanted to come take the children for the day, friends who wanted to come clean my house, and friends who wanted to cook and car-pool. And I said, 'No, no, I can do this all by myself.' My husband still teases me about it and says he hopes I don't ever have to go back in the hospital, because nobody is going to do anything for me. I wish now that I had let them help with the children. It wasn't the house that was the problem. It was the two-year-old. Just to take him to lunch and let him play would have been great. I was exhausted. That was the other thing I wasn't prepared for. I felt good, but I was tired and now I know that the anesthesia takes a lot out of you."*—Lynne

For women who are facing this alone—single, widowed, divorced—asking for help can be complicated if there is no one. Most of us have some form of community, through work, social life, or church. Explore all these options to see if someone emerges who would be willing to offer an ear and a shoulder. Finding a survivor either by word of mouth or through breast cancer support groups can be quite a gift. Often the women who have been there and who have become active in reaching out *want* to be available. Then you must be willing to ask.

Judy D was single and fifty when she was diagnosed. Her brother and her family lived fairly close, but Judy still found she had trouble asking for their help. She also found herself comforting her friends. She finally sought professional help. *"I realized that I had been the caretaker all my life, and now I needed caretaking. They were all willing; it was just very hard for me to ask. But I did, and they all responded beautifully."*

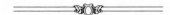

Tip for friends—Don't be put off by the first refusal of help. Drop a line or wait a few days and return the call.

During the first week after diagnosis, friends and acquaintances will be calling to offer help.

TAKE THEM UP ON IT. You may not want to invite casual acquaintances to take you to the doctor, but there are probably one or two friends on whom you can depend.

Think practically right now. How can you relieve pressure? What are the things you have jotted down that you need done? Here are some areas where you might ask for help both before and after surgery.

Research: Hand a friend the list of resources at the end of the first chapter and ask him or her to get the information you want.

Ask friends to find other women your age who have had breast cancer whom you might be able to talk to.

Food: Families still have to eat. Does the church, your company, or your husband's company want to send food? Let them. This might be something they can do if you are facing chemo, when food may not be your highest priority. When people ask what you need, tell them to send food. Many catalogs and specialty stores have prepackaged fruit and cheese baskets. These are great to keep the kids going while you are recuperating. This is also a time when you need to think about eating well. The temptation is to relieve pressure with fast food. Think again. Keep fruit and vegetables handy.

"We had so much food. People would ask how they could help and I would say, 'Bring food.' They wanted to help and I knew they had a need to and because we had a baby it was easy to ask. Some friends from work called to say they were coming to clean the house. I said, 'You can't do that, it's too personal.' They said, 'Sure we can.' I decided I liked that. When they came, I came out in my jammies and no robe. I had a need for them to see me flat."—Jo Anne

Finding a doctor: Ask them to call around and get names of oncologists or plastic surgeons or radiologists.

Shopping for the family: If you can't get it together for a list, ask them to get you the staples you know you will need in the next week: toilet paper, trash bags, milk, cereal, bread, fruit, frozen dinners.

Taxi: Ask them to pick up arriving family members at the airport or children at school.

Child care: Ask for a night of child care so you and your husband or a friend can go out. Have them come to your house. The children know something is going on and will be more comfortable at home.

"All the phone calls I got from people that I knew but didn't really know. They would call up, 'We want to keep your kids.' And I was, 'Oh no. We've got it all worked out.' And now I think, Why didn't I accept some help? I'll take help now. That was one of the hardest things, too, having people do things for me, instead of me doing things for them."—Madeline

Doctor visit: Ask someone to be recording secretary at doctor's visits—the extra eyes or ears.

Presence: Sometimes we need people to be with us. Get together for coffee or lunch.

Shopping for yourself: Do you need something for the hospital? House slippers or a new gown that has a loose top? Or ask a friend to pick up some surprises for your young children for their visit to the hospital room. Prepare snacks or something special for them to do while they visit, to help take the fear out of mom's being sick.

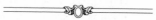

> **Tip for friends and family—Waiting for biopsy information or to check into the hospital can be an incredibly stressful time. Take her for a walk or a slow stroll around the neighborhood or shopping mall. Ask her to talk about what is happening and then shut up and listen. Instead of saying, "What can I do?" say, "I am planning to bring dinner. What is a good night?"**

PREPARING CHILDREN FOR YOUR SURGERY

"My sixteen-year-old son was arrested for shoplifting on the day of my surgery. It was totally out of character for him, and we knew that he was frightened and needed attention."—Harriett

"I had one child who was a senior in high school and one who was a freshman in high school. The senior was very busy all the time. When I was diagnosed he was there for me. He would sit with me for hours; sometimes he would even put his arm around me—just a wonderful presence there. The youngest child had been very close to me and we had spent a lot of time together. I was diagnosed and he became very angry to the point that he didn't even think he could be around me he was so afraid. I think he thought he had to wean himself away from me."—Mary-T

Don't forget to prepare children for your hospital stay. Most of the women in this book who had older children tried to talk to them on the phone soon after surgery and see them as soon as possible. Seeing and hearing from Mom greatly relieves the stress children are feeling at her absence.

A few felt the hospital was too depressing for the children and preferred to just talk by phone for the short hospital stay, but most saw an immediate change when the kids came up for a visit and could see where Mom was and that she was okay.

"I called the teachers before surgery and told them. I thought it was important they know. John came to see me at the hospital. He didn't say anything; he just crawled up on the bed with me. I think he just needed to be close to me."—Kit

"It was wonderful for the children when they came up. They wondered how I looked. I can remember seeing them at the door. Their eyes were huge and here was Mom in a hospital bed. You know moms are not supposed to be sick."—Lynne

In preparing children for your hospitalization, tell them where you are going, what will happen while you are there, and how long you will be gone. If you are planning to have them visit you, talk about what a hospital is and what they will see when they arrive. Tell them where you will be and what you will look like.

Once you are home from the hospital, let the children help care for you. Even a toddler can pat Mom's arm or do little errands. Meaningful work makes children feel like they are helpful. It is also a great message that moms need love and care too. Ultimately, children who are informed and involved in the planning feel a part of the family dynamic and can heal in their own time.

PREPARING YOUR "SELF" FOR SURGERY

Remember during this time to be kind to your body. Take time for yourself and feel good about how you look. What are the little luxuries that you never do? Buy that scented soap or new perfume.

Dottee talked to her body. *"Every day I began to make the affirmation, 'I love you, my body.' After the surgical procedures I knew my body needed all the emotional assurance it could get from its owner."*

Dottee also saw a chiropractor to realign her body after the stiffness from her hospital stay, and she had a monthly massage.

The most important message here is to listen to your body during this time. If it needs rest, let it rest. Pamper it and let it know you love it. *"I would smile at myself in the mirror and then do a complete facial, telling myself with each moisturizing stroke how beautiful and healthy I looked."*

Make time to say goodbye to your breast. Take time to caress and love yourself with the understanding that a part of you is going to be removed. One woman and her husband took a bottle of Champagne to bed with them and toasted her breast as they said goodbye.

> "I remember the night before. I took a bath and it was like I was giving myself that opportunity to look at my body and say, 'You're going to change,' and kind of mourn that. Go through that mourning process."—Diane

> "My surgery was not until 2 P.M. I wanted it on Monday so I could have the weekend. My husband and I went out to dinner on Saturday night, and it was such a bomb. The service was horrible and the food was horrible. Maybe no restaurant could have done anything right that night. A friend came over on Sunday to take care of my son so we could go to a movie, and it was horrible. Nothing was as my fantasy played it out. I had to get up front with my husband later and say this is not working out the way I had planned. I had hoped for some romance here. I remember saying, 'I am going to take a shower now and I would like you to join me.' What an ultimatum. But it was important to me. The next morning before surgery, I showered and said goodbye to my boobs."—Jo Anne

Chuck and Marjorie went to "space," their name for a particular vacation spot in the Caribbean where they could relax and just be together before surgery. Chuck said this was not a time to cry and cope with surgery but rather a time to "suspend reality." "It's like we were in an alternate reality. We really weren't thinking about it."

Joyce took the time between biopsy and surgery to make her own tapes for the operating room and recovery room. "I sat on the floor of my bedroom with my cat curled at my feet and made tapes of my voice telling me things that would help me in surgery. It was self-affirming. My voice speaking to me about my will to live. My blessings and my strength and that I am loved and I am blessed and I am cared for. I had the tape on during surgery, which was fourteen hours. I even had one for recovery. 'Hi. I think I'm waking up.' I'll never forget hearing that."

Joyce also had friends and family positioned outside the operating room with instructions to send good thoughts her way. "I told them to say prayers. I felt they would know what to say. I can't program their love. I just received it. It was a real energy flow. In the operating room I blessed all the doctors and thanked them for all their good work."

Oncology and Grief Crisis Counselor Jan Pettigrew, Ph.D. and R.N., Talks About Women and a Breast Cancer Diagnosis

Jan Pettigrew, Ph.D. and R.N., is an oncology and grief counselor who has worked with cancer patients for thirteen years. Since 1989 she has facilitated a group for women with breast cancer as a service provided through Dr. Sally Knox's practice. She is now in private practice in Little Rock, Arkansas.

What is happening emotionally at diagnosis?

The first word women hear is *cancer,* and they don't hear beyond that. The total focus is on cancer, and the predominant emotion is fear. The major fears of a cancer patient are death, dying in pain, and dying alone. There is also fear of debilitation and disfigurement.

This is when women think, I am going to die. They feel guilty that they are being morbid and not up for the family. They berate themselves for being pessimistic. I think it is very healthy to be thinking about death. Then you can back up and get some perspective about where you really are. If you spend your energy trying to avoid it, you exhaust yourself.

What do women need to know about these feelings?

They need to be hearing that it is okay to be afraid and not to have to fight with the fear, but to go with the flow and let someone be there and comfort them. They need to begin breaking the fear into manageable parts and name the specific fears so that the fear is not so overwhelming.

How do you name a fear?

You name it by talking about where you are. What are you feeling right now? Can you put a name on it?

(continued)

What are some of the other issues women express?

We are inundated with the message that we should be positive and that there are cancer types. There is the pressure when you are diagnosed to do cancer right. "I am onstage and I will pull myself up by my bootstraps and say all is fine and not fall apart." All the mind/body emphasis is really on not denying feelings you are having but letting yourself go with the feeling and letting someone else into that feeling.

How do a wife and husband or two significant people talk about this right now?

Give each other permission to say what is in their hearts. There is a great tendency to try to say the right thing to try to cheer the other person up or to too quickly say, "Everything is going to be okay." It's not just one person who gets cancer; the whole family gets cancer. So the husband is called upon to make just as big an adjustment as the wife, and they need to talk honestly about what they are facing and not protect each other from their fears. To be able to cry together and comfort each other.

What if that isn't happening? The woman is in need and either the man is not there or you are alone?

Your need is still valid and you must activate other parts of your support system, other family members or friends who you can tell how bad it is.

What can friends do or say to help the person open up and then what do they say when she says, "I'm totally terrified"?

The questions are "What is happening to you right now?" "Where are you?" "What is going on?" You can ask, "How can I support you in a way that will be meaningful to you?" You liked flowers and you told your husband that. Some people want cards. It is not so much doing the right thing as being there, being fully present with your heart. Talking is the most valuable thing a while

(continued)

woman can do. It is not so much that your friends hear you, but that eventually you begin to hear yourself. It takes a while.

What does a shut-down person look like?

They are very rigid. They will say things like I am fine, I am okay, I don't need counseling. I can handle this. And then you see a tenseness in their eyes. They are *too* together. That worries me more than someone who is in here screaming.

What about fear? What do we do with it?

Fear manifests itself in depression and anger. I keep saying to lean into your fear. Don't run. Let yourself be who you are. If you are angry, be angry. If you are sad, be sad. Feelings are neutral, even though we tend to label them good and bad. So just allow the experience.

But when you don't have anything to be angry at, how do you vent that?

You get socks and roll them up and throw them at the wall as hard as you can or buy cheap wineglasses and shatter them in a box in the backyard. Get a bat and hit a tree. Get a tennis racket and hit a pillow. Scream in the car. Find a physical response.

What happens after surgery?

After surgery is a time when I see women trying to get it together. They say, "Well, I made it through surgery and now I will get on with my life." There is always a let-down right after surgery—from a few days to a month. It occurs when the adrenaline surge that accompanies surgery cuts out all at once. Then comes preparing for postsurgery treatment and that brings depression all over again. It is a time of uncertainty. They have heard about chemo and it's awful and they are scared all over again. The woman puts a guilt trip on herself that she is not doing well. She thinks, "Oh gosh, I am not coping." But the let-down doesn't have

(continued)

anything to do with coping. The body is worn out and needs a rest and overwhelming emotions always follow the physical state of being worn out.

What is the best source of immediate support?

Someone who has been through it. Support groups or one-on-one with someone who has been there and who is far enough ahead of you to show that you can make it. But someone who will be honest. "I hated losing my hair and I hated throwing up, but that may not be your experience. But you can make it. I did."

When does leaning into feelings become destructive to the person?

That has to do with time and how long it goes on. If there is no release and the woman is just going with the fear over and over and over again, without resolution and release, then that gets destructive. We are talking weeks and months. Being angry is okay, but weeks and months without change means you need help. I see a lot of suicidal tendencies after mastectomy. It is very important that a woman closes the door on suicide as an option for her escape from this scary experience if she is going to live. You have to choose. It is a deliberate choice to choose to live with cancer as opposed to die with cancer. You die by choice. You may live with this disease twenty plus years and yet all that time was wasted because you were mentally dying. You chose to die, not live.

How long does this all last?

I think you are talking years and I can't give you a certain time. It depends on how deliberately the woman has worked through letting herself feel all the feelings. A lot of times women have to get back into taking care of everyone and all the responsibilities. She may also choose to do that as an escape from feelings. Then she undergoes what we call "crash and burn" later and that delays the whole process. Many times women are pressured to hurry up

(continued)

and get to the point where they see cancer as a gift or they see the positive side of cancer so they try to escape the process. I don't think you can get to that point without the struggle.

How do you know when it is over?
The healthiest people are the ones who can be open about all aspects of their experience. That is what you are striving for.

How long does the process take?
Cancer changes a person forever.

REACH TO RECOVERY AND HOSPITAL SUPPORT

When Jo Anne returned home from the doctor's office after receiving word that her tumor was malignant, her first call was to her husband and the second to Reach to Recovery, a national organization in which volunteers who have had breast cancer are matched with women who have just had surgery. They come to the hospital in the days after surgery to show women the exercises that will help in the healing process. They also bring a bra with a cup designed for a prosthesis and a small pillow for propping up the arm. Reach to Recovery is not designed to provide ongoing support. (Although in some parts of the country they are expanding services.) Volunteers will visit once in the hospital and then offer one follow-up call. From then on, you can place a call to the American Cancer Society and the call will be returned.

When you do see someone from Reach to Recovery, you may prefer someone in your own age group. It will depend on your city and the organization whether any will be available to you, so it may take some extra work to find one. Jo Anne's son was six months old when she was diagnosed. *"The first woman was just not a match. Then Lynne called me. She was very empowering because she said, 'You are afraid you will never see your son go to kindergarten.' That was exactly it. That was when we clicked, and I told her I wanted to keep her."*

Reach to Recovery responds to women who have been referred by their doctors—but not automatically. Indeed, volunteers cannot show you the exercises without a prescription from a doctor, although it does not have to be your surgeon. Tell your surgeon or the nurse that you would like a call now, before surgery, and you want someone your age. You can take control and make the call yourself. Tell them what kind of surgery you are having. They match women with similar situations. If you are going to have immediate reconstruction, tell them. This way they will send a woman who has had your experience.

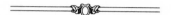

Tip—Call Reach to Recovery yourself and ask for a women who matches your needs. Then call your surgeon (or any other doctor) for the authorization. The volunteer needs this before she can show you the exercise.

Those women I talked with who were visited by Reach to Recovery volunteers in the hospital were divided on the effectiveness of the visit. Usually, it was the age issue that presented problems.

"The woman who came to see me was in her seventies and all dressed up, with lots of makeup. She introduced herself but didn't touch me. She stood at the end of the bed and pulled out this stuffed tit that was made of satin. She said, 'You can sew this yourself.' Well I don't sew; I don't do buttons or hems. The tit was stuffed with old hosiery, and she said I should pin it on the inside of my gown as I left the hospital so my husband would feel comfortable. I thought, You ass. She should have come in with the knowledge that I wasn't married, at least finding out something about me before telling me that I should be concerned about what someone else thinks. I asked to see her incision since she was ten years out and she said that wasn't appropriate."
—Mary H

A number of the women interviewed for this book have become Reach to Recovery volunteers. They say the organization is changing to provide more home visits and that many of the volunteers will talk about emotional issues with women. Indeed, you will find that like most volunteer operated organizations, Reach to Recovery methods and volunteers vary from one part of the country to another, depending on the programs and those in charge.

Teresa M was the coordinator of Reach to Recovery for greater New York City when we talked.

"When I became the coordinator, the woman who had left felt very strongly that breast reconstruction should not be discussed in the hospital and that a volunteer should not discuss whether she had had chemo or how she had handled it, or aspects like that. It was very tightly controlled. And when I came in, I felt that by walking into a room and saying to a patient, 'I had chemo but I can't discuss it' was more frightening than saying, 'Yes, I had chemo and I'm alive today. And it wasn't pleasant but I made it through it and you will, too.' No, we shouldn't discuss the drugs or the individual treatments or things like that, but when I came in, I said, 'I want to have a breast reconstruction program. I want women to come here and talk to those of us who have been reconstructed. I want them to know.' "—Teresa M

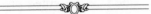

Tip—A number of hospitals have created their own cancer survivor network. Ask.

The proliferation of support groups has also meant many more sources for women who might visit you and talk with you about their experiences. Indeed, many hospitals have created additional cancer visitation groups. Ask your doctor or the floor nurse if the hospital has a group that might send someone to see you.

SURGERY

"Her surgery was delayed about two hours, and it was getting really late in the afternoon. We knew Dr. W had several surgeries, and I

thought he would be exhausted. I was concerned. But he talked to me
before the surgery and he was so high. He was like a football coach,
'Are you ready, let's take care of this problem.' "—Sherry's husband,
Kerry

"*The surgery wasn't bad at all. After four months, you can imagine,*
I was ready mentally. I had prepared myself physically. I felt good. So
I was really ready for that. And I recovered from it really quickly. In
the spectrum of things, it was not that bad."—Diane

"*The hard thing was checking in that morning of the surgery—I*
had to be there at five o'clock, and it was right before Christmas, and
we drove through the dark, dark streets and it was freezing cold, but
everybody had Christmas lights out. And I felt like, I don't want to be
here."—Lise

I don't know when I have been more frightened in my life than the
day my husband and I got up at 4 A.M. to leave for the hospital on the
day of my surgery. I don't remember kissing Kirtley goodbye. It must
be one of those memories that is too painful.

Somehow, driving through cold, dark, empty streets was appropriate
for my state of mind. I was numb with fright that morning. I was
walking and talking but light-headed with fear. My surgery was scheduled for 7 A.M., and after talking to women who waited for hours before
going to the operating room (OR), I think early morning is better. I
tried my best not to really wake up, thinking I would just nap until it
was time. Fat chance.

When we arrived at the day-surgery check-in (in the remote possibility that this was benign in which case I would go home), I was put
in a room and immediately visited by the nurses, who checked vital
signs and drew blood for a last-minute workup before surgery.

The anesthesiologist came and we discussed being put under. If
you have any history with surgery and know you are sensitive to anesthesia, tell him or her. I wouldn't find out until later that I am
one of those people who always throws up after surgery from the
anesthesia. You'll be asked to sign a staggering amount of paperwork
that says, basically, you might die, and if you do, it is not the hospital's fault. Period.

At that early hour, Tom and I were visited by both our pastors and every resident who was awake. It must have gotten out quickly on the floor that I wasn't very modest and was willing to offer up my lump for palpation.

The surgeon also usually stops by. This is a good time to ask some last-minute questions, while your husband, boyfriend, friend or family are there. For example:

1. What will my chest look like when you are finished? Are you using staples or closing with an inside stitch?
2. How many days will I be here?
3. When will I have the results from the pathology report? How many pathologists will see it?
4. Who will tell me the results of the pathology report?
5. What will be done with the tumor when you remove it?
6. Will anyone be assisting you with surgery? What will they do?
7. How long will I be in surgery?
8. What time will I be in my room?
9. When will I see you again?
10. Where will my husband/friend/family be? When will they know something?

Remember, husbands, significant others, and family who are waiting outside the operating room generally will get the news of your condition before you wake up. If you feel strongly that someone not be told before you wake up, be sure to tell your doctor. Sonja was angry that the doctor told her mother, who had a heart condition, of her cancer before she awoke. It will also be our husbands or significant others who will contact family who are not present. You may want to discuss this before surgery.

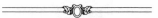

Tip—Ask your surgeon if there will be "call-outs" from the operating room, when the nurse or doctor lets the family know how you are doing.

Many women used music, both in surgery and in their rooms to relax them and facilitate healing. Nancy W discussed at length with her surgeon his talking to her during surgery, an idea he gradually accepted. *"I told my surgeon that I wanted him to tell me the process of healing because I wanted to make a tape to listen to. He wouldn't and I think part of it is that doctors don't really know. Bodies heal, but they don't know how. So I said, 'While I am under the anesthesia, I want you to tell me how I'm going to get better. Maybe not what is happening in my arm and breast, but the stages I'm going to go through and that everything is going to be okay. I don't want the possible good outcomes and possible bad outcomes. I don't want the alternatives. I want you to talk to that real down deep level of me and tell me what's right and what's good and what's going to happen. Even if it is a lie.' He took a deep breath and said, 'All right. I'll do it.' He saw me before I went in and said that he told everybody on the surgical team and that everyone felt like fools and went ahead and did it for me anyway. When I came out, the first thing he said was, 'I talked to you.' "*

Many young women today are making demands unheard of only a few years ago. They want music in the operating room that will calm them. They want the surgeon to say supportive things about healing and wellness while they are under. Many of these suggestions come from Dr. Bernie Siegel's books *Love, Medicine & Miracles* and *Peace, Love & Healing*. Siegel explores the body's responses to music and talk while the patients are under and has found interesting results. Dr. Jeanne Petrek, breast surgeon at Memorial-Sloan Kettering, says the anesthesiologists she works with have become accustomed to turning the tapes over for women during surgery. She says that her surgical team is accepting of anything that will help the patient feel better about her surgery, including accepting a blessing from one patient. "We were ready to put one woman to sleep when she sat up on the table and said, 'I want all of you to kneel down so that I can give you the blessing.' Now, of course, we were all sterile and you aren't supposed to go anywhere near the floor, so we all looked at each other. She repeated, 'Can somebody kneel down, please.' She was very sincere about it, and luckily the nurse anesthetist agreed to kneel down. I told the patient that she represented all of us, and the patient gave us her blessing and then we started."

"The anesthesiologist allowed me to have tapes. I used a lullaby for the first and got a subliminal tape for the second. One side was preparing for surgery and the other side was recovering from surgery. I had earphones on a tape recorder and he flipped the tapes for me."
—Nancy W

After I waved goodbye to Tom and I was being wheeled into the operating room waiting area, a nurse put a warm blanket on me and squeezed my hand. I don't know her name, and she will probably never know what that little human contact meant.

Then a familiar face was there as Dr. Knox came by. Her calm, "this is routine" attitude really helped. I was taken into the OR, where they put the anesthesia in the IV. The last thing I remember was telling everyone to do good work. I woke up in recovery, threw up, and then felt better. Later, I vaguely remember being taken to my room and moved to the bed. When you are trying to wake up from surgery, the nurses are always calling to you from the bottom of the anesthesia well. "We are in your room now and we want you to help us get you on the bed."

I remember having disconcerting dreams. I awoke with the sense that all was not well. Like the typical person who does not like being out of control, I fought the drugs and woke up an hour earlier than anyone expected. Tom had left to tell his mother the news about the clearly malignant lymph node, and I awoke to the face of one of my best friends from church.

Cathy had a degree in counseling, which is probably why she was able to talk with me without telling me that my cancer was worse than they thought and was now in at least one of the lymph nodes.

She called Tom immediately and let me say hi. I know now how terse he sounded, but as far I was concerned, the world looked great. I was alive. I had woken up.

He was back at the hospital in a flash and told me the news. I remember comforting him and promising I would not die and make him rear our daughter alone. Since I am the worrier in the family, I had entertained the idea that the cancer might be worse than suspected. Tom, being the optimist, thought it would be a lumpectomy, radiation, and back to normal. The diagnosis hit him hard. After reassuring him, I slipped into automatic pilot, that state of mind where you function and go through the motions, but nothing really sinks in.

Everyone gives denial a bad name, but I think it is the body's screening mechanism. It's as if the filter on the world closes down like on the end of a funnel. We only hear what we can handle. At some level I knew the cancer was worse than the original prognosis, but I didn't seem to be reacting. I could only deal with minute logistics—the big picture was out of range.

Dr. Knox came by shortly thereafter and confirmed what Tom said and told me they had scheduled the mastectomy for Wednesday morning, just a day away. I felt so lucky to have a surgeon who did not immediately do the mastectomy, knowing that I would wake unprepared for the loss of the breast. She explained that on Tuesday they would do the testing to see if the cancer had spread since there was node involvement.

Spread?

She explained then that lymph nodes are the body's first front against cancer, and when they have been overtaken, there is a possibility that single cells (**microscopic disease**) have also made it past the lymph nodes and are traveling in the body. Therefore, instead of radiation, which kills cells that may have been left locally near where the tumor was in the breast, it was now necessary to talk about chemotherapy, a systemic treatment for cancer, in which the body's whole blood supply is treated and those microscopic cells are searched out and destroyed. But first the radiologist had to check the spots in the body to which breast cancer cells most often spread (or **metastasize**) and form new tumors: the bones, lungs, and the liver. For that reason, I would have a battery of tests the next morning.

I think I said something like, "Oh, okay," as I slipped into a fear-induced stupor.

Frequently, women whose tumors appear large or give other indicators that there may be lymph nodes involved will have the bone scan, lung X ray and sonogram **before** they ever go to surgery.

It amazes me now that I did not know the magnitude of what she was saying or the importance of the results of those tests. The next day I was taken to nuclear medicine for a bone scan, where they injected me with a substance that would attach itself to any cancerous spots in my bones. I then lay on a table while a huge machine moved over me just inches away. It gave a picture of my skeleton.

Next came the liver scan, which was like the sonogram I had had while pregnant—only this time he was looking for dark spots on my liver that could be cancer. The chest X ray was like many I had had in the past.

All the tests were in and negative on Tuesday afternoon. Dr. Knox got the pathology report and gave me the basics on my tumor, which was **invasive carcinoma,** slightly estrogen-receptive and about 2.5 to 3 centimeters in size.

You can have a copy of the pathology report by asking for it. Not being the medical consumer then that I am now, I finally asked to read my pathology report in 1990, four years after my diagnosis. I wish I had seen it then, but this is one of those "when you can handle it" areas.

A couple of the women in this book asked that their slides be sent to an independent pathology lab of their choice. The hospital usually won't give you your slides for fear they will be lost, but they will transport them for you to another lab. Trusting the pathology report, on which all your treatment hinges, is a little scary. Your choice of surgeon again reflects on both the anesthesiologist and the pathologist, both of whom the surgeon will choose.

When Tom called that afternoon, we chatted about bringing Kirtley to the hospital that night. "Oh by the way, all the tests are fine," I said as an afterthought.

"What?" he said emotionally. "Why didn't you call me and tell me?" I remember saying very calmly, "I knew it was okay. What is the matter with you?" Automatic pilot was in complete control.

That night my husband and I bid a fond farewell to my breast.

I have always liked my breasts, seeing them as one of my better features. Somewhere between a B and C cup, they were big enough and not too big. I enjoyed the braless era of the sixties and had a number of antique dresses that I would no longer be able to wear. All I can remember about that night was looking at the bandaged breast and realizing that I couldn't go braless again (little did I know of the wonders of reconstruction then). The magnitude of the loss seemed minor compared to the imminent fear of death, but it would come later.

On Wednesday, I was wheeled again to the operating room where my right breast was removed. I woke that afternoon with two drains hanging from my now lopsided chest. The drains consist of one or two pieces of tubing placed inside the incision that empty into a bulb on the end. I felt fine, and once the grogginess from the surgery wore off, I felt great. It is the famous adrenaline rush that many women experience after surgery. It is that sense that we have beaten this beast. We have won. We have wakened from surgery and the cancer is gone. We are woman and we will survive.

AFTER SURGERY

"I remember recovery and being there a long time and starting to feel real happy. As we were going down the hall toward the room, I could hear the music from The Big Chill *blasting down the hallway. I guess they called to say I was coming. Mark put the tape in and turned it way up. I felt like dancing. I was so glad and relieved to wake up from surgery. I remember transferring from the gurney to the bed. My friend Lynne who was there told me about how hard it was for Mark to see me with the drains. He had to go out into the hall and put his head between his knees. I was euphoric when the resident came in to see me. I had been rude to him earlier and he deserved it. The same resident came in and I asked him to go dancing with me."*—Jo Anne

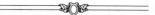

> **Tip for friends and family—Recognize the adrenaline rush for what it is. We are at war and have just won a major battle, but the fight is far from over. Don't be surprised if in a few weeks the positive attitude has been replaced by anger and despair.**

I, along with most of the women I talked to, didn't find the mastectomy painful. Since the nerves have been severed, there is no feeling in the breast.

"I was struck by how nonintrusive the surgery had been. It reiterated in my mind how superfluous these breasts really are. I remember feeling after the surgery how lucky I was that it wasn't an arm or leg or

something I needed to be who I was. The loss didn't have any effect on me. I could do what I had always done."—Victoria

If you are considering immediate reconstruction, the entire surgery process and recovery will depend on which procedure you choose and how long you are under. Marjorie B was in surgery for eleven hours while a section of her hip was removed and reattached to her breast in microsurgery. *"Coming out of eleven hours of anesthesia felt like it went on for years. The first hours were the worst. I would drag my eyes open and it would be three and I would close my eyes and two hours would go by and when I opened them it was only five past three. I was ready to kill myself."*

Some women experienced nerve hot spots, created when one of the nerves sends a signal and it hits a raw end. One woman compared the sharp, quick pain to a cold-sensitive tooth. These last a few days but are sporadic. I didn't have them at all.

Without a doubt, the major complaint from the women in this book about the physical part of the surgery was the drains. The nurses empty them while you are in the hospital and then you will take them home with you and learn to drain them yourself. They don't hurt. They are just inconvenient and a constant fuss.

"I had my own blood and was in the hospital nine days and came home with all kinds of tubes and hated it, hated it, hated it. That was horrible. That was probably the most debilitating, dehumanizing, degrading thing that I can remember."—Joyce

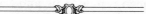

Tip—If you have immediate reconstruction, you may have more extensive pain and a longer hospital stay, depending on the procedure.

Many of the women in the book had friends or family stay with them in the hospital. Chuck spent long hours at the hospital with Marjorie and found that a gift that was most welcomed was food. *"I was glad because you can't do much, but at least she didn't have to eat that hospital slop. Mostly it gave me something to do—going out to restaurants and bringing food back."*

Those of you whose parents are in the city may also want to follow the same guidelines as dealing with children. Of course, most adults know about hospitals, but they will also want information and as much participation as your family dynamics allow. Diane called on her sister to come and care for her during surgery. *"My parents felt excluded. Like I was taking care of them, and they wanted to take care of me. They, from the financial standpoint, had to help, but I probably should have brought them in."*

> *"Oh, it was horrible. My mother and I just really went through a major crisis in our relationship because she is very dominant, and before that time had been very invasive in my life, as far as what I should do and how I should be. When I was diagnosed, it was like she had it. She was really worse than I was. And we really went through a lot of struggles about it."*—Amy

Cindy's mother flew in from out of town and spent the night with her daughter at the hospital. When the doctor came in, he initially asked her mother to leave the room while he changed the bandages. Cindy asked that she stay since she would be helping with the bandages at home.

Make clear to your surgeon and the nurses what you want and who you want in the room. Some doctors ask husbands to leave, assuming that the woman wants privacy. If you want your husband or family member there during doctor visits, say so. Hospital rules about parties and visiting hours have softened considerably in the past decade, but you should use good judgment.

> *"I had surgery on New Year's Eve day and that night at 3 A.M. I had tubes hanging out everywhere and I hear this party coming down the hall of the hospital. My friends showed up at 3 A.M. with hats and balloons and snuck in the room and we had a party."*—Mary H

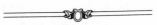

Tip—Hospital rules are softer now, but use good
sense about getting some rest. The nurses can run
interference for you and put a DO NOT DISTURB **sign**
on your door.

Since the surgery is not that painful, most of the women enjoyed
their visitors, and once the surgery and pathology report were out of
the way, they tried to make the most of their hospital stay.

*"The hospitalization was one of the high points of my life. All my
friends were there. I had more flowers than would fit in the room and
lots of cards. In fact, I was exhausted because someone would come by
to visit me and then another person would come in and the first person
would leave and that person would stay until the next person came.
So I had visitors all day long. That ended when I came home. I went
in the second week to get the staples out and the nurse asked how I
was and I said I was really down. She said that was not unusual,
because hospital stays can be good because so many people are around
you. Then you go home, and especially me because I live alone. You
can't work, so you just sit. I had a lot of things to do, but that doesn't
take the place of having someone around to talk to. That was the first
time I started thinking about the future."*—Dana

Tip for friends—Don't forget to call after she goes
home. The adrenaline rush from the hospitalization
is over and the pain from the surgery gets worse as
the incision begins to heal and pull. In addition, the
reality of what has happened has begun to sink in.
Call, go by, or perhaps save your flowers for the
week after she gets home.

The hospital is not the place to begin a campaign for the latest fad cure or books on self-healing—unless she asks for them. Wait until she is home, but still ask first. Unless you have had cancer, you cannot imagine how irritating it is to have a healthy friend bring you the latest cure from a popular magazine. Oh that it were that simple.

I found that friends who visited were uncomfortable hugging or even looking at me. And many cannot help that first glance at your now flat chest. Some of the women were open about this with friends, showing their incision or making jokes about people's tendency to stare.

THE INCISION

"Dr. H had a really good way of showing my husband the scar. He was changing the bandages, and David was in the chair. He said, 'I need some help,' and he was there. I didn't have to prepare myself for showing him and he didn't have to be prepared to see."—Joanne

"The nurse would stand by my husband, and he and the doctor would dress it. Spiritually, he knew that was what I needed. I needed to know that he could look at my body and not recoil."—Joyce

Looking at the incision for the first time is a very personal decision and one that is totally up to you. If you want to be alone, be alone. If you want your loved one there, ask him or her. This is one area where there is no good or bad advice—go on your guts. What do you want to do.

I remember looking down at my flat chest a few hours after surgery. My orientation to the world was now different. I felt a combination of curiosity, revulsion, and calm. It was there and now it's gone. I don't actually remember "looking" all at once. I remember easing into it as I examined the drains and my peripheral vision took in the dimensions of the scar. I definitely think the incision brings home the reality of what has happened to your body, and a strong case of denial will surely crack at the reality of a flat chest.

Mary C couldn't look at her chest for three months. She had a visiting nurse who would come in and empty her drains and change her bandages daily. At the end of the first month, the nurse suggested that it was time. Mary tried to look, but became faint. They put it off again until the nurse's last visit. It took another two months for her to get her courage up. Mary finally looked at her chest when she went to be fitted for a prosthesis, where the owner of the shop provided the additional emotional support she needed.

Joyce found a new dimension to her husband as he changed her dressings every day. *"That was very, very special. He was so meticulous and careful. It was a labor of love. I saw it in his eyes. I watched his eyes. All the time. I don't think I've ever looked into his eyes more, before or since."*

"The day after surgery I kept getting ticked off at my nurse. She would come in and say, 'Well, have you looked at it yet?' and I'd say no. She kept telling me that I needed to look at it. She kept pushing, and it made me mad. Finally, I just ignored her. I didn't want to look at it by myself or with a stranger, like a nurse. I wanted to look at it with John first, so I said, 'I'd really like for you to do this with me,' and he said, 'Sure, whenever you are ready.' So on the third day we looked, and it wasn't that bad. I had built up this fright that it was horrible, that there would be a big hole there—and it wasn't that way. There was an incision and the skin was still there. I forced myself to look ahead and think, 'Well, shoot, once they put stuff in there it'll just pop back out again. So it wasn't as bad as I thought."—Andrea

"My reaction was that it wasn't as bad as I thought. I had pictured grotesque disfigurement, and it wasn't that. It was just a scar."
—Andrea's fiancé, John

"When they were taking off the bandages, Mark walks in the room. I couldn't have asked for it better because there was no time to discuss whether he wanted to be here or how we wanted to handle it. There it was. He could have turned and walked out, but he didn't, and I'll always be grateful for that. He didn't come real close, but he came close enough to look."—Jo Anne

"The day I came home from the hospital was terrible. That was the worst day because I looked at it. Of course, I was in a heck of a lot better situation than a lot of women who don't have immediate reconstruction. But it was there in full, living color what had happened to me. That was just overwhelming, overwhelming."—Ann

HEALING AND EXERCISE

Before you leave the hospital either Reach to Recovery or your surgeon will be by to talk about exercises to restore your arm to full usage. The standard is to crawl up the wall with your fingers, increasing the height every day.

The day after my mastectomy, I felt strange. My chest and underarm were numb and there was a kind of tight feeling. But I could lift my arm almost over my head. I decided this was a breeze.

Two weeks later, when my incision began to heal and pull, I understood the importance of keeping the arm stretched. The scar tissue is much harder to stretch if you have not been exercising. As soon as your surgeon releases you, begin using your arm. I found that standing back in the kitchen to put dishes away gave an extra stretch and, because I had a toddler, I didn't have time to stand around walking up the wall. Instead, I did my exercises in the shower, reaching my arm as high as possible and making a soap mark on the tiles. Each day I went higher until I could walk the arm up the wall by my ear.

Remember, you are not an invalid. I began swimming six weeks after surgery and many women resumed tennis and energetic exercise within weeks.

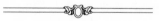

Tip—Don't begin stretching until you talk to your surgeon. Particularly if you have had immediate reconstruction. You may do harm to the implant position or inside stitches.

A great program offered at many YWCA locations across the country is ENCORE, which combines water and floor exercises with peer counseling for postmastectomy patients. Created by a nurse and breast cancer survivor, the exercises can help restore full range of motion in the arm. Call your local YWCA to see if the program is offered in your area.

"That arm is still bothering me after all this time, after two years. Whenever I stretch it in the morning, it's still tight under the arm and I've lost feeling."—Lise

"When I first started, I could just barely get my arm up. And I remember doing those exercises against a doorway. In just two weeks time, I could see the improvement."—Marsha

I remember the strange nonfeeling of my chest and underarm after my surgery. And the good news is that for most women some of the feeling will return after time. My lack of sensation extended almost to my elbow for the first year after surgery. At five years post-op, I could feel to within two inches of my armpit, and in the armpit there is deep feeling. On my breast, I can also feel sensation. When I had the nipple tattooed after reconstruction, I remember wondering why the nurse was deadening it more with a local painkiller. She explained that I had more feeling than I knew, and she was right. When the painkiller wore off, there was a dull kind of pain, like a bruise healing.

I have also experienced in the past year a very deep itching in my armpit. This scared me at first since I had itching as a sign of cancer, but when I asked my surgeon, she said that it was nerve endings and if I would massage my armpit, it would help. Shortly thereafter, I resumed swimming three times a week. Not only has the itching gone, but it seems my sensation is increased. I visualized for a time all the little nerve endings calling out for each other in the dark and then rushing toward each other to reconnect as someone sang "Some Enchanted Evening."

Other women in this book say their sensation has also returned, though none say completely.

The use of the arm after mastectomy should be the same as before unless you have problems with lymphedema, swelling caused by a buildup of fluid in the arm as a result of the lack of lymph nodes. Few of the women who were engaged in active physical activity before the breast cancer indicated they had to stop. Although some, such as Ann, could sense a little weakness.

"There are some things I can't do at the gym, such as hanging from a bar, that I could do before. But I'm able to do everything that I want to otherwise."—Ann

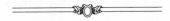

Tip—The mastectomy should not limit any kind of activity as long as you wait until you get clearance from the doctor a few weeks after surgery.

THE PROSTHESIS

"This woman said, 'Oh, you only have one breast,' and I said, 'No, I have about six.' "—Elaine

"Wearing a prosthesis doesn't bother me because I never had large breasts and I wore falsies all the time I was growing up. It's just padding my bra again."—Laura Mae

"You really forget all about it when your clothes are on. It feels so normal. There wasn't a night that I didn't take my clothes off and that thing fell out that I didn't jump. That's how real it felt. Every morning I would say this was not going to happen to me and then at night I'd forget and jump again."—Lola

One of the funniest evenings of my life was in a parking lot after sharing dinner with my support group. Seven of us traveled to the restaurant in my van, and at dinner the subject had turned to prostheses, those charming little chunks of silicone we use to replace what cancer (and our surgeons) have removed. Just as a bunch of guys talking about all the advantages of a new line of cars, we were discussing flexibility and comfort of the newest prostheses on the market. Marilyn, it seems, had punctured hers with her nail while playing with it (to see if it would stick to the bathroom mirror) and was shopping for a new one.

Just as some of us are sports-car types and others go for an all-terrain vehicle, the choice of a prosthesis can take some research.

After dinner, we had barely settled in the van to begin the ride back when one woman, eager to convince Marilyn of the assets of her chosen brand of prosthesis, removed it from its pocket in her bra and tossed it from the backseat to Marilyn's lap in the front. Soon six prostheses were being passed back and forth with much oohing and ahhing as their merits were discussed. Just then a Dallas police car drove by, slowing—I'm sure—in preparation to stop what must have looked like an illegal act of some kind, not knowing that the items being passed around in the dark van were only the various B and C cups of a group of women with a strange bond. The only thing that would have made it better was if the policeman had stopped and demanded we turn over the goods—now comfortably out of sight.

Tip—If you are shopping for a prosthesis, go to a support group and ask who would be willing to do show-and-tell in the bathroom. Also a great place to shop for plastic surgeons. And a lot of fun.

Your first prosthesis and mastectomy bra, which has built-in pockets for the prosthesis, will probably come from the American Cancer Society representative or Reach to Recovery in the hospital. If they don't come by, ask your surgeon or call the local American Cancer Society, but there are a number of other alternatives. One woman used a shoulder pad to get her home. The teardrop shape of shoulder pads in many of today's fashions is actually fairly close to what you will buy.

The Reach to Recovery prosthesis is a soft, fiber-filled form. It is not weighted and is only meant to be used for a few months, while the swelling goes down. Then you can be fitted for a regular weighted prosthesis. I saved my Reach to Recovery form to pin in my swimsuit the next summer. Except for having to squeeze the water out periodically (or let just my right breast drip when the rest of me was dry), that worked fairly well. But, then, I also do not embarrass easily.

When you begin to shop for a prosthesis, take your time. There are many on the market, and some manufacturers make a number of sizes and shapes to fit different body shapes and surgery indentions. If you are in a metropolitan area, you will probably have a shop that specializes in prostheses. In May 1993, I noticed an ad in a Dallas paper for Neiman Marcus's newest addition in lingerie—prostheses. I called and learned that all the sales personnel had been trained to fit the line they carried. Someone at Neiman's saw the market, and, with 1–6 million survivors, I hope other department stores around the country follow their lead.

Evelyn went for her prosthesis and found the model recommended by the clerk to be heavy and uncomfortable. *"She kept saying it was the right one for me and insisted. So I bought it. I don't wear it. It is heavy and I feel lopsided. I knew I wouldn't wear it if it wasn't comfortable, and I haven't."*

Ida Rose had very large breasts and found that a prosthesis to match her other breast was hard to find, so she asked her plastic surgeon to reduce the other side. *"It was fantastic and I found a silicone flesh-colored one that matched great."*

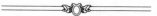

Tip—Don't let the clerk talk you into something. You are the one who will wear it.

The first prosthesis I bought was a large molded rubber form that I had seen at a booth at a Reach to Recovery seminar. It looked like a breast and had a nipple and extensions that fit out from the actual breast. It cost $250 and initially I liked it a lot. But soon I became aware that it just seemed too much for me. I felt like everyone was looking at my chest. Judy W bought two of the same prostheses and loved them; she liked the weight and felt they were very much like her original breasts. I ultimately donated my first prosthesis to a woman who could not afford one and paid $90 for a teardrop-shaped silicone prosthesis that was covered in fabric. It was heavy enough to mimic my breast and keep my bra from riding, but it was much smaller overall.

Those who specialize in prostheses will tell you the forms do best in a bra with a pocket. Most of these bras look like something our grand-mothers wore and to a young woman they can be particularly unat-tractive. I chose my first prosthesis based on the fact that it was worn in a regular bra, and I bought some beautiful and expensive bras to fill. I figured I deserved that. Then, when the first one didn't work for me, I found that the new, smaller prosthesis did just as well. I only wore the prosthesis bra with the pockets after that for particularly strenuous exercise, and that was more so I wouldn't ruin my good bras.

"When I went in to the shop about the prosthesis, she selected a bra for me that would be very utilitarian. It was the neutral skin color and designed to put a prosthesis in either side and very plain. She said this would be comfortable, and at the time I did want something that would be comfortable. But daily, I thought, I can't stand this ugly thing. I'm not going to spend a year of my life in this ugly lingerie, so I spent $150 dollars on panties and bras with the idea that I could have that little piece sewn in. I bought lacy, pretty, sexy-looking things. I took it in and said, 'Sew one of those damn pockets in,' and they did and I had about three of them."—Dot

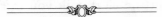

Tip—Before using a prescription to get a prosthesis, check with your insurance company. Some stipulate either a prosthesis or reconstruction. If you want reconstruction later, which is much more expensive, you may want to cover the cost of the prosthesis yourself.

INSURANCE

"I think one of the first things I ever said to my new boss was when I marched in his office and said I needed his help because my health benefits would not help pay for a prosthesis. The insurance company said that a breast was not a functional part of the body."—Elaine

"Why should a woman get a mammogram when she can't afford to do anything if it comes back suspicious?"—Diana

I am convinced that the next riots in the streets in the country will be about health insurance. Indeed, the word is seldom printed without such adjectives as *chaotic, disgraceful, shameful.*

No one questions the United States' supremacy in the medical field. But what good does it do to have technology such as bone marrow transplants and chemotherapy if you cannot afford them?

It is a crime that many cancer patients must fight for their lives while also fighting against financial ruin or inhumane insurance companies. Indeed, women who are uninsured and do not have the cash demanded by hospitals before admission for surgery must take the time to beg or borrow money while they know their tumor is still growing.

While the majority of women I interviewed had major-medical insurance, many expressed some frustration at dealing with their insurance companies. Some women lost their credit standing when the insurance companies paid slowly—sometimes drawing it out to six months or a year.

> *"I had excellent credit before this. Insurance didn't pay as quickly as they should, and they would say a bill had been paid when it hadn't been. It took me several years to get it straightened out and in the process it ruined my credit. The insurance company was supposed to pay 100 percent after a certain amount and they refused, and the hospital wanted me to pay, and I wouldn't because I knew I would never get my money back."*—Sheri

Some women were uninsured or underinsured and had the stress of extra bills added to their situation. Some found their insurance cancelled. Lola's insurance company just issued her a new policy after her mastectomy—with a cancer waiver. Marjorie B called her insurance company when she was diagnosed and was told that because she mentioned that she thought she had felt the lump two years prior to diagnosis, it was a preexisting condition!

As of January 1, 1992, stories were already emerging of doctors who refused to take Medicare patients because of new payment structuring. Indeed, Medicare refused to pay my mother's $100 consultation fee for the initial meeting with the oncologist who carefully discussed chemotherapy. Medicare would not discuss reexamination of the issue, saying that "patient education" should be free.

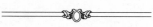

Tip—Insurance companies can do whatever they want. It is the consumers who must then prove they should be reimbursed.

The situation for poor women is appalling. This disease will kill a disproportionate share of poor women who do not have the money for regular care, much less preventive care such as mammograms.

Most private hospitals have a clinic setting, where indigent women can be seen by residents or doctors, within a private pay hospital setting. Many of those will no longer take breast cancer patients because once the patient is accepted, the clinic must continue caring for her. For a breast cancer patient, the cost can run to thousands of dollars.

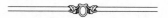

Tip—If your state is one that does not demand that mammograms be covered by insurance, you now have a cause. Establish treatment funds through your surgeon for those women who come after you.

The middle class is not far behind in the health care dilemma, with rising premiums and medical costs. As an entrenched member of the middle class, I found myself only a few months from the kind of ruin many women experience. While I was pregnant with my daughter, the year before I was diagnosed with breast cancer, my husband left his job with a major university to become a consultant. We had a conversion policy, which I thought was the same as a regular policy. Little did I know.

I had never filed a claim for insurance before my daughter was born. Unfortunately, she was early and spent seventeen days in the hospital before coming home. When we finally read our policy, we found we owed some $10,000.

I will have to find the right time to tell my daughter that we paid for her with Mastercard.

Because of this fiasco, I learned how to read an insurance policy. Since I was free-lancing and my husband was a consultant, I found an individual group policy that had out-of-pocket expenses of $1,000 and then 100 percent coverage. It cost us just over $200 a month in 1986, but was a good major health policy.

Two months later I found out I had cancer. If I had not taken out the policy when I did, we would have been wiped out financially and emotionally, trying to cope with cancer and bills. I know now from the stories I have heard that I was lucky.

But a year later, when it came time to renew our policy, we were informed that after the company had covered all but $1,000 of my cancer bills, our premiums would be doubled to $420 a month, because of "escrow balance for our group." We had no choice but to pay what amounted to robbery since I was uninsurable except through a large group.

Luckily, I was offered a full-time teaching position only a month after our new rates were announced. The university's standard insurance carrier wouldn't touch me, but the Preferred Physician Organization (which included all my doctors) would cover us with my preexisting condition. So with not one day to spare, we were covered, although reconstruction presented a minor hurdle.

I planned my reconstruction for the summer of 1988, two years after my surgery, and began interviewing plastic surgeons in the fall of 1987. It took a few "strong" calls to the insurance company—and one of my better letters—to get it to stop calling my reconstruction "cosmetic" and fulfill its obligation to pay for the reconstruction, which was the *one* consideration I made when choosing my new insurance carrier after returning to teaching full-time. I had called, explaining my situation, and the customer representative checked and said that it would be covered. Since then the company had adopted a case-by-case basis for all plastic surgery, lumping reconstruction in with nose jobs and tummy tucks. I offered to show the company in person the difference between cosmetic—which implies elective to improve on something existing—and reconstructive. The company declined, but did agree to cover the reconstruction of my breast, with the clear understanding that it doesn't pay for any modifications to the other breast. That, the company said, is cosmetic.

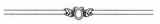

> **Tip—If you are considering a bilateral, take insurance into consideration. Some policies will cover reconstructing both breasts if you are high-risk or can convince the company of the need to remove both, but they won't cover alterations to the remaining breast.**

I am glad I like my job, since I am basically uninsurable. Others have become locked into jobs and marriages because of health benefits.

Elizabeth T's husband, Hugh, realized that a career change after Elizabeth's surgery was complicated by insurance needs. *"I'm limited because I've got to get into a situation that has a group health insurance policy."*

Pat F decided to retire from her job as a school nurse when it became too taxing in the midst of chemotherapy. Her insurance company had been paying 100 percent before she retired.

> *"The teachers' retirement that picks up medical insurance made no bones about it. They said if we wanted to be covered for the preexisting conditions, we had to go with them. So we had to start all over and pay the deductible and get back to 80 percent just to be sure that she would be covered in the future."* —Pat's husband, John

Marjorie's surgeon wanted the swelling to go down before making some adjustments on her reconstruction. Because it was a new calendar year before she was ready for the surgery, she had to pay a deductible out-of-pocket expense of $1,100 for the second time in three months.

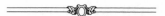

> **Tip—The only way to change the insurance mess is to put pressure on your state officials to control**

such abuse. Write letters and call. Document your situation and let people know. Demand that elected officials take action.

Often, insurance companies will just say no and leave the ball in your court to pursue legal action. For those who can afford it, this often results in a settlement, since insurance companies don't want precedent set in court. If you can't afford an up-front fee, find an attorney who will work for a percentage, or check law schools or legal-aid societies. Diana chose to have bilateral total mastectomies for her lobular carcinoma in situ. Her insurance carrier agreed to pay for the procedure on the left breast but did not want to pay for prophylactic mastectomy or reconstruction on the right side, despite her having provided documentation that this was acceptable and recommended. Even after surgery, when the pathology report showed a precancerous condition in the right breast, the carrier refused to pay. In addition, it greatly reduced the allowed coverage on the rest of the surgeon's fee, saying the charge exceeded "usual and customary" costs, although the company would not say what those were. The carrier said that Diana's policy did not cover reconstruction except following cancer surgery, which it did not consider hers to be. Diana at that point carefully read her policy and looked up medical terms in a medical dictionary. *"The contract used the term* neoplastic, *which by definition can be any new, abnormal growth— benign or malignant. After I brought this definition to their attention, they agreed to cover reconstruction for the right breast."*

Diana and her husband began legal proceedings against the insurance carrier for the surgeon's fees. They settled when it became clear they intended to go to court. In Texas, cases of fraud are eligible to be paid in treble damages, meaning three times the amount of the original claim. If you do have an insurance problem, Diana suggests engaging an attorney. *"But be prepared to have to educate your lawyers about your diagnosis. Don't assume that they know everything. I did some research on my own and was able to provide our lawyer with some critical information."*

There were also occasional stories such as Wendy's. Diagnosed at twenty-six, Wendy soon learned that she would need a bone marrow transplant. At that time, Wendy was only the eighth woman to receive a bone marrow transplant in the state of Texas, and the procedure was still considered experimental. *"The law firm where I was a paralegal was self-insured and I was worried when I found out that the partners had to put up some incredible amount of money—like more than $15,000—for me to get the transplant. They all pitched in and had it the next day."*

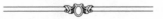

Tip—Be careful on breast assessment for your family members. Some insurance companies are asking about history of breast cancer and then refusing to cover any breast-related issues.

Even those who have insurance must be aware of every bill and every charge, to be sure that the insurance company and the hospital agree.

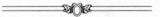

Tip—Keep a calendar that shows where you were on what day and what was done. This will help track insurance receipts that just give the date and the cost. Keep every bill from the hospital and know what each charge is for. Keep all correspondence from the insurance company.

A FEW TIPS TO HELP THE PROCESS ALONG:

1. Become insurance-literate—or if it is too confusing, find a family member who will take charge. It's better if only one person is handling the insurance issues. Keep a log of checks paid and received and calls made and received. Write down dates and the names of the people talked to. Don't throw anything away.

2. Be sure you have read your health insurance policy completely and know what is covered and what isn't. For those areas that are unclear, call the company. Find one person at the insurance company

and always talk to that one person. Some policies require preapproval or second opinions. If you do not follow their rules, you may find you are loopholed in the future.

3. Be sure that your premiums are up to date and that if you are in the hospital, someone is taking care of the monthly payment.

4. If the insurance company is slow to pay, contact your group representative at your office. If you are self-employed, write a letter indicating you have sent a letter to the state insurance board and that the next letter will be to an attorney.

5. If you continue to have problems, contact your state's insurance office. Again, find one person who will help you—this is the only way to get bureaucracy working for you. Often, the insurance companies are just trying to wear you down, thinking you won't actually sue. Create a major paper trail and write letters.

6. Write your representatives and document your problems within the political system.

7. Get an answering machine with a tape-call feature. Just be sure to say that you are taping the conversation.

SURVIVING ON THE JOB

Surviving cancer involves both physical and emotional work and no one going through it needs additional discrimination at work. Yet because of a continuing mentality that equates cancer with death, many cancer patients face ostracism and hostility, at worst, and discomfort and ignorance, at best, in the workplace. Cancer has been called the tuberculosis of the twentieth century, a scourge that labels its holder as unclean. We can't give blood, we can't serve in the military, and some would say we are not employable.

In 1992 there were an estimated 7 million cancer survivors—a figure that is expected to exceed 10 million by the year 2000. Many of these people are young and refuse to have the rest of their lives stamped with the word *cancer* and its associated stigma. They are standing up to insurance companies and employers and demanding to be treated like the rest of the world. In some cases that has meant lawsuits.

In 1990 the Americans with Disabilities Act was passed. And while its very title reinforces the continuation of the stigma, it does ensure that cancer survivors will have specific federal protection against on-the-job discrimination. Under the act, employers cannot screen your medical history and may ask medical-history questions only after you have been offered the job and if they pertain specifically to the performance of that job. The act, which is enforced by the Equal Employment Opportunities Commission, covers private employers with twenty-five or more employees through 1994 and then employers with fifteen or more employees. If you have a problem, call the EEOC at 1-800–872-3362. They will mediate a complaint on your behalf, and if it is found that you have the basis for a discrimination suit, the EEOC will file suit on your behalf.

Women were divided on how much they wanted coworkers to know about their condition. Even in a good work setting, the response of coworkers to a cancer diagnosis can be very painful.

Rula, a nurse, saw the women and men she worked with as her family since her own was in a foreign country. She says her coworkers took the diagnosis hard. *"Starting with when I was first diagnosed, I remember no one was visible. Everybody went into a room and started crying. Then the second day when I came back, everybody was so quiet, and I said, 'Look, guys, we need to talk. Is it better for you if I talk? Or is it easier if I don't?' And they said no, please talk about it, because we don't know what to tell you."*

Leanne and Angela had a very different experience when they returned to work after surgery. Angela: *"People at work, with the exception of a very few, acted like I was dead. People are scared. I didn't realize it then and it was very painful. They don't know what to say, and they are scared to say the wrong things, so they don't say anything at all. They should say, 'Hey, I know you are going through something and I don't really know how to relate but do you want some company?'"*

Leanne went back to work at her day-care job three weeks after her mastectomy. *"I didn't want to think. I just wanted to go to work and do my job and have my mind occupied. My first day back was really hard. They didn't know what to say to me. I expected some support and compassion, and they treated me like nothing happened. It was, 'Hi, nice to see you, I'm glad you're back.' It was a really weird experience."*

"I remember one of the guys at work saying, 'So I hear you have breast cancer.' I said, 'Yes I do,' and he said, 'I am very sorry,' and gave me a hug. It was great."—Jo Anne

Concerns about taking time off from work can add to the stress of a bad job situation for someone going through cancer. Cindy found her coworkers and employer concerned and caring until she began radiation and she missed a number of days' work. *"When I started doing radiation, they were like, 'This should be over.' It has changed my attitude a lot about the work force and people who are having a bad time. They need to be much more educated about what we are going through."*

Cindy remained locked in her job until her reconstruction was finished in mid-1992, knowing that she could not change jobs and expect to find insurance that would cover her reconstruction surgery. When she scheduled her expander reconstruction, she learned that her company would not allow her to work part-time, requiring that she leave for three months. While the company guaranteed her job would be waiting, she returned to find she had been replaced and is now working on projects throughout the company—at the same pay, but under much more stressful conditions. An infection in one of her incisions that required she take off additional time after returning to work was met with irritation by her new superior, who didn't know her history and with whom she had no relationship. *"It's hard, when you have been through so much, not to lose your temper when they say something like, 'It's hard on everyone when you are out.' Does this man think I want to be sick again? I could only say, 'Well, it's hard on you, but it's harder on me.'"*

Gale was simply fired from her job as manager of an event management company—on the last day of thirteen months of chemotherapy. *"I'd been to work every day for thirteen months. At the end of that thirteen months, with my final chemo, my boss and his family had just gone skiing, and when he came back he said it was time for me to go. He offered me two days' severance pay after thirteen years."* Gale says she turned her anger to profit by opening her own company, which is doing very well.

What we must do as cancer survivors is make our voices heard. The Americans with Disabilities Act was passed in part because of lobbying by the National Coalition for Cancer Survivorship, a very active organization that works for survivors in a number of areas. Think about joining. Ten million voices can be 10 million votes. In its winter 1992 newsletter, the NCCS listed which concerns it sees as critical in exploring new health care options: exclusion of coverage for preexisting conditions; denial of benefits for experimental drugs or treatments; job and marriage lock; employment discrimination; difficulty securing payment of clinical trials; experience- or family-history-based ratings of insurance premiums; caps on out-of-pocket expenses; patient's right to choose health care providers.

RESOURCES

ORGANIZATIONS

National Coalition for Cancer Survivorship, Fifth Floor, 1010 Wayne Avenue, Silver Spring, MD 20910; (301) 650-8868. A nonprofit organization whose goal is "to generate a nationwide awareness of survivorship." Much of the focus is on insurance and job-related issues. A $25 donation will bring the quarterly newsletter. The NCCS also offers a number of booklets. Also available from NCCS is *Charting the Journey: An Almanac of Practical Resources for Cancer Survivors.*

PUBLICATIONS

CompCare Publishers, 2415 Annapolis Lane, Minneapolis, MN 55441; (800) 328-3330. CompCare is a small press that has a catalog with a number of fine books about coping with cancer and breast cancer specifically. Call for a free catalog.

Coping **magazine,** 2019 North Carothers, Franklin, TN 37064; (615) 790-2400. *Coping* offers a range of articles for cancer survivors, including new research, complementary healing issues, political and research updates, and organizing National Cancer Survivors Day. Ads include those for products and prostheses as well as treatment centers, conventions, and books. At publication the quarterly magazine was $17 a year. Call for current rate. Back issues can be purchased.

Chapter 3

TREATMENT

STAGING

"I think the only thing you learn about breast cancer is that the more you learn about it, the more you realize that there's a lot more to understand, because there are so many variables in this disease."

—Robert Mennel, M.D., medical oncologist

After surgery you may be struggling with the emotional loss of the breast and the disruption to your life, but few women feel physically sick aside from the tenderness on the chest wall. Indeed, most feel good to have survived the surgery and to be on the other side of the diagnosis.

Now comes the "what next" appointment. What you know at this point is that your tumor was malignant and it has been removed. Now you begin to look at whether further treatment is needed. While the surgeon may be able to tell much from the biopsy, it will not be until the tumor, breast tissue, and lymph nodes have been examined after surgery that the complete picture will begin to form.

You may have already heard the word *chemotherapy* and be somewhat prepared that there will be follow-up treatment. For those women still in denial, the word is sure to be a blow—for no other word is more synonymous with cancer—i.e. "this is serious"—than chemotherapy.

You will get the news on whether you will have additional treatment in a consultation with an oncologist and/or surgeon within a few weeks following surgery, when the complete pathology is back from the lab.

If you have not yet contacted a medical oncologist—even if your surgeon assures you that you don't need to—see one. Again, take a tape recorder. This meeting may bring up even more statistics and jargon than the original diagnosis consultation with the surgeon. Be sure you understand what is being said.

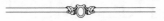

> **Tip—When you make the oncology appointment, ask about the transfer of any necessary paperwork, such as the pathology report and surgery report. Ask also who is leading the team for your cancer treatment from this point forward—the surgeon or oncologist.**

At this meeting, the oncologist will "stage" your cancer. This is a clinical and somewhat arbitrary scale that rates the seriousness of the cancer. I have left off the stages in the bios of the women in this book because they do not tend to be what a woman remembers. In addition, two women with similar staging factors may receive different treatment plans due to pathology findings.

The stage will depend on a number of factors:

- if the tumor was invasive (infiltrating) or in situ (intraductal, or inside the ducts or lobules)
- if any nodes were involved
- the size of the tumor, and whether there is any indication that the cancer has already spread to other locations in the body.

The pathology of the individual cell and whether it was aggressive or slow-growing are factors also taken into consideration for treatment and prognosis.

Because of earlier detection, the majority of women being diagnosed today fall in the early stages, meaning that when the tumor is removed, there is no evidence of any remaining cancer in the body. They are NED (**N**o **E**vidence of **D**isease). Follow-up treatment at this point is called

adjuvant, which means the cancer is gone and the focus now is on preventing its return by searching for any stray cells and eliminating them. The stages, according to the American Joint Committee on Cancer and International Union Against Cancer:

Stage O is in situ carcinoma, intraductal or lobular carcinoma, or Paget's disease of the nipple with no tumor.

Stage I is a tumor no larger than 2 centimeters (about the size of a grape) that has not spread outside the breast.

Stage II is a tumor no larger than 2 centimeters that has spread to the lymph nodes **or** the tumor is between 2 and 5 centimeters and may or may not have spread to the lymph nodes **or** the tumor is larger than 5 centimeters but has not spread to the lymph nodes.

Stage III is divided into **A** and **B. A** is smaller than 5 centimeters and has spread to multiple lymph nodes. **B** is cancer that has spread to tissue near the breast and/or to lymph nodes near the collarbone.

Stage IV includes inflammatory breast cancer or a tumor that has already spread to other organs of the body, most often the bones, lungs, or liver.

In addition to the stage, the pathologist and oncologist will look at the cell type, using DNA indicators to determine aggressiveness when determining a treatment plan.

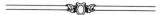

Tip—In treatment options there are many factors to be considered. If you have questions or feel indecisive, remember that you can get more than one opinion.

The surgeon and oncologist are going to recommend a treatment plan after surgery that also takes into consideration your age, general health, and if you are pre- or postmenopausal.

Treatment options may range from no additional treatment needed to some or all (in varying combinations) of the following standard treatments.

Radiation therapy, using X rays to kill cancer cells locally around the affected area. Radiation is almost always coupled with lumpectomy. Often it is used with mastectomy when the location of the tumor is near the chest wall or outer edges of the tissue that has been removed. Radiation may also be used on metastatic sites such as bone.

Chemotherapy, a systemic (throughout the body) chemical treatment in which drugs are injected into the bloodstream to search for and destroy microscopic cancer cells before they settle somewhere else or to arrest an existing tumor.

Hormone therapy, a form of chemotherapy using one of a number of drugs that reduce hormones or affect their interaction with cancer cells. This may be an estrogen block such as Nolvadex (tamoxifen).

Bone marrow transplant, a treatment reserved for women with high risk of recurrence who are clear of disease. The patient's bone marrow is removed before she is given high-dose chemotherapy to kill cancer cells. The marrow is then reintroduced to the body.

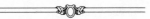

Tip—Doctors tend to quote studies, clinical trials, and percentages. Ask for consensus papers, which are the nationally agreed upon approaches presented at conferences. Ask the doctors if they have had patients with indicators similar to yours.

Be aware that many women are still not getting the most up-to-date treatment options from their doctors. To ensure you are receiving the most up-to-date care, follow these guidelines from NABCO (National Alliance of Breast Cancer Organizations).

1. Be sure your physician is board-certified in that specialty.
2. Seek physicians who are involved in national clinical trials of new cancer treatments, because they tend to be the best informed.
3. Ask the treating physician to consult a PDQ (Physicians Data Query), a computerized database, sponsored by the National Cancer Institute, of state-of-the-art treatments for all cancers at each stage. *Ask for a copy for yourself.*
4. Don't be afraid to ask questions, and when in doubt or when unsatisfied with the physician's answers, get a second opinion.

Bridie found, when she asked for a copy of the report from the cancer team that met to discuss her case, that the tape had been lost. The team had determined that adjuvant chemo was unnecessary in Bridie's case. *"This great news was relegated to Post-it notes and contained an aside that stated if I were anxious about my condition, they could begin a series of chemo treatments to relieve my ANXIETY. I informed them that Valium and/or scotch would be a more pleasurable alternative, thank you very much."*

When she asked for copies of the records and found that the transcript from the original tumor board was not included, Bridie asked that the board reconvene and do it again. *"I now have a specific, signed profile of my medical history since diagnosis and a statement which definitively states that I did not need additional therapy."*

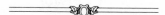

Tip—After the "what now" meeting with your team, ask for a letter restating everything that was said, the suggested treatment, and the reasons for it.

CHEMOTHERAPY

"I kept saying, 'I'm not interested in chemotherapy.' And my doctor of thirty years was on my case every day. 'We're going and I'm going with you to hold your hand.' And my husband was saying, 'You know, we can't not do this.' I was still absolutely adamant that there was another way, with a positive attitude and nutrition, that we could avoid the horror stories of chemotherapy. I just didn't have time to hang around the commode all day. We were lying there in bed one night and Gerry just looked so tired and so stressed out and so awful. And he said, 'I can stand anything unless I lose you.' And I thought, Oh shit. I'm going to be in the middle of chemotherapy no matter what."
—Gale

"Dr. X said the size of my tumor was kind of the deciding factor, and he never said that I had to have chemo, because my nodes were negative and my estrogen receptor was so high. But he said, 'The size of your tumor . . . if it were me, I would have it done.' I said, 'Well, that's what I want to hear.' Because if he had told me they weren't going to give it to me, I was just going to keep going around until I found somebody that would."—Madeline

"It never entered my mind that I might die until I entered chemo."
—Cindy

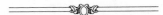

Tip—All reference to drugs in this chapter are to the commonly used brand names.

WHY CHEMO?

"He found what he said was an almost microscopic amount of tumor in one lymph node. He said if I hadn't been in such a good medical center, they probably wouldn't have even found it because it was so small. But because of that, he wanted to go ahead with the chemo. I was just devastated. Chemo—all the horror stories you have ever heard

hit you. So I was really frightened of that. But that was really not bad. I took it in stride."—Dot

"Chemo was hell. After the result came back from the lab in California, the doctor said that ordinarily, with everything I had, no, I would not have chemo. However, my anueploid factor indicated a higher incidence of recurrence. With that, he elected chemotherapy, which I'm glad about now, of course."—Julie

"I don't know what made me go back, because it was all voluntary and they didn't even know if I needed it. I didn't have any lymph nodes involved; I had forty-six removed, which was a world record, they told me. I guess having a four-year-old, I felt like I had to give it one extra good shot. I mean, you look at your children's faces, and I think that's what kept me going."—Lise

When I was diagnosed in 1986, the standard treatment for Stage I node-negative women (which it appeared I was until surgery) was removal of the tumor by either lumpectomy or mastectomy, followed by radiation, which would take care of any remaining cancer cells locally in the breast area. I had already seen the radiation oncologist before surgery and made an appointment for my first radiation treatment.

All that changed in the operating room when it became clear that I had at least one malignant lymph node, meaning there was a good possibility I had cancer cells in my bloodstream. Now we were talking Stage II and plan C for chemotherapy.

I never thought I would say this, but I am almost grateful now for that one node. Chemotherapy is a bitch, but it's the best we've got right now in the fight against breast cancer. It is now standard treatment for the majority of Stage I and II breast cancer diagnoses.

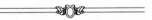

Tip—In January 1992, a major study released in *Lancet,* **a British medical journal, confirmed that women with early-stage breast cancer do live longer when they have adjuvant treatment of chemotherapy, Nolvadex (tamoxifen), or both.**

Why chemotherapy has become standard treatment is not very re-assuring and underscores how little is known about individual cancer cells.

Basically, removing the tumor and following with radiation is going to cure an estimated 60 out of 100 node-negative women with early-stage breast cancer. The 40 women who will suffer recurrence is de-creased to 15 or 20 by **adjuvant treatment,** such as chemotherapy. Adjuvant treatment is used when there is no evidence of cancer re-maining in the body—but there may be microscopic disease in the bloodstream.

So while statistics indicate 40 of 100 women with early-stage breast cancer would have recurrence without any adjuvant therapy, only 10 to 15 will have recurrence with systemic treatment. The problem is that oncologists don't know yet how to determine who are the 25 to 30 who will benefit—so everyone gets zapped.

It's a nasty lottery and one that will change as more prognostic factors (such as those provided by DNA and hormone tests) become available. In the meantime, it becomes the route we love to hate. It may make you sick, at worst, or be merely unpleasant, at best, and the long-term effects of many of the therapies have yet to emerge.

On the other hand—it may also save your life.

As a patient, the best you can do is ask that all your options be laid before you, with their benefits and risks outlined to the best of the doctors' abilities. Understand what is being said to you—and keep ask-ing questions until you do—and then decide what you want to do. Be sure that you understand clearly what the doctor is recommending for your case. Some women are clearly at risk for recurrence without che-motherapy. For others, chemotherapy may be suggested. For some, it is a personal decision based on their desire to be as conservative in their treatment as possible.

Emelda refused chemotherapy. She had no nodes involved but had a 4-centimeter tumor, for which she demanded a lumpectomy instead of a recommended mastectomy. *"He really tried to frighten me, and went on and on. He was kind of upset with me when I said no. But there's nothing wrong with my heart, my lungs—to damage all of my body, my organs. I worked for an insurance company and we had to look up all these drugs for payment. So I just looked things up for my own information. Every drug for chemo had bad side effects. I asked if there was something I could take that didn't have these side effects, but there wasn't. With everything God has given us, surely he has given us a way to cure ourselves without having to mix and mingle all these drugs. So I heard about this herbalist and bought a plane ticket and did that for six months."*

Unfortunately, Emelda suffered recurrence in her bones in late 1992 and began chemotherapy at that time. Whether adjuvant treatment after surgery would have prevented her recurrence is unknown.

Sylvia was diagnosed with in situ carcinoma with microscopic invasion at age thirty-nine. Her surgeon said she had a 95 percent cure rate with the modified radical mastectomy and no follow-up treatment. *"He said I would get my 5 percent chance of recurrence down to 1 percent with chemotherapy. I had five-year-old twins and a nine-year old, and 4 percent sounded like it was worth it. I told him I wanted the most conservative treatment possible, so I had six rounds of chemo. Of course, afterward, then he said we could watch me for twenty years to see what it may cause. I said that was fine. I wanted the twenty years to raise my boys. I really chose to do it."*

Clearly, chemotherapy is the original good news/bad news treatment. The good news is that it seeks out and destroys cancer cells that may be heading for another, more vital, organ where they will settle and begin multiplying and eventually impede function and cause death. Pretty scary thought.

The bad news is that on this search-and-destroy mission, the drugs have been developed to attack anything that looks remotely like a rapidly dividing cancer cell. Unfortunately, the drugs are not able to distinguish between the bad cancer cells and the good rapidly dividing cells, which include white blood cells and those cells found in the intestinal track and hair follicles. The destruction of these good cells leads to chemo's nasty side effects of nausea, hair loss, and fatigue.

As a college professor, I ask my students for evaluations at the end of every semester. My favorite evaluation came a few years ago and it sums up how I feel about chemotherapy, with a few editorial changes. It read: *The best class I ever had and I never want to do anything that hard again.* For me chemotherapy was the best choice at the time, and I hope I never have to go through anything like that again.

The chemotherapy used most frequently on breast cancer patients uses aggressive drugs and usually is given intravenously or in combination with oral drugs.

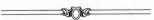

> **Tip—When Aunt Gert wants to tell you about the chemotherapy she had for her cancer, it may not be the same drugs or dosage.**

While hormone therapy is also considered chemotherapy, it is addressed separately.

QUESTIONS TO ASK ABOUT CHEMO BEFORE IT BEGINS, FROM THE NCI (NATIONAL CANCER INSTITUTE) AND OTHER SOURCES

1. Why do I need chemotherapy?
2. What would be the most aggressive treatment I could take?
3. What would be the most unaggressive treatment I could take?
4. How successful is the treatment for the cancer I have?
5. What are the benefits and risks?
6. What is being done in studies across the country that may provide an alternative?
7. When will I begin chemo?
8. Where will I have it (ask to see the room)?
9. Who will give it to me?
10. What drugs will I be given? Can I see the package inserts?
11. Can I go back to work?
12. What kinds of tests will I need and when?
13. Can I eat before a treatment?
14. What will I experience physically from the drugs?
15. What side effects are normal and which ones should I call about immediately?
16. Can I continue taking current medication? (Give drugs and discuss interactions.)
17. Can I drink alcohol?
18. Is there anything I shouldn't do during chemo?
19. Will these drugs affect my ability to conceive or have children after cancer?

MEDICAL ONCOLOGIST DR. ROBERT MENNEL, TEXAS ONCOLOGY, TALKS ABOUT BREAST CANCER TREATMENT

What is an oncologist?

The medical oncologist is an internist who subspecializes in the diagnosis and treatment of patients with malignancies.

What is a radiation oncologist or radiation therapist?

A physician who is board-certified in radiology, who specializes in the diagnosis and treatment of patients with malignances with the use of X-ray treatments.

When a patient is looking for an oncologist, what should she consider?

You want someone who has the credentials and is board-certified, but then I think you also need to find someone you relate to. I think that you can have the best credentials in the world but not be a good doctor because of the lack of interpersonal relationship skills.

Just as in choosing a surgeon, it's good to shop around?

Yes, although that's a very difficult situation. A woman doesn't have the luxury of a couple of months to decide on treatment. I think if you know a physician or if you relate well to your surgeon, you can ask which oncologist they feel you would best relate to. Then it is important to sit down at the initial visit and decide if you hit it off with him or her.

Explain the surgeon/oncologist relationship.

Let's say that we're talking about a surgeon who really knows what he or she is doing with breast cancer, who's up on things and is really on the forefront of what should be done. In that situation, most of the surgeons who know that the woman needs chemotherapy beforehand, or feel that the woman may be high

(continued)

risk for recurrence, refer her to an oncologist immediately. We would usually see the patient before she actually has any surgery, or right after she's had a biopsy, so that we can talk about our treatment possibilities. Then we would see what evolved as far as the tumor itself and what stage it turned out to be and what the various markers are.

Is there a trend in oncology toward looking at pre- and post-menopausal breast cancer as two different diseases?

I think all of us have always felt that breast cancer in a pre-menopausal woman is a much more aggressive disease as a whole than it is in postmenopausal women. That is primarily anecdotal information, but there are a few papers that address it. Now, among young women, there are clearly women who have all of the poorest prognostic features you could have but who do very well with their breast cancer for a very long period of time. And there are other women who seem like they're going to do rea-sonably well, who may be postmenopausal, be estrogren- and progesterone-positive, who have a terrible course with their breast cancer. This points out our lack of complete understanding of the biology of breast cancer.

When a woman walks in here and she is Stage I, what do you look at to determine if you will do adjuvant chemotherapy?

Up until about ten years ago, basically, the only things that we had to really look at to determine whether to use chemotherapy was whether there were positive nodes and the size of the tumor. We knew that if there were positive nodes, there was a risk of recurrence. If there were no positive nodes, we looked at the size of the tumor. And then, about eight or nine years ago, we started realizing that there were a lot of women who were Stage I and had tumors less than 2 centimeters, no positive nodes, no meta-static disease, and whose cancer recurred. We saw about a 40 percent risk of recurrence in that group of women that was re-duced by chemotherapy to about 20 percent. So we realized

(continued)

that some node-negative women would benefit from chemotherapy.

Who are those Stage I women who do not get chemo?

A woman who has a tumor of less than a centimeter who has markedly positive estrogen and progesterone receptors, who has a diploid tumor and a low S phase. Her risk of recurrence, if you put all those things together, is less than 5 percent. You would have to argue whether to reduce the risk to 2 to 3 percent is worth the chemo and the side effects. We would have to study thousands of women to answer that question. And you would have to balance the complications from chemo for the 2 percent difference.

Explain why particular drugs are used for breast cancer chemotherapy.

When we are talking the best treatment for adjuvant treatment the answer is that no one knows which treatments are better. There are studies that look at different combinations, but the two most commonly used combinations around the country are CMF, which is Cytoxan, methotrexate, and 5-FU or fluorouracil; and FAC, which is 5-FU, Adriamycin (also known as doxorubicin), and Cytoxan. If you ask physicians which is the best of these two treatments, many would say that FAC is better than CMF. However, if you asked them to prove it, no one could do that, because there has not been a study that compared them head-on. The reason why most physicians think FAC is better is that there have been studies of women with metastatic disease in which the cancer has already spread to the lung or liver, which show that the response rate, meaning at least a 50 percent regression of the tumor, is 5 percent higher with FAC. The way the thinking goes for the physician is that if that is true for metastatic disease, it would also be true if you are trying to prevent a recurrence. The answer is, that is not necessarily true. Because when you have visible disease, the drug may not work the same way. But many physicians carry

(continued)

over information and suppose it to be true. So, if a physician is making a recommendation of FAC or CMF, it is on more of an emotional basis.

It sounds like it's not very clear-cut.

That's true, and it's not to damn the system. I think one of the problems is that there is so much information coming at us about what to look for. It is like information overload. If you treated only in the situation where you had clear-cut data that something was beneficial, you would probably not treat half the people who walk in the door. The physician realizes that these are uncharted waters and it is his or her choice to do nothing or something that would be beneficial. Unfortunately, I think most people feel that medicine has all the answers to all the diseases. The problem is that every time you answer one question, you usually raise three others that you have to attempt to look at.

Explain exactly how chemotherapy works. Why is there hair loss and nausea?

Well, I think in a very general way, all the chemotherapeutic agents work by affecting DNA. They either cross-link the DNA so it can't unwind, or they may make it askew, so the DNA cannot unwind properly. The replication of the cancer cell is a very, very orderly process. If you happen to disrupt it during a time when it's going through a division, what you've disrupted is coding for a chemical or protein that's important for the survival of the cell, and the cell dies. As a general basis of how it works, you have to realize that every cell in your body has DNA in it. So every cell in your body is potentially susceptible to the chemotherapeutic drugs. Now, cancer cells divide quickly and the drugs are targeted to those cells that divide quickly. Also, it stands to reason that any normal cell in your body that multiplies quickly is at high risk for the effect of the chemo. And the cells in your body that multiply quickly are your skin, your gastrointestinal tract, and your bone marrow. The major side effect related to the skin is the hair loss,

(continued)

because those cells in hair growth turn over quickly. The nausea and vomiting, which everybody relates to that effect on the DNA of the stomach, really isn't from that effect. It's from the chemo receptor trigger zone in the brain stem. But there are other gastrointestinal effects, like women who get fever blisters or women who may get diarrhea. But that can be an effect on the rapidly proliferating cells of the mouth and the gastrointestinal tract.

RECEIVING CHEMO / IV VS. CATHETER (CENTRAL LINE)

"At the end she had to inject in my hand because I have no veins. But I didn't want another surgery to put in a catheter."—Sandy

Chemotherapy drugs can be introduced into the body in a number of ways and combinations. By the time this book is published, those may have changed yet again. In 1992, and for the women in this book, adjuvant chemo was usually given once every three weeks, beginning a few weeks after surgery. Those who receive chemo intravenously will do so at the oncologist's office. Most doctors have a special room. The one I was in reminded me of the orthodontist's office where I took my stepson for his braces during adolescence. There are six or eight reclining chairs, with a partition between each one. At Texas Oncology, each chair has a small television, and in the middle of the room is a large saltwater fish tank. (Watching fish has been shown to have a calming effect.) You will be hooked up to the IV, and then a number of drugs will be introduced over the next forty-five minutes to an hour.

Before you begin chemo you will have some tests, particularly a heart scan if you are taking Adriamycin, a very strong drug that has possible cardiac side effects. In the heart scan you are injected with dye that will make it possible to measure the strength of your heart muscle. The scan will be repeated to be sure that the drugs are not damaging your heart. If you did not have a bone scan, liver sonogram, and chest X ray before surgery, your oncologist may order those—or a CAT scan, which gives a picture of the overall body and would show anything suspicious. As with everything else, when a test is ordered, ask why and what it will show.

Bill and Lise decided for a lesser regimen of chemotherapy that would eliminate the more toxic Adriamycin.

> *"Her tumor was very small, with no lymph node involvement. And the pathologist was very extensive. She sectioned forty-six lymph nodes, and none of them were positive. And normally, they'll do a much smaller sample. So we felt very confident. And Adriamycin has its risk. Physical activity is very important to her and you're going to give a drug that's cardiotoxic. She could be in congestive failure and never exercise, never be able to do any of this again. There's a certain quality to life that would be lost, and was that really worth it? If it had been much more severe, we probably would have considered it."*—Lise's husband, Bill

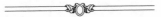

Tip—Ask what drugs you are being given and in what dosage. Ask to see the list of side effects (written in the package insert) if they are not clearly presented to you by the nurse before your first chemo.

The method for transmitting the chemo varies, depending on the number of treatments, dosage, and treatment protocol. For those women facing fewer than six treatments, the chemo is usually delivered intravenously every three weeks. For women who are facing more treatments—or as a preference of some oncologists—there are also catheters or shunts (also called ports), small devices that fit under the skin near the collarbone. The catheter gives direct access into a vein and provides a permanent port for the IV needle, making finding new veins unnecessary. Some catheters have to be cleaned daily, and some varieties have an external line that is taped against the chest when not in use.

The pros and cons of the catheter are many. Some women rejected another surgery to have it implanted. Some begged for a catheter to save their veins. Some felt the slower infusion made possible by a catheter was better for their tolerance. In a few instances, women had major difficulties with catheters. Leanne had by far the most serious complication and one that was truly a worst-case scenario. The tubing from her catheter detached and traveled into her heart. It was located by X ray and removed through a vein.

If you have a preference, be sure to discuss it with your oncologist. Because of the problems I have had with my veins since surgery, I wish I had insisted on a catheter. Remember that it is wise not to use the arm on the side where you had surgery for any medical procedures, including blood pressure and drawing blood, because of the risk of infection. This leaves only the other arm for all future sticks for blood.

Joan had a direct line inserted at the time of her mastectomy for chemo infusion. She had had a lumpectomy and suffered from lymph-edema (swelling of her arm) when another small tumor was located in the same breast, necessitating a mastectomy and chemotherapy. *"I think that was a better way to go. They couldn't use the left arm because of lymphedema, and Dr. B said, frankly, veins in the other arm weren't that great. He said he was afraid that after the first time that they'd tell me to put it in, and he said it was easier to put it in when we did the mastectomy."*

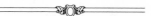

Tip—Those who have had catheters inserted recommend marking your bra line before the insertion, to be sure the catheter is not irritated by your bra strap.

Veins become a big issue for women who have had chemo. We know where they are and where they aren't. Chemotherapy does make your veins hard and scarred. The arm on the side where you had your surgery cannot be used for any medical procedures because of fear of infection due to a lack of lymph nodes. Some women know that they have small, inaccessible veins.

Even those of us who had good veins finish chemo with fewer veins, and that makes drawing blood painful and difficult. I now know to tell the techs I have no veins and to ask for the best on the staff. There is usually one tech who has worked on children and will get a small "butterfly" needle (needles come in different sizes). The techs don't mind being asked. In fact, I have had more than one tell me she appreciated my directness and wished all patients did the same.

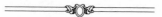

Tip—Heat helps veins expand, making them easier to find. Keep your arm warm before the blood is drawn. If you are a very hard stick, there is a trick, used by one ingenious tech, that helps dramatically. He applied an Infant Heal Warmer, a little plastic bag of chemicals that become hot when smashed. He gave us a handful when we left the hospital, but to find your own supply call the maker, Baxter Healthcare Corporation, in Valencia, California.

A catheter also allows the slow infusion of chemotherapy drugs. This means you go to the doctor's office and the drugs are attached to the main line and then you can leave. The drugs will be infused slowly, over hours or days. The patient actually wears a little pouch of the drug in a sling against her body with a battery pack that has a little pump. Oncologists who prefer the catheter contend that it allows for slower infusion of the more toxic drugs, minimizing possible side effects, and allows, in those women with more aggressive tumors, a higher dosage of drugs. Some women wore their chemo pouch to work and were infused during the day.

"They gave it to me in a drip. I wore a line connected to a little bag of chemo drugs, and I made little ultrasuede pouches that looked like my clothes, and stuck the pouch of drugs in there. I slept with it plugged into the wall on the third night, so it would have enough energy to run the fourth day."—Gale

In Dana's case, a central line was inserted to allow for slower infusion due to uncontrollable nausea. *"I had the first treatment and came home and felt okay. I made a big plate of nachos that night after the treatment and ate them all, and that's the last time I've eaten nachos—boy, I saw those nachos for a while. I woke up at 6 A.M. the next morning and threw up every hour on the hour. At 1 P.M. my friend called and she picked up from my voice I wasn't doing well, and she said to try to get to the door and unlock it. She took one look at me and called the doctor and said, 'She is dying here. She hasn't eaten, she has had nothing to drink, and she is the color of her sheets. Something is wrong.' They put me back in the hospital to rehydrate me. I went back Sunday. The second one was the same, and they put me in emergency room and gave me an IV again. So the third time they put in a central line. I would go to the office and they would attach the little blue tube to it. I would go home wearing it."*

Tip—In some cities there are companies that will come to your home to infuse you through an IV or unplug your slow infusion drugs. Ask your oncologist.

WHAT TO EXPECT FROM CHEMO

"Chemo was not as devastating as I thought it would be. I was lucky. I did not get very sick. After the treatment, for the next two or three days it was just like morning sickness, and the thought of food would just gag me."—Sandy

"When I thought of somebody on chemo, I thought of somebody who was thin, pale, horrible-looking, and I think you need to know that you can go through chemo—that chemo isn't a lot of fun and it isn't real easy, but you can survive it, that a lot of people continue to work."
—Joan

The women interviewed for this book had many different reactions to chemo. Some tolerated it well physically but suffered severe depression and psychological distress. Others had nausea and vomiting and were very ill as a result of their treatments but handled it well psychologically.

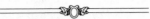

Tip—Most of these women were interviewed about chemo before the introduction of the new drug Zofran, which has reduced the numbers of women who experience vomiting.

By reading women's individual reactions and responses, you must sense that this is a highly individualized experience. Some of us are more chemically sensitive than others. Each body is unique in its tolerance. Chemo threw some women into early menopause. It regulated others. While the majority stopped menstruating for a few months, some remained regular. There is no common reaction or right or wrong or better or worse way to handle it. The only good thing to say about chemotherapy is that it will end.

With my chemo treatments, I began to recognize a pattern. After being sick to my stomach for a few days, I began to feel better very quickly. Then in the middle of the cycle, about a week and a half out, I would have flulike symptoms—low-grade fever, body ache and general malaise—as my white count plummeted. These symptoms could come on with such speed it was astounding.

About ten to fourteen days after each chemo treatment, your white blood cells will plummet as they are attacked by the drugs. Before you can receive your next treatment, they will have to recover adequately. For this reason you will give blood at each visit before receiving your chemo treatment, to be sure your "counts" are high enough. If they aren't, you will be asked to wait a few days before returning.

"I went once every three weeks or when my blood count would allow me to. They put me below the level of being alive twice when I was on chemotherapy—my counts were so low. On two different occasions, they said, 'You can't be moving.' I said, 'I feel fine.' "—Gale

During all of chemo you will be more susceptible to infection, but particularly during this midpoint of treatment. It is during this time that you must be very careful you don't catch something. A low white blood cell count means you are particularly vulnerable to infection, and in your weakened state, this could be serious. Your doctor should warn you to call at the **first sign of infection or fever.** Believe him or her.

> *"I went in for treatment, and apparently, they test your blood that day, which I didn't realize. And my counts were at 800 and needed to be at 1,200. He put me on antibiotics to keep me from getting something."*—Anne

---

Tip—If you have a small child who will be getting vaccines while you are on chemo, check with your oncologist and pediatrician. Many vaccines work by giving the child a mild case of the disease, to which he or she will build immunities but to which you might be susceptible.

Tip—If you have any dental work done during chemo, including having your teeth cleaned, tell your oncologist and your dentist. Most prescribe penicillin as a precaution to infection.

> *"By 2 A.M. my temperature had shot up. I called them and they said, 'Take Tylenol. Come in and do a blood test in the morning.' The next morning they sent me directly over to the hospital. They wouldn't even let me go home. I was going out to lunch with a friend. I thought, No. I'm going to lunch, and I'll be back. And they're like, 'No you're not.' And we went over and they stuck me on antibiotic IVs and I was on that for five days. That was a real scary time, too."*—Diane

During the time I was on chemo, I was a free-lance writer and could take the luxury of collapsing for a few days right after chemo and then in the middle of the cycle. Had I been working at a regular job, I would have been unable to get to work for about a week of that time. Most women interviewed in the book took their chemo on Friday afternoon and were back at work on Monday.

Perhaps the hardest news to hear is that the effects of chemo are cumulative. And whether the oncologists will say so for the record, there were few women I spoke with who said they felt better as they went along. Most reacted like Sheila.

"It's like you've had an awful accident that goes off in your body. The way I felt toward the end . . . I just kept feeling worse and worse and worse—you just kind of die . . . you're just killing more cells and killing more cells. I probably didn't have a really good grip on what was happening until it was all over."—Sheila

Like myself, most women found the surgery itself a breeze compared to chemo. But many made peace with the necessity of chemo, knowing at its end that they had done all they could do medically against this disease. In their experiences is a wealth of information about enduring this time. They want to share them with you. Remember when reading these firsthand accounts that adjuvant chemo usually lasts from six to twenty weeks—but the side effects are limited to a few days of each three-week cycle. If you are being treated for metastatic disease, your regimen and drugs may vary, depending on the location of the cancer and your response.

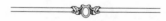

Tip—Be sure you are not alone for the first twenty-four hours after chemo.

COPING WITH CHEMOTHERAPY AND ITS EFFECTS

COPING EMOTIONALLY

"Chemo was very, very hard psychologically. Physically, it wasn't that bad. I kept having to tell myself over and over and over again: Think

about what actually goes on. Don't blow it out of proportion. Don't give it more power than it deserves. Think about what actually happens. But it was so easy to get very scared and just let it overwhelm me."
—Sherry

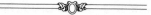

Tip—Don't make any assumptions about chemotherapy and how you will respond. Every woman is different.

"I'm very much against losing control, and on the first treatment they gave me Benadryl IV, and that was like I was floating up to the ceiling and lost the feeling in my legs and stuff, and that scared me more than anything, and I said I would not do that again. So they gave me an antinausea drug by mouth an hour before the treatment, and that would hold me until I got home, and then I would start throwing up a couple of hours later. But it didn't give me that weird floating out-of-the-space feeling."—Lise

"I had one period after I started chemotherapy, and I've never had another one since. There was a woman at work who's in her early sixties, and I'd say to her, 'I feel real hot. Is it hot in here?' 'Oh, you're having a hot flash.' But I never had the terrible night sweats and all that stuff women talk about."—Marsha

"I've missed two periods since August. Actually I didn't miss them, but one time I was two weeks late, and I've been regular to the day since I was fourteen. The other time I was three weeks late. But my oncologist said he was surprised that my period was even that regular during chemo."—Melissa

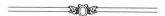

Tip—If you are having severe problems with your menstrual cycle, you may want to consult with a gynecologic oncologist.

I can remember lying in bed after my third chemo treatment and ten hours of vomiting. Tom had been in and out frequently to ask if I needed anything. If there is a universal truth, it is that no one can help you vomit.

When he suggested that I might want to consider going in the hospital for my next treatment, I was crushed. Being sick for hours was horrific, but being at home made it bearable. Tom saw that my feelings were hurt and sat on the side of the bed.

"I feel so helpless when you are this sick," he said.

Helpless I could understand. I felt possessed by chemicals and out of control. The only thing that kept me going was the knowledge that there was an end and that the chemicals were killing the cancer cells. I was not in a support group during that time, and with what I know now, it was the biggest mistake I made. It would have made such a difference to see and hear from women who had been so sick and lived.

My emotional needs during chemo were generated by how violently ill I became. Many women I talked to had what could be called a good physical response but experienced psychological difficulties that ranged from mild depression to paranoia and suicidal tendencies.

Getting through chemo remains a very personal journey. But from the women who have been there comes a list of how-tos. Take what works for you.

Commitment: Decide you are going to do this and that it is the best route to go. Believe in it.

Ritual: Many women had a system. Some made it a point to do something nice for themselves on the day of chemo. Others had a ritual that helped them cope. Theresa always wore her bunny house slippers for chemo. It made her feel better and added a little humor.

"On chemo days my friend would take me to lunch or plan something special. I always enjoyed seeing her, and it made it easier."
—Marsha

Personifying chemo: Many women referred to chemo as an "it" and addressed it directly as an adversary or friend.

Support: Have somewhere you can go and scream and/or be praised. Tell friends the dates of treatment and ask for cards or flowers or whatever will make you look forward to the date if not the treatment.

Humor:

"I did silly things. My friends gave me a hat that had a fan in it because I was always complaining in the summer about how hot the wig was. It had a big badge on it that said, Just say no to drugs. While I was waiting on the doctor, I changed wigs and I put this wig on and this hat and I would prance around. I was never really a comical person or a funny person. I guess I wanted everybody to feel more comfortable around me. Then I realized by doing this I felt better."
—Mary-T

Remember: Weird is normal during chemo.

"I developed an aversion to the color red because that is the color of Adriamycin and I watched it go in. I actually walked out of the office that day and saw a red car and gagged. Red anywhere—cars, clothing, hot sauce—made me nauseous."—Judy D

Some hospitals around the country have begun using complementary techniques, such as visualization and relaxation techniques, before and during chemo. If your oncologist doesn't offer any, suggest that he or she look into it. Then take the initiative and find out on your own. Many women took tapes to listen to while they received chemo.

Remember to tell people how you are feeling. No one, unless they have done it and maybe not even then, will understand the strange feelings the chemicals cause. Try to describe them to your friend, partner, or support person. Identifying your particular pattern with chemotherapy may provide a sense of control. The women I interviewed seemed to develop an understanding of how it would go by the second treatment.

"I do remember throwing up. I said then that any man who can take care of you when your head is over a toilet has got to love you. He took me home after every chemo, which was on Friday and nursed me until Monday. My ex-husband took care of the children."—Kit

Total recovery after the end of chemotherapy is again an individual timetable. I think it took me six months get my energy back. Other women said it seemed like a year. Others were back to "normal" in a matter of months. Just remember not to beat yourself up if you can't run a 10K three months after finishing chemo. Know that it may take months before you have your energy back.

Coping with Hair Loss—Wigs and the Ice Cap

They say it's our crowning glory, but when it comes out by the handful, hair is a mess.

During interviews, I always asked women what had been the worst part of the breast cancer experience. Emotionally, they answered, the worst part was usually the fear; physically, the worst was always chemo, if they had it, and hair loss specifically. When our hair starts to fall out, it is yet another violation of our bodies and one that most women felt was much more visible and hard to conceal than the loss of a breast.

> "I washed my hair and it was a spring day and I was out in the garden; Dick was in the garage. I took the towel off and there was just hair everywhere. And I started brushing and then blow-drying and watching my hair blow away in the spring breeze, and it was okay. I went in to my husband and said, 'You're not going to believe this. I just stood on the deck and brushed my hair out and I'm not hysterical! And I'm letting you see me because you know what I look like with just a few strands here.' "—Sandy

> "The loss of hair was one of the most traumatic things I had to go through. My hair was down to my waist for years and then I had to cut it to my shoulders. When it started falling out, I had my hairdresser come to my house and cut my hair. I bought wigs and had my hairdresser cut them because my job is very visible so I had to look good." —Cindy

> "I lost all my eyelashes, which made me look much stranger. It's really funny, because most people never know what their head looks like. I had a mannequin head. I could have gone without a wig. I had these big eyes anyway. And my head looked like a sanded mannequin. There were no knots, bumps, veins, bruises, nothing."—Gale

"I also found that sleeping on a satin pillowcase helped a great deal to reduce the loss of hair. Plus, when you wash your hair in the shower, I didn't scrub it like I normally would. I lost only about 15 percent of my hair."—Julie

"When you have cancer, people tell you that losing your hair is minor; you shouldn't be thinking about that. Don't be vain. But when you're twenty-eight years old and you go completely bald,—I mean, nothing. I was completely bald. It was hard to deal with."—Leanne

Some women had success with the ice cap, a plastic cap that looks like an inflatable swim cap and is filled with a frozen substance. It is worn from thirty minutes before chemo begins to thirty minutes after. According to the doctors, when it is done right, the ice cap can prevent hair loss.

Right means putting it on at least thirty minutes before chemo on a wet head so the cold gets to the roots. The cold constricts the vessels to the scalp, which shuts down the blood supply, thereby preventing the chemicals from reaching the hair. But I found that the majority of women could not tolerate it.

Knowing that I am one of those people who gets a headache from eating ice cream too fast, I valiantly tried the ice cap for about four seconds. There was no contest between the ice cap and the hair loss. I could not tolerate the cold. It was the worst pain I have ever felt.

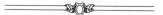

Tip—There is also a theoretical argument that says the ice cap should not be used because it keeps the chemicals from the blood supply in the scalp, where cells may be lurking.

"The only thing I could compare it to was sticking my head in a snow bank. I think I would opt for total loss of hair. All I did was wet my hair in preparation for the cap and I got nauseous. For a year I could not pick up a glass of ice water because it made my head ache. I hated the ice cap."—Kit

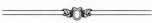

Tip—To keep as much hair as possible, use a gentle shampoo and don't shampoo as often. Don't brush your hair. Use a wide-tooth comb to gently untangle.

When a former breast cancer patient suggested I shave my head before my hair started falling out, I was appalled. I couldn't do that, I thought. Just let nature take its course.

When my hair began falling out, I saw her reasoning. There was hair everywhere: on my pillow, in the tub, on my clothes, in the sink, in food. I walked around with a halo as my hair left my head. I had fairly thin hair. I couldn't imagine what someone with thick hair must be facing.

So on the day before Thanksgiving 1986, my husband and I met in the bathroom and he shaved my head. At the time, I didn't feel much about it. But I know now that it had an impact on both of us. It was simultaneously intimate and traumatic, but more than anything, it created a bond between us. We were in this together for the long haul.

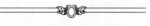

Tip—Buy a cheap turban to wear while your hair is falling out. It catches it and keeps it from getting all over.

I bought the standard three wigs from a store that catered primarily to cancer patients. The total cost for all three was around $200. Three seems to be the magic number for women.

"Larry said, 'Let's go today and we'll pick out the wigs you want.' We bought three. I got one short, one shoulder-length curly, and one shoulder-length really curly for my glamour look. I had a work look, a glamour look, and a fun look."—Cindy

We buy the first one for what we think we look like, the second for what we want to look like, and the third for what we really look like. I wore the first two for fun and the third every day at school as I taught. It was permanently curly and required only a good shake before I put it on. I hated wearing it, but being bald in the winter means having a cold head. Around the house, I didn't wear it unless my teenage stepson was home. He didn't like seeing me bald. Somehow the baldness was a much larger indicator of illness than any other aspect of the disease.

Tip—Don't wait to get a wig. Buy one before your hair starts to fall out. You might want to get your hair cut, since the weight may cause it to fall out faster. Check with your insurance company about its regulations before you buy a wig. Most require proof of need, which your doctor can supply. Ask for a prescription for a cranial prosthesis.

I wore my wig from October until May, when I had enough dark fuzz to cover my head. It was getting hotter and I was debating if I had enough hair to go natural when my mother-in-law said I looked very exotic. That was enough of a compliment for me to decide that exotic was better than scratchy.

I also lost the majority of my eyelashes but none of my eyebrows. The rest of the hair on my body just stopped growing.

My hair came back in darker, thicker, and curly, but it didn't stay that way. It is a little thicker now and seems to have more body, but the color has returned to mousy brown and the curl left after the first cut. But one thing I did get that stayed was a blond streak on my temple. It's about a half-inch wide and my hairdresser says it is really blond, not gray.

The women interviewed for this book adjusted to and adapted to hair loss in a variety of ways. Some bought expensive wigs; some wore turbans or scarves. Check with your local American Cancer Society to see if the Look Good Feel Better program has arrived in your city. This

program offers women cancer patients a workshop that teaches apply-
ing makeup, styling wigs, tying scarves, and buying lingerie. Major cosmetic companies donate samples, and professionals show the women
how to apply the makeup to help with skin and hair problems during
chemotherapy. To find a program in a community or hospital near you
call 1-800-395-LOOK.

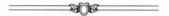

**Tip—Hair dryers and curling irons can damage re-
maining hair. Try air drying and using styling gel
or spray.**

Anne couldn't tolerate the wig and wore hats the entire time. *"I
intended to wear the wig, but I started wearing hats when my hair was falling
out. Then when I wore the wig I found that I had to hold on to it to keep the
wind from blowing it off. I just had nightmares about that wig. I could not
look at it. Finally, I put it away."*

There is no right or wrong. Indeed, I have noticed at the oncologist's
office that the new, fashionable, very short "boy cuts" are catching on
with women going through chemo. At the oncologist's recently for a
checkup I noticed that four young women had chosen not to wear wigs
but instead had their hair cut in a boy cut and then used mousse or
high-powered hair spray to make it stand up in front like the old burr
our brothers wore. It looked great and was in style.

Nancy S, an African-American who straightened her hair, discovered
that she looked great with the natural look. *"I call it a chemo cut and
have kept it this length since it grew back. I get lots of compliments and never
would have known how good it looked if I hadn't lost it."*

> *"I got two wigs—a conservative brunette one and one that was
> frosted curly, that I never wore. I had my hair cut short. It was hard
> having it fall out. I would pull it out in the shower and lay it on the
> side of the tub so it wouldn't go down the drain. I didn't cry about it,
> but I didn't like taking showers that week. I would joke about it at
> work. Something would come up and I would say, I could just pull my
> hair out and then people would look at me. So I joked about it, but it*

is awful having that happen. No one saw me without my hair except my sister."—Dana

"*I had a good friend at the time who was a hairdresser, who had been doing my hair at his house. And he was great. He ordered my wig for me. Once again, I was planning ahead. They said, 'Well, maybe 40 percent hair loss.' Ha ha. I mean, after the first two weeks it was coming out all over the place. I mean, everywhere. We all went out to dinner and came back and took off the scarf and shaved it off. My friend says, 'You look like that actress that just made the movie and shaved her head for what—$5 million or something.' And they wouldn't put me in front of a mirror. So I went and looked, and I damn near passed out. I couldn't believe it. I was just like, 'Oh my God. I look like a freak.' But it was the best thing for me to do because I couldn't stand seeing the hair everywhere."*—Diane

"*It was like my hair stopped growing. It just stayed the same, and it thinned out. Then it was, 'Oh, I'm not losing my hair. Maybe it's not doing the trick. It's not really killing those cells off.' So that was kind of a strange worry."*—Marsha

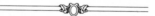

Tip—Remember that if your hair doesn't fall out, it doesn't indicate that the drugs aren't working. You are just lucky.

"*I bought a wig, but I wore a cotton bandanna because the wig hurt my head. If I ever do this again, I'm going to buy a $300 wig. I mean, I'm going to get a good one made for my head."*—Marilyn

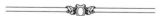

Tip—Wigs can be cut and styled like hair—even the cheap synthetic wigs, which some women preferred because they were much less trouble.

I actually lost two pounds on chemo. But that was because I was one of the 5 percent who had severe vomiting that, in 1986, could not be controlled. I also had a rather uncommon side effect, shared only with two or three others I interviewed. About six weeks into chemo, which would have been the third treatment, I developed a mouth full of ulcers and walked around with a mouth full of liquid painkiller during my waking hours. It made eating (and conversation) out of the question.

Indeed, my reaction to chemo was so severe that my oncologist reduced my dosage for my last three treatments. I began chemo in October 1986 and finished in February 1987. In January 1987, with two chemo treatments remaining, I resumed teaching a full university load at Southern Methodist University. Like many of the women I interviewed, I had chemo on Friday and was teaching the next Monday. This alone is proof that as sick as you can be, the body does bounce back with time.

"I reacted really badly to the chemotherapy. I mean, it just made me terribly sick. Then my aunt told me about Nembutal, but the doctor said they didn't like giving it because I'd get addicted. I said I really don't care about sticking a suppository up my ass to get addicted. It's not because I think I'm gonna like it. I just don't want to be sick. So they said, Okay, we'll try it. It would knock me out for like three days totally, day and night. I'd wake up, I'd get sick, I'd pop another one, and then I'd pass out for another three days. It was like going into a sleep, a deep sleep, and you didn't have to be bothered by anything. But you had to have somebody there, because if you got sick in the night, you would die by choking on your vomit."—Angela

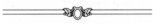

Tip—For severe problems, you do have an option of being hospitalized for chemo treatments. In some instances this allows slower infusion; in others, you can be monitored more closely.

Be aware that you can become dangerously dehydrated from vomiting. Be sure that someone is checking on you if you remain alone.

Tip—The drugs given for chemotherapy for women with breast cancer should be accompanied by increased fluid intake, to prevent kidney and bladder problems.

Most women found some kind of system that worked for them to help control the nausea. None of these have been studied. Indeed, I wonder if it isn't the sense of control that comes from you deciding what will help you that makes the difference. For your information, these are the tips women offer.

Diane found that marijuana worked best for her nausea, but she reminds those who are going to use it that it has to be in the bloodstream before you receive the treatment. She preferred to smoke hers, but the doctor also offered the pill form. *"We talked about the marijuana, and he said, 'For some patients, it works well. I don't even bother to recommend it to my older patients because they flip out at the idea. You know, they're like, "We're going to be busted." But if you want to try it, go ahead.' So I did, but he didn't tell me to smoke it two to three hours before I go in for the treatment because it has to be in your system. So I would come home and I'm like smoking this pot, and I'm starting to feel a little bit nauseous and stuff, and I'd wake up and they'd bring marijuana in to me to smoke and finally I was like, 'Get it the hell away from me.' The last thing you want when you're sick to your stomach is to smoke. It was terrible. So then we find out later, it was like, 'Well, you did it all the wrong way.' So that didn't work. But later on, he prescribed it and I went back to it and it worked the best of anything I had."*

Cindy, a skin diver, used acupressure bracelets for chemo nausea. Acupuncture theory holds that there are pressure points on the wrist that control nausea. The bracelets can be purchased at shops that sell skin-diving equipment and they will explain their use.

Kit ate an egg every day and found that helped her nausea and her white counts. Her doctor also put her on prenatal vitamins during chemo.

Nancy S found that the Cytoxan pills were making her nauseated, and she asked that it be given in the IV with the other drugs. The nausea stopped. *"I'm one of those people who hates to take pills. I can't even take aspirin every four hours. So I think it probably was the Adriamycin that made me sick, but because I hate pills, I blamed them."*

RADIATION

"I think the idea of the radiation bothered me more than anything. I kept thinking, I'm lying under this huge machine zapping my body with whatever. I just kept thinking this thing is doing all this bad stuff to me and I'm supposed to understand that it's good stuff. It is supposed to be helping me, yet I'm thinking, this is radiation, something that we have always feared."—Dot

The same radiation used to create an X ray, when used in high-energy doses and aimed at a specific part of the body, has the capability to destroy cancer cells locally.

After lumpectomy, external doses of radiation are used on the remaining breast tissue and, depending on the location of the lump and whether there were positive lymph nodes, on the area from your underarm to your collarbone and over to your sternum. The radiation will kill any remaining cancer cells in the breast tissue adjacent to the tumor site. Radiation may also be used in conjunction with other therapies, such as chemo and hormones after mastectomy. This will depend on the location of the tumor and other diagnostic factors.

Depending on your diagnosis, you will begin radiation immediately after surgery, immediately after chemo, or in the middle of chemo. Radiation is also used to slow a metastatic cancer site and to reduce pain in these areas.

As with any cancer treatment, women facing radiation should be sure that they are in an accredited facility and are being seen by a board-certified physician. There have been significant improvements in radiation equipment in the last decade, when the cobalt machines began being replaced by linear accelerators, which are capable of more accurate application of radiation that prevents irradiating other organs or the spine. The use of such high-energy equipment has revolutionized how radiation is administered and has offered doctors much more control in delivering the radiation. And while most locations have the newer equipment, some do not. You must ask.

You will meet with the radiation oncologist before treatment, and he or she will go over the routine. Ask about the dosage you will receive and the specific area that will receive the radiation and what possible side effects you will have. You will probably have pen markings on your chest to indicate the borders of the area that will be irradiated. These should not be washed off. Some radiation oncologists use a tattoo that will be permanent after radiation. If you have freckles, it may not be noticeable. Discuss this option with the doctor.

Lise suffered from claustrophobia and found lying under the radiation machine particularly difficult. "*I had to tell myself to overcome that. I visualized women I knew who had breast cancer and lived forever. I would repeat their names inside my head when the light came on, and then the treatment would be over and they would open the door and change the field and go out and close the door and start again.*"

As with chemo, the physical reactions to radiation vary from woman to woman, with some complaining of mild itching and others of a condition they likened to a severe case of sunburn that lasted a few days to a few weeks. But consistently, the major complaint from women was the time commitment. Radiation for breast cancer is usually one treatment a day for five days a week for twenty to thirty treatments, meaning a daily visit to the hospital for four to six weeks. Those women who have lumpectomy will also have a booster dose after the full course of radiation has ended. And while the treatment visits are usually only twenty or thirty minutes long, the reminder of why you are there can be distressing.

"*I would go in there and have to wait maybe five or ten minutes sometimes, and they would bring in people on gurneys that were coming over from the hospital to get treatments. I would sit there and think how lucky I was to be able to drive here, have the treatment, and drive to work. Then I would get to work and someone would be griping. I would want to tell them how lucky they were.*"—Marsha

"Radiation was when it really hit me. I was like, No, I don't want to do this anymore. I'm sorry. The chemo was different because I would deal with it for two or three days and get better. I wouldn't feel great, but I'd get better and go on about my business. Radiation therapy was different; it was every day."—Theresa

Dottee also found visualization worked well to cope with the radiation treatments. *"Suddenly the monster machine began to whine and click as its shutters opened. I closed my eyes but still felt the splashing of the energy rays as they hit my body. From out of nowhere an inspiration came. I would visualize the light as a good guy entering my body to seek out only the cancer cells in order to destroy them, like seeing a movie of the heroes of light battling the foes of darkness. Comforted, I continued to affirm with my inner sight the light beams attacking the diseased cells, and then watched as they disintegrated into flames. Four times each treatment, the huge machine growled and spit its light at me, and each time I silently watched the fire as it continued to burn away all malignant cells."*

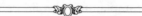

Tip—Don't use any home remedies for the itching or burning associated with radiation. Ask the doctor. Many off-the-shelf creams have ingredients that can interfere with radiation or worsen the effect.

Radiation often results in changes to the skin. Some women said it felt thicker; others said it remained sensitive, particularly to heat, for a number of months.

In more than one instance, I have been in a group of women when half said radiation was a breeze, while the other half said it was painful and emotionally draining. Be aware that as with any therapy, you may have a unique reaction. A few women said the radiation caused their ribs to become brittle. Leanne broke a rib after radiation during a coughing spell.

"Dr. G said they did a wonderful job on my reconstruction. She cringed when she heard I was going to have radiation. She was afraid that it was going to harden the tissue. But she said they did such a good job of zooming in on the site that it kept it soft."—Melissa

"As a reaction to the radiation, my chest filled with fluid and that was a downer and they put me on prednisone for three months."
—Elizabeth P

"One thing about radiation, you cannot stand any heat. I could be outside ten minutes and the heat is just incredible."—Betty

"I've got really sensitive skin, so I still have scarring left from radiation therapy, and I got really severe burns. I got to the point where I'd walk around without any clothes on because I couldn't stand to have anything touch my skin. And I guess that's the first time when I got really angry."—Theresa

"Once it started blistering, it was mainly a deep burn. I had one section in particular that was blood-red. It was tremendously painful. I worked and put aloe vera cream on and then it got bad and I went back in and they gave me sulfa cream and it was immediate relief."
—Cindy

RADIATION ONCOLOGIST DR. JOHN W. GEBERT, WEST COAST RADIOLOGY AND WESTERN MEDICAL CENTER, TALKS ABOUT RADIATION

Explain the difference between a radiation therapist and radiation oncologist.

A radiation therapist is a board-certified technologist who actually does the hands-on treatment of the patient. They align the radiation beam to hit the target, which is designated by the radiation oncologist. The radiation oncologist is an M.D. who first goes through medical training and then one year of internship and usually three years of residency. The radiation oncologist supervises the work of the radiation therapist.

(continued)

What should a woman look for in a radiation oncologist?

There are basic guidelines to look for with any physician, depending on his or her field: Reputation is very important, whether the doctor did his or her training at a reputable institution, and board certification. The physician is either board-eligible or board-certified. Board-eligible means the physician is ready to take the written examination, which a radiation oncologist usually takes the last year of residency. This is followed by an oral examination the next year. After passing both of these examinations, a physician is board-certified. Consequently, if a physician is board-certified in radiation oncology, the patient can be assured that the radiation oncologist has passed all the scrutiny of his or her peers following training.

So a woman finds a board-certified radiation oncologist. What else is important?

The equipment used is important in the sense that equipment has evolved to higher technology in radiation oncology as it has in all practices in medicine. Cobalt machines, although still in use by many cancer centers, in my opinion are not the preferred equipment to treat breast cancer because the skin reaction is more severe than with use of a higher linear accelerator, which generates high-energy X rays that penetrate deeply and subsequently spare the skin from being overly irradiated. Consequently, the skin reaction is less severe with the linear accelerator than with a cobalt machine. This is especially important if the breast is extremely large, because you would have to give more radiation to the surface to penetrate deeply and this can cause severe skin reactions at times. A higher-energy machine can penetrate without excessive use of X rays on the external surface.

Anyone undergoing radiation therapy might consider inquiring about the equipment used and the side effects of more outdated equipment compared with the newer linear accelerator. Most accredited cancer treatment centers do indeed use linear accelera-

(continued)

tors. The patient, via use of medical libraries or just by calling the facility, can find out what machinery is being used, what the potential side effects will be to her body, and what organs could potentially be affected by the use of X rays when she receives the radiation. It only makes sense in this day and age to be as educated as possible when you are the patient receiving radiation therapy. It is also important for the patient to understand what organs will be affected as there are maximum limits of radiation doses to various organs—and those limits vary.

Explain exactly how radiation works and the standard treatment for breast cancer.

The radiation works by keeping the cancer cell from multiplying and consequently killing it. The cancer cell cannot repair the radiation damage in a twenty-four-hour period of time and therefore dies when it goes through cell division. Normal cells can usually repair themselves because they are genetically intact.

The standard course of radiation therapy is determined by the stage of the woman's disease and her surgery choice. Once the pathologist looks at the specimen and a woman is appropriately staged, which means the extent of the disease is measured, the mode of therapy can be determined. In many instances the patient will have a choice between lumpectomy or breast-conserving surgery coupled with external radiation therapy, or a mastectomy. She should discuss these options with her physician. When she is eligible for primary breast radiation for breast conservation, the standard course is external radiation therapy for five weeks, followed by a boost to the area where the tumor was removed—or the lumpectomy site. This boost can be adequately achieved with either electron-beam therapy to the area of tumor removal or with the placement of an implant. The implant involves placing tubes at the lumpectomy site under general anesthesia and then, after the patient has recovered from anesthesia, placing actual radioactive material in these tubes. The tubes constantly emit X rays,

(continued)

which will bring the local site up to the dose anticipated by the radiation oncologist.

Explain why the boost dose is given and the difference between the electron beam and the use of implants in the breast for a boost dose.

The boost dose would apply only to a patient who has had a lumpectomy followed by external radiation to the entire breast. The boost dose is given to boost the area of lumpectomy, which theoretically would be the site of most likely recurrence. We feel that the electron beam, which is one of the beams generated by the linear accelerator, gives a better cosmetic effect and also saves the patients time in the sense that they are not required to stay in the hospital as they are during the implantation of the rods. They also don't have the puncture sites involved with the implantation, and they are not subjected to the isolation that is required during the hospital stay to avoid radiation exposure to other family members. Usually, the electron beam is administered on an outpatient basis and the treatments last only several minutes. They are painless and the whole process of radiation therapy does not cause nausea, vomiting, or hair loss. The main toxicity is the irritation of the skin, which can usually be eased by placement of emollient or topical steroids. And this is only a potential side effect and not the case in every patient. It is also important that the therapist is trained in the use of the electron beam prior to administering electron-beam therapy to the boost site.

Why is radiation used when the breast has been removed?

Depending on the extent of the disease, sometimes radiation therapy is used following a mastectomy. Factors that determine whether the radiation oncologist is going to administer radiation therapy on a postoperative patient include the size and location of the cancer as well as the proximity to the chest when the tumor was removed. Also, whether or not the cancer had invaded the

(continued)

lymphatics or small blood vessels. If, following the surgery, any or a combination of these factors is positive, then radiation therapy may be indicated. Historically, we know what dose of radiation it takes to kill cells that may be left behind after surgery that may tend to cause a recurrence on the chest wall after mastectomy. This dose is approximately 5,000 of our radiation units. We administer our radiation units at 180 to 200 units per day, which is fairly standard.

When do you recommend beginning radiation?

It varies from institution to institution, but the primary limitation in beginning radiation therapy is appropriate healing of any wound. If the patient has had a mastectomy, the surgical incision must be healed before postoperative radiation is begun. If the patient has had a lumpectomy, the incision site must be healed before we begin. Depending on the stage of the initial breast cancer, frequently radiation is used with concomitant chemotherapy or radiation is cycled following two to three cycles of chemotherapy treatments. Following a mastectomy, the most likely place for a tumor to recur is on the chest wall, because the scar tissue, which gets reduced blood flow, appears to be a sanctuary for tumor cells.

Do you mark a woman's chest with a pen or tattoo?

We use a pen to initially mark the area. Following verification of the radiation oncologist of the correct area being treated, many radiation oncologists use tattoos to permanently mark the skin. They are small black dots that go under the skin and are permanent. Some women who have oily skin and who do not retain their temporary marks are candidates for tattoos. The tattoo will also help identify the area in years to come should the patient have a recurrence. I have heard the comment by some patients that the permanent tattoos remind them of their treatment and of their disease, and they request not to be tattooed. It is my feeling that we should respect the wishes of the individual and document

(continued)

in the charts where the radiation has been applied. With good documentation, verification of previous radiation therapy can be interpreted.

What are side effects from radiation?
There are two categories of side effects in general. There are the acute side effects, which we see during the course of radiation, and the long-term side effects which come months or years after radiation. The acute side effects include itching, which can be treated with emollients; some skin reddening, which can be treated with emollients such as aloe vera cream and vitamin E cream or, if the radiation reaction is severe, sometimes the radiation oncologist may prescribe topical steroids. In addition, the patient may feel some fatigue from the radiation treatments and, depending on which beam is being used and the areas being treated, some difficulty in swallowing.

The long-term side effects again depend on the individual, but may show up as firmness of the breast being treated, which we call fibrosis. This is the major long-term side effect.

HORMONE TREATMENTS

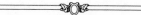

Tip—Tamoxifen is the generic name for Nolvadex.

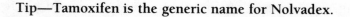

"He put me on something that threw me into menopause. And I felt great. I felt wonderful. I didn't have the mood swings like I get right before my period. Because that's when I would have my worst depression about all this is as I went through the mood swings for the month. Even my husband commented. He said, 'This is great. You're so much

easier to live with.' It took a couple of months for my periods to come back once I stopped taking it."—Madeline

"The sexual desire isn't there. People say it's mental, but it isn't, because I still have a good sex life. I have always had a good sex life. It's not that I don't want sex. Mentally, I want it, but physically, the body's not there. That's irritating. I think it is the combination of the loss of the estrogen and taking Nolvadex more than the loss of the breast."—Pat H

In the past decade a drug has arrived in the fight against breast cancer. An anti-estrogen called tamoxifen, trade name Nolvadex, was accepted into general usage in the late eighties and has since then been heralded as a miracle—when it works.

The drug acts effectively in a number of ways against cancer, particularly those cells that have estrogen receptors. While some researchers contend that it competes for estrogen for binding sites in the breast, thus causing the body to throw off estrogen, it is also thought to neutralize an enzyme that is part of the cancer-causing process. Others describe the process as cell starvation, tamoxifen starves the cell of estrogen it needs to grow. But it is more complicated than just the flow of estrogen in the body.

While the argument continues over how and why tamoxifen does what it does, it is being shown to be effective in preventing recurrence in women both young and old. It is therefore being prescribed liberally to young women with breast cancer, many of whom are given the entire scope of treatment—chemo, radiation, and tamoxifen—to, as one doctor told a patient, "Go for the cure."

Tamoxifen, which is taken daily in pill form, differs from other chemotherapy drugs in that its toxicity is minimal. But to hear doctors talk about the drug, it sounds like there are no negative side effects and those few that are present are insignificant.

A twenty-eight-year-old women who has been thrown into menopause may not agree. For other women the drug had an opposite effect, regulating an irregular menstrual cycle. Still others had no noticeable side effects at all. Diana was given the option of taking tamoxifen. Her oncologist said there would be no side effects, but Diana visited her gynecologist about the pregnancy issue. *"When I told her he said there would be no side effects, she rolled her eyes. She said that since he sees women die of breast cancer, he doesn't consider the side effects an issue."*

Diana decided not to take tamoxifen after conferring with her mother's oncologist. Her mother had died of endometrial cancer six years before Diana's diagnosis and the doctor said there was some evidence that there was an increase in the incidence of endometrial cancer with tamoxifen. It was not a risk under normal circumstances for those women who would benefit from the drug, but since it was not highly recommended, he advised against it. Diana is also still undecided about pregnancy, but her ob said that if she does decide to start a family after a year, she could discontinue tamoxifen and get pregnant. Debra did just that after a year on the drug. At twenty-nine, she was also much younger than Diana.

Chemotherapy and hormone treatment together are almost assured to throw a women into premature menopause, which is more likely to become permanent in women over thirty-five even after treatment has stopped.

While it is true that, compared to other therapies, tamoxifen's side effects are minimal, those who do suffer from the negative side effects of an induced menopause—hot flashes, vaginal dryness, and mood swings—can find yet another set of emotional and physical hurdles as well as another obstacle to intimacy.

Judy D said her hot flashes were so intense they steamed up her glasses. *"I would be sitting in a business meeting and have to casually remove my glasses and clean them so I could see."*

Tip—Ask to see the insert from the tamoxifen box and any other printed information provided by the manufacturer. If you still have unanswered questions about this or any other drug, call the manufacturer directly.

"He recommended tamoxifen, and I didn't mind about the menopause. I figured I was close to menopause, anyway. There's early menopause in my family. My mother was forty-one when she went into menopause. I think, oddly enough, this medicine may have stopped that process, because I don't have hot flashes, and I did have them before. But I'm sure I have depression from it."—Elizabeth T

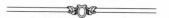

Tip—There are preparations on the market for vaginal lubrication. Ask your ob about Replens, an over-the-counter vaginal lubricant.

"I still have periods, but they're irregular. I had one almost every month up until about three months ago, and now when they come they're very light."—Leanne

Tip—Some women have found natural products that reduce their hot flashes. Cindy uses Royal Jelly, and others recommend 800 units of vitamin E a day. If you find a natural concoction you want to try, be sure to confirm it does not contain some form of estrogen.

Tamoxifen is also being prescribed for older women such as Sadie, who says that the emotional side effects reminded her of menopause. *"You just think of something and you cry at the drop of a hat. That has been the only way it has affected me."*

Gynecologic Oncologist Dr. Allen Stringer, Texas Oncology, Talks About Tamoxifen, Hot Flashes, Menopause, and Estrogen

Define a gynecologic oncologist.

As a gynecologic oncologist, I treat malignancies of the female reproductive tract exclusive of the breast: cervical cancer, endometrial cancer, fallopian tube cancer, ovarian cancer. I will often see breast cancer patients for the management of issues that may or may not relate to their cancer treatment. For example, the patient who has breast cancer who has been treated with chemotherapy may have abnormal menstrual function as a result. Another example is a patient who has been treated with Nolvadex who has symptoms or a dry vagina that will require management by a gynecologist.

How do you address the assertion that Nolvadex has no side effects?

Chemotherapy as a treatment for breast cancer certainly has more side effects than Nolvadex, but Nolvadex is far from being free of side effects. I see patients who have hot flashes, dry vagina, sexual dysfunction, and occasionally a woman will have abnormal uterine bleeding that could indicate endometrial cancer.

The most common side effect from Nolvadex is hot flashes. Is there anything that can be done to stop or control them?

There are a number of drugs available but none that work in all cases. Many women have tried Bellergal and gotten good relief. But for some it didn't help at all. Another drug that has benefited some women is clonidine, which is an antihypertensive. But clonidine can cause side effects related to its antihypertensive properties and some patients decide they are better off dealing with the hot flashes than the side effects.

There's an herbal root called cohosh root that one patient found

(continued)

at a health-food store. She said it worked well controlling her hot flashes. I contacted the company that made it because I was concerned that it might contain some estrogen. They were very nice and replied promptly explaining that the root had been around for centuries. They said that though it had some estrogenic properties, it didn't contain an estrogen as such. For that person it worked and I don't discount it, but it makes me a little bit nervous that it functions as an estrogen and may therefore represent a risk factor.

Isn't estrogen forbidden for women who have had breast cancer?

Most of the concerns about estrogen-replacement therapy in women with breast cancer are theoretical concerns, based on observations that anti-estrogen-type therapy is associated with a response in patients with recurrent disease. And based on our observations, it's not clear to us that estrogen-replacement therapy is clearly contraindicated. I know for sure that many women with breast cancer have been given topical estrogen that is absorbed systemically for vaginal dryness or bladder symptoms. Yet there hasn't been any clear evidence of increased recurrence rate for these women. So the whole issue is up in the air.

It's important to understand that there have been some mandates passed down about when you can and can't use estrogen-replacement therapy, based on *theoretical* concerns rather than clear evidence. I'm not saying we ought to start treating everybody who has had breast cancer with estrogen-replacement therapy, but there's no question that cardiovascular disease is still the number one killer of women. And there's also no question that estrogen deprivation significantly increases a woman's risk of a fatal heart attack, and that it can be avoided with judicious use of estrogen-replacement therapy. So I think that it's reasonable to ask if there are subsets of women who have had breast cancer who would benefit from estrogen without undue risk.

A lack of estrogen also materially affects the quality of women's

(continued)

lives. Without estrogen they are at greater risk for osteoporosis and for cardiovascular disease, and they certainly have the burdensome local effects of estrogen deprivation, including lower genital tract atrophy and dryness and hot flashes.

What about the emotional effects of Nolvadex? Loss of sex drive? Moodiness?

Estrogen deprivation can certainly cause depression and sleep disorder and loss of sex drive. Dry vagina and discomfort with intercourse will certainly contribute to that and reinforce it. I think how well they function sexually in the face of those problems is determined in large part by how healthy they were sexually before the diagnosis. Breast cancer has a huge impact on a woman's sexuality and sexual function before you even begin Nolvadex. In fact, the emotional impact of the diagnosis on sexuality has never been thoroughly studied, and that's something that we know should be looked at in detail. One study looked at sexual dysfunction in women with gynecologic malignancies, and it showed a very dramatic impact on sexuality.

When you begin with the understanding that a diagnosis of breast cancer will affect sexuality, it's difficult to say how the Nolvadex will affect the situation. Chemotherapy can also have an impact on sexuality, especially if it causes hair loss. What is the psychosocial and psychosexual effect of hair loss? All those things are connected, and none have been looked at in any detail. I believe that a really healthy sexual life with a sensitive, caring partner before treatment is the single most important factor in a patient's maintaining a healthy, gratifying sex life after a malignancy.

What do you do for vaginal dryness?

Topical estrogen is the treatment of choice, but I'll treat patients with it only after I've discussed it with the medical oncologist. For the patient for whom it's not appropriate, the only thing left is lubricants such as Replens. It's a conveniently packaged, non-

(continued)

greasy, water-soluble lubricant that really works well for some women. I think it provides a good lubricant for sexual intercourse. Some women who have dryness and irritation from undergarments carry a little K-Y jelly or Replens, and when they urinate, they'll lightly apply a small coating of lubricant to the external genitalia.

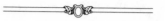

Tip—In 1993 two separate studies began looking at using estrogen-replacement therapy for women who had had breast cancer.

DIAGNOSIS DURING PREGNANCY

The fear I felt when diagnosed was overwhelming as I digested the knowledge that I might die of this disease. It seems unimaginable to me that I could have been more frightened. Talking to women whose diagnosis came in the midst of a pregnancy has given me a glimpse of a new dimension to the dilemma of breast cancer.

As breast cancer strikes younger and younger women and the incidence of breast cancer rises, more women of childbearing age are being diagnosed with breast cancer. According to statistics compiled at Sammons Cancer Center at Baylor University Medical Center in 1991, between 2,000 and 6,000 women will be diagnosed in 1993 with breast cancer during pregnancy.

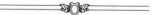

Tip—According to an article in *Oncology* magazine in November 1991, while there is often delay in diagnosis for these women, patients with breast cancer during pregnancy have the same prognosis as nonpregnant patients. The most important predictor of survival is the stage of the disease.

While they are a small percentage of the overall breast cancer cases, pregnant patients present a number of complications in diagnosis and treatment.

In July 1991, "The Management of Cancer in the Pregnant Patient" was published in *Baylor University Medical Center Proceeding*. The paper was the joint effort of Stephen E. Jones, M.D., Director, Clinical Research at the Charles A. Sammons Cancer Center at Baylor; C. Allen Stringer, M.D., Obstetrics and Gynecology; Robert T. Dorr, Ph.D., Departments of Medicine and Pharmacology/Toxicology, University of Arizona College of Medicine, Tucson; and Neil N. Senzer, M.D., Radiation Oncology, Baylor University Medical Center.

According to the article, pregnant women face delays of two to five months from the first awareness of a breast lump to diagnosis.

"Physicians contribute to this delay for a variety of reasons," the article states. "Such as a reluctance to biopsy the breast of a pregnant woman. Even if mammograms are performed with fetal shielding, mammography may be negative."

They cite in the article one study that reported negative mammograms in six of eight pregnant women who subsequently were proven by biopsy to have cancer.

The article continues by explaining that while it used to be thought that terminating the pregnancy would slow the growth of the cancer, it is now believed that because these cancers are often high grade, it is the delayed diagnosis and more advanced staging at diagnosis that lead to the growth, meaning that as with nonpregnant women, early detection is essential.

Yet the article's more positive note is that breast cancer during pregnancy can be managed. It states:

"Considerable experience has been gained with mastectomy in pregnancy-associated breast cancer. Anesthesia is safe and local control is achieved for operable cancers by mastectomy. Locally advanced cancers or inflammatory cancers pose special problems because the standard approach is now to give preoperative chemotherapy for these lesions. More patients are opting for breast conservation (lumpectomy, axillary dissection and breast irradiation). This too poses a special problem as one would like not to administer therapeutic radiation to the pregnant patient."

The article concludes that women with breast cancer can undergo mastectomy and, in most cases, wait until the baby is delivered to undergo radiation, and that chemotherapy can be given during the second and third trimesters of pregnancy, probably with relative safety, stressing that all the risks associated with chemotherapy and pregnancy are not known.

The issues of delayed diagnosis and staging inability are complicated by treatment decisions to ensure the safety of the fetus in those women who decide to continue their pregnancies, a difficult and perhaps heartbreaking decision.

Two of the women interviewed for this book were diagnosed during pregnancy. They both chose to continue their pregnancy, although that is a very personal decision and one that must be made by the woman, her husband, and her doctor. All factors—both physical and emotional—should be taken into consideration, including length of gestation and all available information about the tumor itself. The fact that these women continued with their pregnancies is in no way a suggestion that you do the same. It does present some evidence that healthy babies can be born to women who have breast cancer and who have undergone chemotherapy.

BETTY B (38)

Betty B and I first talked in August 1991, ten months after her diagnosis and six months after the birth of her daughter, Kelsey. She and her husband also had a six-year-old son.

Betty found the lump before she became pregnant. Her obstetrician pointed it out to her in March at the beginning of what would be regular appointments while he counseled her in fertility. In June, after a month on a fertility drug, she became pregnant. *"The lump got bigger, but you know my breasts were getting bigger since I was pregnant. I had the ob feel it and he reassured me. My husband could feel it, and he was very concerned. He went with me on one visit specifically to ask about the lump. The ob reassured us again. The next month it was larger and my husband insisted he feel it again. This time he referred us to a breast surgeon."*

When the breast specialist could not aspirate the lump, he ordered a mammogram with fetal shielding. Betty was still not worried, thinking it was a going to be a cyst. *"He came in after he had looked at the mammogram and said he was 99 percent sure it was cancer."*

Betty says that despite her mother's diagnosis with breast cancer at age forty-eight, when Betty was a teen, she was totally unprepared since her mother never shared her feelings or the experience with her—including any cautions. *"My mother has told me since, that after her surgery a friend came by who told her that the way she and her husband had dealt with it was to never talk about it, and that was the route my mother took."*

Betty did call her ob with the news that the tumor was malignant. She said that despite some feelings that he should have suggested a surgeon sooner, she decided to stay with him for the delivery of her child.

Betty underwent a modified radical under general anesthesia, at which time a catheter was placed in her chest area above the other breast. Surgery revealed that Betty already had three positive lymph nodes.

The fetus came through the surgery fine, and when a second surgery to correct the catheter was required, Betty recalls she was more frightened. Betty began chemotherapy the next week. *"He said the Adriamycin and vincristine are large enough that they won't pass the placenta, but the Cytoxan could. So I told him I wanted to wait until the last trimester for the Cytoxan. I went in and got the Vincristine through the Hickman catheter. Then I came home and they put the Adriamycin in a pouch, which I carried for four days so it was really slow infusion by pump."*

Betty says her exhaustion from chemo was indescribable. Because her husband is disabled, Betty's parents cared for her son and the house so Betty could return to her job as an elementary school teacher part-time a month after chemo began, a necessary decision since hers was the health insurance for the family. Betty relied on a home health service, which made house calls to disconnect her pump and for complications with the catheter, which she recalled as endless. *"What happened was that my blood had thickened as it does toward the end of a pregnancy so you won't bleed to death when you have the baby. And it had formed little webs over the top of the catheter. So they had to take it out and put a new one in."*

In the midst of all this Betty was trying to focus on the new life in her body who was going through this with her. *"I just wanted her to be healthy. My husband and I had had a real battle over whether to have amniocentesis before the cancer. I didn't want to do it because of the risk to the pregnancy. He wanted to know because if I had to be off work, we needed to know since he is disabled. We knew she was a girl and we knew she was healthy. But then they started doing all the tests. I was convinced that she was going to be sick when she was born and I was bonding to a sick infant."*

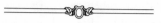

Tip—Betty refused to sign the permission for a cesarean because she wanted the option of the TRAM reconstruction.

After five treatments of chemo, Betty gave birth to Kelsey in natural childbirth one week before her scheduled due date. Kelsey weighed six and a half pounds and had a full head of hair. Her mom was bald. *"She was fine. I was feeling great and the doctor was trying to get the placenta out and it got real quiet and I said, 'This is not going to work. You're going to have to give me something.' They took her away and I had to have a saddle block and it took three hours to get all the placenta out because it had disintegrated from the chemo."*

The emotional adjustments were difficult. Betty resented not being able to breast-feed Kelsey, and her son was having behavior problems at school due to all the upheaval at home. Betty had two more chemo treatments after Kelsey was born and began radiation two months later. Her Sunday School class brought food once a week for seven months.

Soon after Kelsey's birth, Betty began to struggle with the emotional impact of the previous months. She recognized that her entire pregnancy was crisis management. The anger came six months later. *"I think when you are going through it, you don't have any emotions left to be angry with. I was just sad. I cried all the time. I am in counseling now with a woman who specializes in postnatal depression. I started seeing her when Kelsey was a month old. I wasn't bonding to her like I did with my son."*

Betty has also dealt with some strong feelings of disfigurement. A friend called a few months after her surgery to tell Betty she had found a lump, and when the friend discovered that it was cancer and needed only a lumpectomy, Betty found she was angry and jealous. She began taking a mood elevator and continued with weekly therapy sessions. *"I dread dealing with the loss of my breast. I'm resentful of the time I lost with my daughter. And it's still hard for me to bond with her."*

Yet while Betty attests to the negative feelings, she also says the experience has had some positive aspects. She says her faith is stronger and she has found new friends in her church who provided support. She also found it was time to ask her parents for some distance from their constant disapproval of her life-style and—literally—of her home, which they constantly criticized. *"I am beginning to get some control. I am taking more time to be with the children, playing. I don't care so much if the house is neat."*

Betty is also clear that her daughter will know about her experience and be more in touch with her body.

When I checked back with Betty in January 1992, she had begun attending a support group regularly and had found a new relationship with her daughter. *"I'm glad now that I didn't find out about the lump before getting pregnant,"* she said, *"because I would not have gotten pregnant and I would go through the whole thing again to have Kelsey."*

TERESA C (28)

Teresa C maintains that she does not feel like an inspiration, but few who have heard her story would agree.

In 1972, at age twelve, Teresa lost the majority of her right leg to bone cancer. Two recurrences in her lungs, surgery, and four years of chemotherapy later, she was clear of cancer. She was then nineteen and a freshman in college, after spending her entire adolescence in hospitals.

She went on to earn her degree in business administration and accounting and began law school. She had graduated and married and was practicing business litigation when in March 1988 she learned she had breast cancer. She was also five months pregnant with her first child.

Teresa found the lump after noticing a discharge from her left breast that was slightly tinged with blood. *"I had just had a sonogram, and we could tell he was a boy. I saw in the pregnancy books that the discharge was normal, but the tinge of blood made me call my ob. He looked at it and said it was probably a clogged duct, but he wanted to make sure, so he referred me to a breast surgeon."*

The reassurances from the surgeon that it was probably nothing did little to calm Teresa. *"After what I had gone through my whole life, I'm going, 'Not me. This is going to be cancer.'"*

The confirmation of the malignant diagnosis after a biopsy led to suspicions of the high-dose radiation Teresa had received for her lung tumors twelve years before. While there is nothing conclusive, Teresa and her oncologist feel certain that the two were related. The tumor was in the exact spot that had received radiation. *"One of the first things I remember the surgeon saying was, 'We'll have to terminate the pregnancy.' I don't remember what my response was, whether it was a simple no or what, but we'd had a sonogram and this was a baby. This wasn't a pregnancy."*

The surgeon recommended a Dallas oncologist who had treated pregnant women, and the same day, Teresa and her husband met with him. There was little study material to follow. *"He basically said we could take this one week at a time and try to get as far as we could with the baby. As long as the tumor stayed the same or shrank, we could do that, and he didn't think I'd be in any danger, but there was the risk that by continuing, those pregnancy hormones in my body would make it grow."*

Two days later Teresa had a Hickman catheter placed near her collarbone. The oncologist spent a considerable amount of time with Teresa's doctors from her childhood poring over chemo records to see how much Adriamycin she had received, since there is a lifetime limit for the drug. The other chemo drugs chosen were those that were believed not to cross the placenta. *"They decided to treat me with Adriamycin over a three-day period for each treatment, rather than just an injection all at once. That meant no cold cap and hair loss. I felt really ugly. Pregnant and hairless."*

And during this time Teresa and her husband were worrying about their unborn child and the effects the drugs would have on him and whether he would be born prematurely, with the accompanying problems. Teresa continued to work, taking time off for the three-day infusion. The doctors, meanwhile, were working together for the next event: the birth of the baby, followed by immediate mastectomy. *"I began chemo in April and the C-section was scheduled for July 13. We had a sonogram the week of the 4th that showed the placenta was dying off, probably from the chemotherapy. Then on July Fourth weekend I went down the Brazos River on a boat for the day and that night didn't feel too good. My husband got a movie and he put it in and I heard a balloon pop, but there wasn't one in the room. I began having pain and didn't know it was contractions, but I called the doctor and they said he was en route. It was 11 P.M. and Jake was born vaginally at 2:30 A.M."*

Jake was five weeks premature and weighed in at 4 pounds and 13 ounces. His lungs were fine, probably a result, the doctor said, of the early dying of the placenta, which stressed the lungs, causing early development. He also had more hair than his mother.

Jake went home from the hospital ten days later, the same day his mother had a modified radical, which indicated Teresa had two positive lymph nodes. Teresa elected to have the other breast removed before reconstruction in 1990. *"The pathology showed links to the former radiation treatment, and while I just had that one pinpoint radiation, I had also had radiation to my entire lungs. My plastic surgeon was saying that cosmetically she could do a lot more if she started from scratch than trying to match the other."*

In August 1992, Teresa learned that her cancer had metastasized to her lung, liver, and bones. Because her tumor was hormone-receptive, she immediately began tamoxifen and had her ovaries removed. Scans in October showed the tumors were dying, and Teresa is hopeful.

HIGH-RISK DIAGNOSIS

"When she got her records, she read through them and the statement that a '50 percent survival is being optimistic' sticks in her head. She probably repeats it hundreds of times a day."—Leanne's husband, Craig

Those women who find their cancer after they have multiple malignant nodes or who have other clear indicators that they are at high risk for recurrence must live with statistics that say they might die from this disease. With breast cancer there is no truth in statistics, either. Theresa and Nancy S were two women interviewed for this book with excellent prognoses. Both were node-negative; both took adjuvant treatment. Both had recurrance when their cancer metastasized to their lungs and bones within two years of diagnosis.

You have to battle your own "what if" and come to some kind of peace.

But the good news is that for clearly high-risk women there are new treatments and new hope that they can beat this disease. I always remember something Dr. Jan Pettigrew likes to say. *"When the oncologist says 80 percent chance of recurrence, there are those patients who make up the high end of that statistic who do well."*

These women are real and they are out there, and you may be one of them.

Lona had ten malignant nodes when she was diagnosed in May 1986. She had chemotherapy and radiation and began taking tamoxifen. When we talked in 1990, she was cancer-free and had just banked her bone marrow in case she needed high-dose chemotherapy and a bone marrow transplant. When I called to check on her in February 1993, seven years after her diagnosis, her husband explained she couldn't come to the phone—she was at her Jazzercize class. Still cancer-free, Lona had beaten the odds.

Sadie had twelve nodes involved when she underwent a mastectomy in May 1989. At four years out, she is fine and feels great.

I wish I knew what Lona and Sadie had in common. Lona says she just decided she wasn't going to get it again. *"I consider myself cancer-free,"* she wrote in her survey. *"I plan to die from something else."* Lona started counseling as soon as she was diagnosed and said that the message she got was that she had a choice whether it came back. She just decided it wouldn't.

Sadie expected she would have a recurrence and says that a serious infection in the incision may have helped her immune system begin killing cancer cells immediately after her surgery. She had chemotherapy and tamoxifen. *"The doctor said there isn't anything scientific to prove it, but maybe the infection threw my immune system into high gear."*

For Lona and Sadie and the rest of us who live with a fear of recurrence, there is the knowledge that new techniques offer more hope than ever before that we can beat this disease. Indeed, during the two years that I researched this book, it seemed that every month something new appeared about breast cancer research.

BONE MARROW TRANSPLANTS

In the late eighties a new treatment for breast cancer began to move from experimental to accepted procedure—autologous bone marrow transplant, a procedure that allows a very high dose chemotherapy for those women who are clearly at high risk for recurrence with only standard treatment regimen.

Chemotherapy can kill cancer cells, but doctors also know that in those women who are clearly at high risk for recurrence or have metastatic breast cancer, the doses needed to clear their body of cancer would also wipe out the bone marrow, leaving the woman open to deadly infections, with no natural defenses.

Autologous bone marrow transplant involves removing about a quart of bone marrow from a woman before blasting her with chemotherapy. Then the bone marrow is reintroduced, allowing it to rebuild the blood supply. It is, as one woman said, "taking a woman to the brink of death and then bringing her back with her own bone marrow."

When it was introduced, the transplant procedure was dangerous and involved a lengthy hospital stay in sterile surroundings while the body recovered. It is still quite expensive, but insurance companies have begun to accept that it is no longer experimental and is the best option for women who are at high risk. The discovery of growth factors, which can help the bone marrow recover at a much faster rate, has shortened the hospital stay for women undergoing the treatment, which is now offered at a growing number of cancer centers around the country.

For women such as Rula and Wendy, it has been a lifesaver. Rula was twenty-eight and single when, in March 1990, she discovered a massive tumor in her right breast. With twelve nodes involved, her risk for recurrence was very high. She chose to undergo a bone marrow transplant, which involved three hospital stays and months of recovery. I last talked to Rula in spring 1993. She was still cancer-free and volunteering with new breast cancer patients.

Rula began the process when about a quart of her bone marrow was removed from her body and stored. She then entered the hospital and was given high-dose chemotherapy, which essentially wiped out her immune system and, hopefully, any remaining cancer cells. Her own bone marrow was reintroduced, and she spent the next three weeks in a sterile environment as her bone marrow worked to rebuild her own immune system. *"When I was first diagnosed, they said, 'Chemo.' So I went through chemo. And after chemo, the tumor stopped shrinking and that's when they said, 'Okay, we're going to go for a mastectomy.' So we went through a mastectomy, and they said, 'Just radiation and that will be it.' And after a month, Dr. M called me into his office, and he said, 'Listen, this is not going to work. We need a bone marrow transplant.' And he said, 'Sleep on it, think about it.' "*

Rula began a series of tests, including kidney function, bone scans, and X rays, to confirm she was eligible. *"They wanted to make sure that I would tolerate the chemo because the mega-doses of chemo that they give you* are *experimental, and there was the risk of dying."*

After harvesting her bone marrow, Rula entered the hospital a month later and was given massive doses of chemo over a period of days. A week later her own bone marrow was reintroduced to her body. *"I missed a whole week and a half. I don't remember anything. My brother said I would get up and was short of breath and wanted to go to the bathroom and shower, and the nurse would want to help me, and I'd say no."*

Rula spent the next weeks recovering after her bone marrow was reintroduced. Because of her susceptibility to infection, she was isolated in a room with its own ventilation. *"You live for the numbers. They come and weigh you in the morning and take your vital signs and you take a shower and come back and say, 'Are my numbers back? Is my count back?' And they would tell me, and I had the little schedule on my wall."*

It was not an experience Rula wants to repeat, but her chances of disease-free survival have risen from around 10 percent to 85 percent with the transplant. *"I have it very strong in my family. My mother passed away with breast cancer at thirty-two. My aunt passed away with breast cancer, my uncle with leukemia. It's all from one side of my family."*

Rula wants other women to know that bone marrow treatment is possible despite the slow recovery and distress involved. *"I lost twenty-five pounds and you really can't walk for a while. I mean, you're short of breath, you have to build up little by little and go back. I finally started walking my five miles again now after a year, but it took forever."*

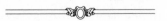

Tip—Some women who are at high risk for recurrence are having their bone marrow harvested in case they need it in the future.

Wendy was twenty-six and single when she was diagnosed in May 1989. The tumor, which was estimated at 10 to 12 centimeters, did not respond to preoperative chemotherapy. *"I had a mammogram and the radiologist said they couldn't see anything. Well, the reason was that the tumor was so big it encompassed my whole left breast. The whole left breast was tumor."*

After her mastectomy in August, which revealed four malignant lymph nodes, the doctors recommended to Wendy that she consider a bone marrow transplant because of her age and the aggressiveness of the tumor. She was given a 90 percent chance of recurrence within eighteen months without it. *"When I was first diagnosed, it was like I was in a movie. I was removed from the whole situation, looking down on it."*

Wendy said the first meeting with the transplant-team doctor was only somewhat reassuring. He told her that she would be the eighth breast cancer patient to be transplanted and that of the women they had done, all were doing well, but that it had only been two years. *"So he was basically saying that the best he could project was two years. They didn't know the life expectancy, but he said I could have two years. It was either that or die. But I knew I would do it and come out fine. I'm just that kind of person."*

Wendy had her bone marrow harvested. She then entered the hospital and received high-dose chemotherapy for three days. She spent the next six weeks recovering. *"You are hooked up to a number of different fluids. I had terrible nausea. I lost my hair. And then they started me on high-dose antibiotics and they were just as bad as the chemo. I had a rash all over my skin. It moved up my body, from my feet to my legs and chest. I just didn't want it on my face. Because every day I would get up and shower and give myself a little facial. I tried to pamper myself as much as I could. Another of the antibiotics caused me to have fever and chills. The nurses call it shake and bake."*

Wendy was back at work six weeks after being released, but she says it took two years for her to feel totally well. *"I'm five foot eight and used to model and I wind-surf and used to lift weights. I was in such good shape that you could see the muscles in my stomach. The doctor said the reason I did so well in the hospital was because I was so strong and so muscular. I did physical therapy on the unit every day."*

The year following her transplant Wendy was a visible presence in the Dallas area in breast cancer causes. She spoke at high schools about the importance of education. After losing three friends to breast cancer, Wendy decided it was time for a change and moved to Florida with her fiancé. *"I just decided to get away from Dallas. I needed to move and be near the sunshine and water."*

Wendy returned to Dallas in the fall of 1991 for reconstruction, using her tummy muscle. *"It was a piece of cake. It was very painful, more painful than the bone marrow transplant, because I had never been cut on my stomach, but after the first two weeks of pain, I wouldn't trade it. I love being able to wear a bathing suit."*

Wendy accepts that with her diagnosis she will live a life of constant vigilance. *"I'm getting on with my life. I'm planning to live, and if I don't, I've got everything in my will. But I can't sit and think I've only got five years or whatever. I'm just glad it's over and I'm glad to know I could help other girls, to educate them about breast cancer and how to do monthly self-exam. And that's exactly how I found mine."*

MEDICAL ONCOLOGIST DR. JOSEPH FAY, DIRECTOR OF THE BONE MARROW TRANSPLANT PROGRAM AT BAYLOR UNIVERSITY MEDICAL CENTER, TALKS ABOUT BONE MARROW TRANSPLANT

Dr. Joseph Fay established one of the country's first bone marrow transplant units, at Duke University in the late seventies, after working with the National Institutes of Health. In 1982 he moved to Baylor University Medical Center, where he established its bone marrow transplant center.

Explain how bone marrow transplant works and what it means for breast cancer.

There is a dose response relationship between chemotherapy agents and breast cancer-cell kill. For example, if the dose of chemotherapy agents is doubled or tripled, one may see an increase in cancer-cell kill. A major toxic manifestation of chemotherapy agents is bone marrow suppression. Thus, bone marrow trans-

(continued)

plantation allows the administration of high-dose chemotherapy, resulting in an enhanced tumor cell kill.

What is different about the chemotherapy drugs used in bone marrow?

Most chemotherapy agents used in marrow transplantation protocols are alkylating agents. They have the property of killing malignant cells regardless of where they happen to be in the cell cycle. For example, they will kill malignant cells if they are dividing or not dividing.

Who is eligible for the procedure?

The first group of patients are those whose cancer recurs, meaning they have developed metastatic breast cancer despite previous treatment with surgery, radiation and, usually, adjuvant chemotherapy. A major criterion for being treated with a bone marrow transplant protocol is that the patient must have responsive disease. In other words the tumor has responded to chemotherapy before. These patients often respond to additional chemotherapy but essentially are never cured. The principle behind high-dose chemotherapy and bone marrow transplantation for this group is obtaining a remission with additional treatment, then using intensive chemotherapy to destroy residual breast cancer cells.

So you want someone who responds?

Correct. For patients with metastatic lung and liver disease who receive an Adriamycin-containing regimen and experience no response—that is, the tumor grows in spite of chemotherapy—high-dose chemotherapy does not significantly prolong life. Remissions achieved with intensive chemotherapy are short-lived. For this category of patients, we recommend clinical trials examining new chemotherapy agents.

(continued)

So they have already responded to chemotherapy when they are chosen?

Correct. After having a successful reduction in the size of the tumor metastasis, patients are treated with a well-designed high-dose chemotherapy regimen and autologous marrow transplantation. Preliminary results are good. For example, with this approach, approximately 80 percent of patients with metastatic breast cancer have experienced a complete remission, in contrast to 10 to 15 percent of patients achieving a complete remission with conventional-dose chemotherapy. Thus, high-dose combination chemotherapy treatment and autologous bone marrow transplantation results in a much higher complete response rate than seen with conventional treatment programs. What is even more exciting is that a substantial number of these patients—that is, about 40 percent—remain in complete remission with several month's follow-up.

A second group of patients who are being treated with high-dose chemotherapy and autologous bone marrow transplantation are women who are diagnosed initially with advanced local regional breast cancer. These patients have a primary breast tumor that is greater than 5 centimeters, often multicentric—or throughout the breast—and have axillary lymph node metastasis. A subcategory are patients with primary breast tumor of any size who have ten or more axillary lymph nodes containing breast cancer at the time of initial surgery. The tumor size and the lymph-node status are strong predictors for the development of metastatic disease despite surgery, local radiotherapy, and conventional-dose chemotherapy. With standard treatment approaches, the majority of these patients—between 50 and 90 percent—will develop metastatic breast cancer. Accordingly, this group of patients is being treated with intensive combination chemotherapy and autologous bone marrow transplantation.

(continued)

Talk about the process. What happens when you come in for high-dose chemotherapy?

All of the patients enter these clinical trials voluntarily. Patients must satisfy certain protocol entry criteria, including normal cardiac, pulmonary, and renal function studies. Careful staging is done to determine whether metastatic disease exits. In the case of patients with metastatic disease at the start, an assessment is made regarding disease responsiveness. The marrow is obtained with standard techniques of harvesting. This consists of a brief period of anesthesia, during which time marrow cells are aspirated from the pelvic bone. This marrow is then cryopreserved—or frozen. After all of the workup has been completed and the patient has signed informed consent, she is hospitalized and receives a combination of high-dose chemotherapy agents, followed by marrow transplantation. In other words, her marrow is reintroduced after the chemotherapy.

So after the patient is chosen and the marrow is harvested?

The patient enters the marrow transplantation unit and receives treatment with high-dose chemotherapy. The chemotherapy is given intravenously, with careful attention to intravenous fluids, blood electrolytes, and other blood chemistries. Our current regimen is a three-day program involving high-dose thio-TEPA and cyclophosphamide. For our patients with metastatic disease, carboplatin is added to this regimen. After chemotherapy is completed, the marrow cells that have been stored earlier are thawed at the patient's bedside and given intravenously. From this point, patients are managed with blood products, antibiotics, and growth factors until marrow function recovers. After patients are discharged, some will require radiation and tamoxifen following the transplant.

Explain growth factors.

Growth factors are products of recombinant DNA technology. These factors are small-molecular-weight proteins that stimulate

(continued)

the bone marrow cells to proliferate and differentiate and have increased qualitative functions. They enable faster marrow engraftment after transplant, and that reduces the hospital stay.

What do you do for the patient's emotional needs during bone marrow treatment?

The transplant program employs a team approach. Our patients are seen by our social worker and dietitian, and patient volunteers on a regular basis. Physicians, nurses, pharmacists, and the dietitian make rounds on the transplant unit daily to see all the patients. Careful assessment of their emotional needs are made prior to their being admitted to the transplant unit.

What other experimental treatments for breast cancer have emerged?

In the early eighties, research involving breast cancer began to involve other treatment modalities in addition to chemotherapy to control cancer cell growth. Encouraging results have been seen in biotherapy, a generic term used for immune therapy and other measures to specifically impair cancer cell growth.

Biotherapies take advantage of studies at the cellular level to determine which factors are responsible for cancer cell division and proliferation. By doing this, one may determine how to interfere with cancer cell division, leading to effective treatment. These research studies involve such things as cancer cell growth factor receptors and cancer cell biology. If one could interfere with cell division, that would be sufficient. A patient could live a normal life span, free of symptoms, with a few breast cancer cells if we could simply devise ways to prevent cancer cell division and proliferation.

How is that different from immunotherapy?

Immunotherapy is based on the principle of killing cancer cells by an immune mechanism. This can be accomplished using antibodies or by specifically or nonspecifically enhancing a patient's

(continued)

immune system to destroy cancer cells. A recent interesting development is the use of antibodies that have a toxin biochemically linked to the antibody. This antibody is given to patients, which in turn delivers the toxin to the cancer cells specifically. There are a number of other cellular growth factors under study to stimulate the patient's own immune system to attack cancer cells.

IMMUNOLOGIST AND ONCOLOGIST DR. AMANULLAH KHAN, ST. PAUL MEDICAL CENTER, TALKS ABOUT IMMUNOTHERAPIES AND THEIR USE WITH BREAST CANCER

Dr. Amanullah Khan, an oncologist/hematologist, specializes in clinical immunology. Dr. Khan's research has centered on ways to enhance the immune system so that it might aid in the body's fight against cancer.

What is immunology?

The immune system is our first line of defense against any cancer. The body's immune surveillance is made up of many components. We have T cells, complement system, antibodies, and macrophages. T cells have the ability to secrete certain substances that are toxic to the target and can destroy it. B lymphocytes produce antibodies that can attack the target. All of these components work together in the immune system. One component initiates another or interacts with something else and the whole cascade comes in to destroy the target.

We have learned a great deal about immunology and cancer in the past few years, but even as early as the fifties the pathologists commented on women with breast cancer whose tumors were surrounded by a lot of lymphocytes. These women did better than those who didn't have many lymphocytes. We also know that if you test the immune system of patients with cancer, those with

(continued)

better immune systems have a better outcome. Therefore we know that the immune system has a definite role in controlling cancer.

How can the immune system help in fighting cancer?

We are now dissecting the immune system to try to learn about each component of immunity and its role in fighting cancer. A number of areas are being studied, such as interferon, which is a product of the cells in the immune system and had some early enthusiasm for treating breast cancer. But the studies done with the purified interferon produced by genetic engineering have not borne the same results that were seen earlier. Recent studies indicate it increases the effect of 5-FU, which is a standard drug of breast cancer treatment. This effect was seen in the treatment of colon cancer.

Another area of interest is the tumor necrosis factor, a substance manufactured by the body in response to certain infections and stimulation of macrophages. It has been shown to be very destructive to the tumor, and in animal models it looked promising. But there have been problems in humans because we cannot deliver it to the tumor site effectively. Work is in progress to circumvent those problems.

Interleukin II, a substance that is in essence the driving force behind the immune system, stimulates and proliferates certain cells, makes cells produce other substances, and turns cells into killer cells. It has been shown to be effective in certain tumors such as renal cell carcinoma and melanoma. Since Interleukin II can change the lymphocytes into killer cells in the test tube, we take a patient's own lymphocytes and stimulate them in a test tube with Interleukin II to become killer cells and give them back to the patient. Again, encouraging results have been seen in other tumors but not in breast tumors.

Are there any new areas of exploration?

There is a lot of momentum in developing the monoclonal antibodies. This is a way to create an antibody in the laboratory that

(continued)

will seek out and destroy a target. In the past we made antibodies against diseases by creating serum in cows and horses. Immunologists had long desired to make them in a test tube, where you take human cells and have them produce the antibody. This process requires taking a cell that knows how to grow in the test tube and combining it with the cell that knows how to make the antibodies. The antibody-producing cells are taken from mice that have been injected with the antigen, such as breast cancer. The hybrid cell knows how to grow in vitro and also knows how to make an antibody. Then you select the cells that are producing the specific antibody you want, and grow clones of the cell. These antibody-producing cells are known as monoclonal because they are cloned from one cell. They produce very uniform antibodies. These monoclonal antibodies when injected into the patient will seek out and bind to the target. They localize to where the tumor is. You can put a label on these antibodies such as a chemical or radioisotope and use them for delivering those substances to the tumor site. These procedures are being investigated for treating or localizing tumor in the patient. Those antibodies are also being used extensively in diagnostic tests. Trials with monoclonal are also under way.

Are these substances being used?

At present we are in the investigational stages with many of the immunologic substances. Two such substances, Interleukin II and interferon, have been approved for treating patients. Combined action of interferon with other chemotherapy agents is being used successfully. But in the next few years we will be seeing many more combination studies. Presently for our patients with breast cancer, we give the standard regimen. But with recurrent disease we are trying different approaches because we know that the outcome is not good. Therefore we are incorporating immunological approaches. For example, we have used interferon and chemotherapy with success in some patients. These are anecdotal experiences.

(continued)

We don't know if the patients who respond were destined to have a better survival with just chemotherapy, or if the interferon made a difference because it was not part of a large study.

In what other ways do you incorporate the immune system in your cancer treatment?

We encourage patients to do those things that will build the immune system: eating a healthy diet and staying away from alcohol, tobacco, pesticides, and toxic chemicals. We also encourage a healthy life-style, the use of vitamins, such as vitamin C, which we know enhances the immune system, and trace elements. There are many sources for information on this and doctors are offering more and more. But the patients must also participate and learn about the disease, be educated.

We also incorporate the patient's circadian rhythms to determine when they receive chemotherapy.

The body goes through physiological changes and rhythm in a twenty-four-hour period. At certain times of the day we are more active, while at other times we are asleep. Our body temperature varies during the day, and the body is constantly changing and adapting. Studies show that chemotherapeutic agents are less toxic during certain times in this cycle. Circadian rhythm is being used to minimize toxicity. Similar studies are being done that address performing surgery during certain periods of the menstrual cycle and the suggestion is that it will affect the possibility of metastases.

RESOURCES

These are all NIH publications and can be obtained by calling 1–800-4-CANCER:
- *Chemotherapy and You: A Guide to Self-Help During Treatment*
- *Radiation Therapy and You: A Guide to Self-Help During Treatment*
- *Eating Hints: Recipes and Tips Better Nutrition During Cancer Treatment*
- *Answers to Your Questions About Metastatic Cancer*

BOOKS:

Coping with Chemotherapy, by Nancy Bruning (Ballantine Health, 1985)

Everyone's Guide to Cancer Therapy, by Malin Dollinger, M.D., Ernest H. Rosenbaum, M.D., and Greg Cable (Somerville House Books Limited, 1991)

Choices, by Marion Morra and Eve Potts (Avon, 1987)

To find experimental programs, check the clinical trials portion of the PDQ (Physicians Data Query) from the NCI. To obtain this, call 1–800-4-CANCER or Physicians Data Query Service at (301) 496-7403. For a list of cancer treatment centers offering immunotherapy or biotherapy, call the national cancer hotline or write Public Inquiries, National Cancer Institute, Room 10A24, Building 31, 9000 Rockville Pike, Bethesda, MD 20892.

Chapter 4

RECONSTRUCTION
(or, It's a Lot Harder to Put It Back On Than It Is to Take It Off)

CHOOSING RECONSTRUCTION

"When I saw it for the first time, I was flabbergasted. It looked so beautiful I cried like a baby. The doctor thought I didn't like it because I was crying. I just hugged her and thanked her and thanked her. I was surprised it looked so good."—Linda

"No matter what they tell you about the reconstruction, you expect it to look real. They told me that it would look real as it could from one view. But it's not the real thing, and it's not going to be the real thing."—Lola

"I am very pleased with my reconstruction. It has been a positive experience because I felt that I was in control this time—not the cancer. It was the first step in putting this behind me."—Leanne

"It's not a breast. It's a fine approximation. If you are the kind of person who wants the perfect body, you're not going to get it, but you know, you're not going to get one as you get older anyway."—Marjorie's husband, Chuck

"Since I've had my nipple on, my husband just looks at it and says, 'I can't believe it. I just can't believe it. How did he do that?' "—Madeline

"I think that reconstruction was very, very helpful to her because it put the daily visual reminder somewhat behind her. You can never put it all the way behind you, but the visual stimulus is less."—Lynne's husband, Norm

"I did chemotherapy for my husband; I did reconstruction for me."—Gale

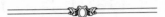

Tip—Many women have the option of immediate reconstruction. This chapter addresses information that will be needed at the time of initial surgery to make that decision—and information needed for future reconstruction.

RECONSTRUCTION GLOSSARY

The lingo for reconstruction, like that for breast surgery, involves new words and phrases. Here are the basics. The techniques listed will be addressed more specifically and thoroughly in the remainder of the chapter.

Augmentation: When an implant is placed under existing breast tissue to increase the size of a normal, healthy breast. Augmentation is not reconstruction, because the breast tissue is not removed.

Capsular contracture: The most common complication from any reconstruction that involves an implant. The body forms a hard scar tissue sack around the implant, resulting in a hard breast. Capsular contracture can be corrected by replacing the implant and removing the scar tissue. New implants have textured surfaces to reduce the chances of capsular contracture, but it still may occur. Some women have capsular contracture repeatedly. Others do not experience it at all.

Delayed reconstruction: Reconstruction is delayed months or years after initial breast surgery.

Expander reconstruction: A type of reconstruction and the name of the device used. A modified radical mastectomy removes the skin of the breast in addition to the tissue. In some cases the remaining skin can be stretched to a size large enough to match the existing breast. This is done by inserting an empty silicone sack under the skin and muscle and then gradually filling it with saline solution over a period of weeks, during which time the skin stretches. The sack is replaced by a permanent implant.

Flap: The skin moved from another location to create the new breast.

Immediate reconstruction: The reconstruction is begun at the same time the breast is removed. Not all women are candidates for immediate reconstruction.

Implant: The sack placed under the skin and chest muscle to fill out the reconstructed breast. Implants can be filled with silicone gel or saline fluid and come in various sizes. Some surgery techniques, in which body fat and/or muscle is moved from another location, do not require an implant.

Implant reconstruction: The simplest reconstruction that can only be used on a woman with small breasts who has adequate skin remaining at the mastectomy site. In this instance the plastic surgeon can simply insert an implant under the muscle and skin at the mastectomy site. A nipple can be added later.

Latissimus flap reconstruction: Also called the back flap. The latissimus dorsal muscle and an eye-shaped wedge of skin are moved from the back to the chest wall and sewn in place, leaving the tissue attached to the original blood supply. Depending on the size of the breast the surgeon is trying to match, an implant may be added under the muscle.

Microsurgery reconstruction: Also called free flaps, because they are cut free of their blood supply and reconnected to the breast blood supply. Reconstruction procedures that move muscle and fat from other places on the body, such as the hip or abdomen, may require microsurgery to reconnect blood supply. Those procedures that move tissue that is close to the breast, such as the latissimus flap, can leave the blood supply attached. When fat and/or muscle and skin are taken from the stomach area, it may be left attached to the blood supply or it may be completely severed and moved externally to the breast, in which case it has to be reattached to the local blood supply with microsurgery.

Mound: The term for the new breast before the nipple has been added.

Necrosis: A problem that can occur with any reconstruction surgery is skin necrosis, which means skin death when there is inadequate blood supply and the skin dies. Every woman has different blood supply to the skin. Necrosis is a serious problem and when it occurs, the dead area must be removed, often meaning reversal of a procedure or removal of an implant to allow healing. Smokers tend to have greater problems with necrosis because of constriction of circulation. The surgeon may request that you stop smoking before surgery.

Nipple reconstruction: A new nipple can be created in a number of ways. The existing skin can be pinched and tacked to create a nipple and then the areola tattooed, or skin can be taken from another place on the body, such as behind the ear or the groin, and attached to the breast mound. It may later be tattooed to match the color on the other breast.

Prophylactic removal or reconstruction: Those women who have a single mastectomy may choose to have the other breast removed to prevent possible problems in the future—prophylactic removal. A woman who has had a modified radical for breast cancer may choose a subcutaneous mastectomy on the other breast. This procedure leaves the skin and nipple and replaces the breast tissue with an implant. A prophylactic reconstruction technique where there is a precancerous condition would go one step further, such as the total glandular mastectomy, in which the nipple is actually removed and cored or studied to be sure there are no cancer cells, and then replaced.

Prosthesis: The external breast-shaped form that fits in the bra to approximate a breast. Prostheses come in a variety of sizes and shapes.

Total glandular mastectomy reconstruction: Removing the breast tissue and leaving the skin. The nipple is often removed and cored and then replaced.

Transverse Rectus Abdominis Myocutaneous flap reconstruction: Also called the TRAM. Also called the tummy tuck. In this procedure, the woman's fat, skin, and muscle are taken from the abdominal area and moved up to form one or two new breasts that are totally the woman's own tissue. The tissue remains connected to the woman's own blood supply and is tunneled up under the skin of the abdominal area to the breast. The stomach is then closed (often using mesh insertion for additional strength if the muscle is taken) and a new belly button is fashioned. The TRAM leaves a horizontal scar that can be significant.

TO BE OR NOT TO BE

The decision to be reconstructed or not be reconstructed is very personal and is generated by a number of factors and emotions. Some women do it because they hate the prosthesis. Some do it because they want to wear clothes again without concern for a low neckline or how much is revealed. Some do it because they spend a lot of time in a swimsuit, one of the more difficult pieces of clothing to wear with a prosthesis. Some do it for when the lights are out and the scars don't show and balance is important. Some do it for when the lights are on and the feeling of being whole is important for sexuality. Some do it because they simply want their breasts back. They had two and they want two again. Some are ambivalent and ultimately just say, "Why not?"

When cost is not a factor, those who choose not to reconstruct generally weigh the positives against one thing—more surgery, which means more anesthesia and more hospital time, more scars, and just more messing with your body. These women refuse to have reconstruction either from a personal desire not to have further surgery or because they just don't think it's that important.

Marjorie S decided against reconstruction specifically because of anesthesia. *"I have always been sensitive to it, and I have always needed three doses of anesthesia to be put out. It takes a long time for me to come out of it, and I just felt my head and brains had had enough."*

> *"I am knife-shy. My attitude is that as long as it doesn't bother my husband, it doesn't bother me."*—Kit

> *"If someone said that I would get the feeling back if I had reconstruction, I would go through the whole operation. But for decoration, no."*—Pat H

There are also women who see reconstruction politically and feel that to reconstruct somehow trivializes the loss of the breast. Yes, there are those women who feel that to reconstruct—or even wear a prosthesis—somehow diminishes the reality of this disease. They feel that women who reconstruct are, at some level, responding to what society dictates and not to what they really want. In May 1991, I took my oncologist the story from New York's *Village Voice* about breast cancer. Mostly, I wanted to show him the full-spread picture that opened the piece. Here was a woman, arms flung wide, with an elaborate tattoo where her left breast used to be. I loved it. She looked so free and at peace with her loss. I prefaced showing my doc the picture by telling him that some women had approached the loss of a breast with a new kind of acceptance that I hadn't seen in Dallas. He said, "Naw." I showed him the picture, and he quietly agreed. I also took the picture to my group and was surprised by the painful expressions. Few saw the same freedom I did. Most of the women in my group thought the tattooed woman was nuts.

I saw the same kind of freedom on the faces of the women I met in Washington, D.C. in October 1991 who had gathered to testify about the importance of the availability of silicone implants for breast cancer survivors. About ten of us from across the country had gathered in one woman's hotel room after a long day of testifying. The discussion centered on the importance of reconstruction in our emotional recovery from breast cancer. We had undergone a variety of techniques in being reconstructed, and it wasn't long before blouses were unbuttoned and dresses dropped as one woman after another said, "Well, if you think that's something, look at this." We laughed and cried at the bond that had brought us together and complimented the artistry that had restored our bodies. Every woman there had fought some kind of personal battle for her reconstruction, and the reasons for each woman's reconstruction were as varied as the regions we represented.

I embrace any woman's feelings about her breasts and her desire to reconstruct—or not reconstruct. It's a personal decision that should be unencumbered with projections from others about what is important and what isn't. After a recommendation that she have her other breast removed, Mary H decided against reconstruction, nor does she wear prostheses, explaining that her breasts were small to begin with and she just didn't want to mess with it. I believe that the important thing is to find a cure for breast cancer, and one can be an advocate of that with or without a reconstructed breast.

"I was unbalanced, and it bothered my back. I hated the prosthesis. If I didn't get a light bra, it would always hit and I would always have a bruise. And I was just always concerned when people would hug me,

especially men, that they could feel it. And it would make a suction sound. So I really wanted the reconstruction for a lot of reasons, and now I can forget a lot of times—you know, unless I really look at myself and concentrate."—Mary-T

"I have gone from elation to disappointment to elation and back again."—Theresa

"I just don't think it's important. Maybe if I were younger I would feel differently."—Betty L

I don't remember when I decided to have reconstruction. I think it was always in the back of my mind and moved to the front after I had finished chemotherapy and could plan for the future. My daughter was getting old enough to be aware of my body, and I wanted to look like all the other moms—both with and without my clothes. Tom's attitude was that if I wanted to go through with it, fine, but I shouldn't do it for him.

When I woke up after undergoing a back flap procedure (where my latissimus dorsal muscle below my right shoulder blade was moved to the front with a wedge of skin), I was in a tremendous amount of pain and hooked to a morphine pump—God's gift to reconstructed women.

Actually, the pump allows you to administer your own painkiller and is regulated so you don't overdose yourself. Research has shown that patients tend to use less pain medication with the pump.

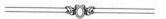

Tip for family and friends—Don't forget her during reconstruction surgery. She will probably be in more pain and more debilitated than after the mastectomy.

When I could focus on my chest, I saw the "mound," which had arisen like a Phoenix from my chest where there had been nothing. Even with the bandages on it, I would see that it was there. My perspective on the world was right again. I cried. It wasn't vanity. It was something much deeper. A breast was there again. I didn't realize how much I had missed it until it returned.

I had the nipple attached a few months later in day surgery. They took a little piece of skin from my groin (not the vagina, as people suggest, but the crease). The next year I had it tattooed a darker shade to match my existing breast. I still have a concave area above the breast, and the scars are always there. But I am amazed at how used to them I have become. The best thing is that in clothes and naked, I am balanced again. It feels great. And in the dark it's as good as the real thing.

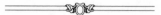

Tip—The skin for the nipple can be taken from a number of locations. My surgeon now prefers the earlobe rather than the groin area.

WHO WILL DO YOUR RECONSTRUCTION

"He has an ego as large as any, but the guy is a straight shooter. The guy is good. He puts his skill where his mouth is."—Lynne's husband, Norm

Whether or not you are having immediate reconstruction, shop for your plastic surgeon with the same intensity you would an architect. The plastic surgeon is an artist, and you are going to have to live with and look at his or her work every day for the rest of your life. Go to support groups and ask about plastic surgeons—and ask to see their work. Talk to women who have had the procedure you are considering—more than one. Ask what was the worst thing—and the best thing—about the procedure. Make up a list of plastic surgeons you are considering and then begin the same process as when choosing a breast surgeon. Then create your list of questions and make an appointment with a board-certified plastic surgeon. Watch out for the "come-on" by the receptionist. One woman was told by the receptionist that the surgeon did reconstruction "all the time." She learned he had done twelve in a five-year career.

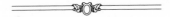

> Tip—If your cousin is trying to sell you on the guy
> who put in her implants when she had her breasts
> enlarged—and he is so cheap—proceed with cau-
> tion. Many surgeons call themselves plastic sur-
> geons and do cosmetic surgery and are not
> board-certified. And the skill level required for re-
> constructing a breast can in no way be compared to
> what is required for inserting implants for breast
> augmentation.

Get out your list of questions from your surgeon. Before going, think about other considerations you may have involving the other breast.

1. Do you want to consider prophylactic removal of the other breast in conjunction with reconstruction? Do you want to reduce the other breast?
2. Will the surgeon have to adjust the other breast to match? When would this be done? What is the cost, since few insurance companies will cover it?
3. How many steps are there in the procedure? How long until completion?

"I found a lump in the other breast six months after my mastectomy and got totally hysterical. It was benign. So when I decided to have reconstruction, he said I might want to consider having a subcutaneous on the other side. He explained that if I were sixty-five he would feel differently, but at thirty-five and with cancer in one breast, it wasn't worth the risk. I have never regretted it. I had the mastectomy in December, the subcutaneous the next November, and then reconstruction in February."—Lynne

The plastic surgeon cannot begin to discuss reconstruction options without seeing your mastectomy site or discussing the surgery options with your breast surgeon. The plastic surgeon must consider the size of breast to be created; how much skin you have; if you have had or will have radiation; and the quality of your skin.

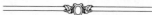

> **Tip—If you know you have scarring problems or are a slow healer, tell the surgeon when you go for a consultation.**

Debra decided that she wanted an expander, a procedure during which the remaining skin is stretched slowly by filling a sack that has been placed under the scar. When the skin has stretched adequately, the sack is removed and a permanent implant is put in its place. She kept looking for a plastic surgeon who would do the procedure after two told her that her skin was not good for expanding due to radiation. She finally found a plastic surgeon who would do the procedure. Then, a few weeks after the surgery, she woke up one morning to find that the incision had split. *"It wouldn't hold the stitches, and they had to take the whole thing out. I should have listened to the first two."*

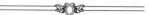

> **Tip—A good plastic surgeon should have a video-tape and/or literature that describes the different procedures as well as pictures of different procedures—both before and after.**

When the surgeon has made his or her suggestion for the best procedure, ask how many he or she has done. Be aware that only highly trained plastic surgeons can do the microsurgery procedures that require moving body fat and skin from the stomach and hip and reattaching it to the blood supply. If your doctor suggests one of these procedures, ask how many he or she has done. Ask to talk to a patient who has had this surgery. Then go see a second surgeon for another opinion. If the second surgeon disagrees or presents another set of problems—go see number three, and so on, until you are comfortable that you have explored all the options and found the surgeon who is right for you.

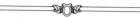

> **Tip—Plastic surgeons, even more than general surgeons, have strong opinions on the best surgery. A friend of mine in California said her plastic surgeon will not do the TRAM procedure, period, calling it too invasive.**

"Dr. A didn't think the tummy tuck would work for some reason. And he didn't like the idea of the expander, and what he wanted to do was move the back muscle over. Well, after I had the lymphedema, I said I didn't want anything else done anywhere near those lymph nodes in that area. I decided to have the other breast removed at the same time, and he was talking about three steps: the mastectomy on the breast with the tumor, putting in an implant, and then waiting three months and doing the other side. The impression I've been getting all along is that this can all be done at one time. So then we went to Dr. B, and his first choice of methods was to do the tummy tuck and bring it all up and do it all at one time. His second was the expanders and then go back in and put the implants in. He was at opposite ends from Dr. A, and we walked out of there and looked at each other and said, All right, now what? So I asked my oncologist and I told him what the deal was, and he thought a minute, and he said, 'Go see Dr. C. I think he'd be a real good one for you to sit down with.' He was in there with us from 2:20 until 4 o'clock, and other than two five-minute periods when I changed, he was in there the entire time. Finally, he said he didn't think I would be happy with the results unless tissue was moved from someplace, and he agreed about the lymphedema, so then I decided to go ahead with Dr. B and it's been great."—Joan

WHEN TO HAVE RECONSTRUCTION

"I had immediate reconstruction. The surgeon and plastic surgeon worked hand in hand. I had tissue expanders, with fourteen weeks of

expansion before putting permanent implants in. I had absolutely no problems. I talked with women who lost implants and had infections. Just horror stories. But in defense of the implants, if you go back and talk to these women who had infections and couldn't heal, they had generally at one time in their life, or recently, been smokers. That is not a problem I had."—Joyce

"The surgeon asked me if I wanted immediate reconstruction. I said, 'Absolutely not. I've got enough to handle and deal with because of chemo.' "—Linda H

"Because I woke up from surgery with the mound, it helped initially. It really helped psychologically, and that's why it took me a year and a half to finally think I'd lost something, because I didn't really feel that way."—Kim

"I had a six-month-old baby and I knew I couldn't lift him after surgery. I did a lot of reading about reconstruction very quickly and the plastic surgeon wanted to wait six months, because he found better results when some healing had taken place. Now, in hindsight, I wish I had had it done at the same time because I wasn't in touch with my fear of surgery, and now I won't go back."—Jo Anne

Factors in the past decade have greatly increased the number of women who choose to have breast reconstruction: The refinement of reconstruction techniques has resulted in more natural-looking reconstructed breasts. The elimination of the radical mastectomy—which removed the chest muscle as well as the breast tissue and was much more complicated to reconstruct—and techniques that allow for the creation of larger breasts—by moving skin and body tissue from other sites—have meant that women with a large remaining breast can get a better match.

Those women who choose to have immediate reconstruction at the time of their mastectomy often find the psychological impact is lessened—although some argue that it only delays the sense of loss.

If you are a candidate for immediate reconstruction and choose to do it, your surgeon will have to work in tandem with a plastic surgeon during your surgery. This necessitates securing another professional before surgery. If you don't have immediate reconstruction because you are facing other treatment or want to know pathology before deciding, you can plan for reconstruction as soon as the mastectomy site is healed. This will give you time to find a surgeon, discuss your options, and plan for surgery. You may also choose to have reconstruction at a later time.

Choosing when to have reconstruction can involve a number of factors that you may want to consider. Here is a list of pros and cons with regard to immediate reconstruction, as presented by the women interviewed for this book.

Pros
1. You wake up with a mound.
2. It eliminates another surgery down the road.
3. It lessens the sense of loss.

Cons
1. Depending on the technique chosen, your surgery may be much longer and involve a number of body parts, meaning a longer recuperation.
2. If you need adjuvant treatment such as chemotherapy or radiation, you will be facing a longer recovery and more treatment.
3. It lessens the sense of loss (yes, this is a positive and a negative in terms of emotional healing!).

WHICH RECONSTRUCTION IS RIGHT FOR YOU

"I had a reduction on the other side before reconstruction, and I don't even have on a bra. If I wear something heavy or a camisole, I can get by without a bra. Before I looked like I had jugs. It's so wonderful not to have that weight."—Kitty

"I think the scar on the back is not worth it. I would rather have had the TRAM, but he didn't want to do that. He said it was too much trouble at my age. I wouldn't have cared. I would rather have had a pretty back. I probably didn't talk to as many doctors as I should have."—Gale

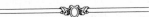

Tip—In most instances reconstruction requires more than one surgery, with the creation of the mound being the major surgery and the creation of the nipple and insertion of implants being day surgeries.

Be aware when reading about your options that **you** cannot decide what surgery you want without conferring with a plastic surgeon. The plastic surgeon must look at numerous factors before offering you options that will work for you. Every woman brings a unique set of problems—and a unique body—for reconstruction. Your emotional needs and fantasies must mesh with medical possibilities such as scarring, circulation, skin type, whether you have been radiated, desired size, and a number of other factors.

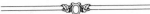

Tip—a good rule of thumb to remember: The more complicated the surgical procedure, the better the result and the greater possibility of complications.

Tip—Be aware that in most surgery options involving implants, the breast will not take on its final appearance for a number of months.

EXPANDERS

Tissue expansion can be used when there is enough existing skin to stretch to the size for the desired reconstructed breast. This is accomplished by placing an empty silicone sack under the skin and muscle in a surgical procedure that may involve an overnight stay. The sack will then be filled with saline solution over a number of weeks (usually, six to twelve). The sack is filled with a syringe that is inserted in a "port" in the sack, which may be under the arm or at the nipple site.

When the breast is expanded to the point that the skin is large enough to accommodate an implant, the expander sack is removed and the implant is inserted. The nipple is attached later, in day surgery. One woman compared the expander to having a pregnant breast that grew by the month. A new option on the market is the expander sack that is filled and then, instead of being removed, is plugged and remains in the breast as a permanent implant.

> *"It's a big bore to get pumped up. You know I am squishing all over."*—Bridie

> *"It's been a year now, and I am more pleased with the way it looks. For a while I just cried all the time because it was so much higher than the other breast. It's dropped a lot now and there is more symmetry. Now in clothes, you would never know. But without clothes, it will never be the same."*—Amy

> *"I was three times as big on the reconstructed side when they finished filling the sack. I couldn't wear anything and it hiked all up and it was terrible. I hated going to get more saline. I was trying to do it as quickly as possible, so they were putting as much as possible in there every week and it hurts, and as soon as it starts feeling better you have to go again in a couple days."*—Lola

When the breast skin has been "pumped up" with the saline solution to the point where it is large enough, the reconstructed breast is usually much larger than the other breast (usually, about 50 percent larger than the implant that will be used), to allow for natural droop when the implant is inserted. In day surgery, the saline bag is then removed and a permanent implant is placed beneath the skin and muscle.

Andrea had immediate reconstruction with an expander. She found the pumping up very painful, but she chose not to try the other techniques. *"I couldn't go for the other options because it was too much at the same time. Too much scarring, too much operation, too much to do. The surgeon is becoming more optimistic because he says I am doing well. It's stretching well. When it drops, it will look better."* For her wedding a year after reconstruction, Andrea found a dress that would show off her new cleavage.

TRANSVERSE RECTUS ABDOMINIS MYOCUTANEOUS FLAP (TRAM FLAP)

A popular reconstruction technique for the women in this book, the TRAM is affectionately called the tummy tuck. The TRAM moves the fat, skin, and muscle from the abdominal area to form one or two new breasts, resulting in breasts that are the woman's own tissue, with no implants. The abdomen is closed, often using a mesh insertion for additional strength, leaving a significant scar.

The TRAM resulted in both the strongest positive and negative feelings about reconstruction from the women interviewed. The ones who had no problem loved the procedure and the resulting natural-looking breast. The ones who had problems, which ranged from herniated incisions to necrosis of the incision to extensive recuperation time in order to stand upright, loved it after they hated it.

Debra and Leanne both herniated their TRAM scars by lifting their children too soon after surgery.

> *"I should have waited to have the reconstruction until she was older so I wouldn't have had to lift her. My stomach is pretty messed up with the hernia, but I don't want to go back to the hospital again."*—Debra

Mary-T, who had bilateral TRAM, said she still hurt a year later, which her plastic surgeon said was not unusual. But she loved the reconstructed breasts. *"They took fat, skin, and the two muscles. The first operation took nine hours, with three plastic surgeons working on me. It was horrible, let me tell you. It was the worst thing I went through."*

LATISSIMUS FLAP

"I didn't realize how old the mastectomy made me feel until I was reconstructed. I felt like a new person. In fact, people said, 'What have you done to yourself? You look great.' "—Chris

When additional skin is needed for the reconstruction in order to match the remaining breast, the surgeon may suggest the latissimus flap (back flap) procedure, in which the back muscle that is behind your arm is moved along with a wedge of skin to the chest area. The blood supply to the flap remains intact. An implant is then placed under the muscle for additional size if needed. The surgery requires a four- to five-day hospital stay. The nipple areola is completed later, in day surgery.

> *"They put the muscle on top and put an implant underneath. Because the radiation had made the skin contract and it was hard and tight, they had to work a long time to get it to loosen up. Then I had a staph infection in the incision and they had to open it up and clean it out. It still seems that it's too bulgy under my arm."*—Doris

This is the procedure I had, and when I could finally see my back, I have to admit that I was surprised by the size of the scar, which is about eight inches long. It has faded now, and I have no sense that I am weaker physically. I swim frequently and have had no loss of upper body strength for usual activity. The only time I am physically aware of the loss is when I have a massage and forget to tell the masseuse that the muscle is gone. I have come off the table in pain a few times when they hit that spot.

The advantage of the back flap is that it is a good choice for healing, in that there are fewer problems with necrosis and loss of blood supply. The disadvantage is yet another scar.

Chris had a Halsted radical in 1974, which left few possibilities for reconstruction. But when the back-flap surgery became available in 1980, she had the surgery and loved it.

MICROSURGERY TRANSFERS (FREE FLAPS)

> *"They literally cut the muscle and the tissue loose in the stomach and flip it—they do from the left side to the right, from the right to the left, and then they reconnect the blood supply with microsurgery and you've got little marks so that they know where to listen, and they use the Doppler every hour for three days. They come in and listen to the blood flow to make sure it's going."*—Joan

"I love it. Especially after the implant controversy. I mean I have my own tissue and I have no further worries in that regard."
—Marjorie

Unlike the TRAM and the latissimus flap procedures, which leave the blood supply connected to its original source, microsurgery techniques involve cutting free skin and fat and moving it to the breast location before surgically reattaching the blood supply. This can be done with the abdominal tissue or tissue from the buttocks or thighs.

Free-flap surgery offers the woman her own tissue, without an implant, and what many plastic surgeons say is a more natural-looking breast than those in which an implant is used. The negatives are longer surgery, more cost and, in some cases, finding a plastic surgeon who is willing. The advantage of the abdominal free flap over the TRAM flap is that only a patch of stomach muscle is taken, thus preserving abdominal strength. The disadvantage of the free flap is that the surgery is longer and there are greater risks of failure when the blood supply is reconnected.

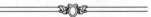

**Tip—Another positive for this "all-natural" breast
is that it responds to weight gain and loss naturally,
while an implant will not.**

Marjorie chose to have microsurgery to move tissue from her upper hip to her chest, where the blood supply was reattached. She also had to "convince" her plastic surgeon to do the operation when he tried to cancel. *"He had done the same surgery two days beforehand and it had failed, and had that not happened, I think he would have taken less skin and I would have a smaller scar, but he tried to overcompensate. He had to go back in and reduce the breast."* Marjorie says there is a noticeable crease in her hip from where the tissue was removed, but overall she is pleased with the result.

NIPPLE RECONSTRUCTION

A number of women I talked with were so tired of doctors and surgery that they never returned for the nipple reconstruction and continue with the Barbie look. But even if you wait a year, you might want to think about it. Sheila had significant problems with the TRAM. She healed slowly and could not stand upright for ten weeks. She wanted nothing to do with the nipple. *"The surgeon really wanted me to do it. He said that after what I had been through, I deserved it."*

Lola said she had a number of friends who didn't get the nipple. *"I thought, well, that's crazy to go through all that and not get a nipple."* Lola even bought an artificial nipple from a medical supply while waiting for surgery. *"The whole reason I went into this thing was to look better with my clothes off. That was one thing the surgeon asked, Did I want this to look better with clothes on or off? I said, Definitely off."* Lola wore a nipple pastie until surgery. Now she makes up her new nipple in the morning when she does her face makeup. *"It's not the same color as the other. They can't really do that. So I put makeup on it. I am so vain. I am terrible. But I don't do that for anybody but myself. First I put that tanning lotion on it and it darkened a little. Now I put eye makeup on top of it and it looks fine. It's kind of fun."*

The nipple tissue can come from a number of places. If you are lucky, you have a large areola on the other breast and half of it can be harvested to create a new one on the other breast. Most of us are not that lucky and have to have a transfer from another place on the body that has skin that approximates the texture of the areola. The most common site now is the back of the ear. When I had my reconstruction done, the skin came from the crease in the upper thigh. I found that this was relatively painless. In fact, the biggest problem is the hair that continues to grow.

"I told the doctor that there was hair growing out of my nipple. Everyone laughed, because we all know what kind of hair it is. I think it's funny. At least I know it's alive and well and can grow something."—Doris

Debra had electrolysis on her nipple. I just pluck mine when I do my eyebrows. I also had my nipple tattooed so the color would match, but I have found that the color has faded significantly. People are working on these techniques, and by the time this book is published they may have come up with new, longer-lasting color. For now, I am following Lola's advice and using makeup on the nipple for those times when I want to know they will match.

PLASTIC SURGEON DR. FRITZ BARTON, JR., UNIVERSITY OF TEXAS SOUTHWESTERN MEDICAL SCHOOL, TALKS ABOUT CHOICES IN BREAST RECONSTRUCTION

Dr. Fritz Barton was head of Plastic Surgery at the University of Texas Health Science Center Southwestern Medical School from 1971 to 1991. Today he continues to teach there while maintaining a private practice.

In light of the silicone implant controversy, what are the problems with saline implants?

They deflate. We have deflation reports that are anywhere from 6 percent over fifteen years to 40 percent in seven years. It depends on the style of implant, the type of implant, and when it was made. What is true is that they require more reoperation than gel implants.

What are the advantages and disadvantages of immediate reconstruction that you see in your patients?

Advantages of immediate reconstruction are that the skin flaps on the breast after mastectomy are more pliable. It may save a patient a step because the flaps are more manageable. You have to realize that immediate reconstruction is really a bad name because it makes it sound as though you are completed immediately. In reality, you're only started immediately. Every reconstruction requires more than one procedure. The advantage to doing it after the patient is healed from the mastectomy, which takes about

(continued)

three months, is that the patient has more time to make a good decision about options, because it's sometimes overwhelming to decide all the options of treatment and reconstruction at the same time.

Do you notice a difference in satisfaction level with immediate as opposed to delayed?

Sure. Delayed patients are happier. I think there's less psychic trauma if they're reconstructed in the first year, and there is a study that actually has shown that. Having lived with the deformity, women are better able to accept the compromise in quality. They are comparing a reconstructed breast with the memory of nothing, as opposed to comparing it with the memory of a natural, normal breast.

If you know a patient's going to have chemotherapy, do you look at treatment that's coming up afterward before you consider doing immediate reconstruction at time of mastectomy?

The only thing that influences that decision is her state of health, the state of skin flaps at the time of surgery and whether she's going to need radiation. I don't want to radiate the skin flaps that have just been moved from the back or stomach. It compromises the artistry. There's really no reason why the reconstruction would delay or interfere with any of the treatments for the tumor unless she gets into healing problems.

How does radiation compromise the artistry?

The skin flap will sometimes get firm, like a radiated breast. Fat that's radiated is damaged. You should have radiation if you need it. You've got to be alive to look good, but radiation does significantly compromise the quality of the skin for later stretching. It makes it stiff and nonexpandable. It influences your reconstruction significantly. It's very unlikely to get a good

(continued)

reconstruction with an expander without additional tissue if you've been radiated.

When a woman comes in to you and you're discussing recon-struction after mastectomy or delayed reconstruction, how do you help her try to make a decision of what kind to choose?

There are two categories I discuss. The first consists of the technical limitations and considerations. The other is her goal. Those are frequently at odds with each other. The technical limitations mean the aesthetic discrepancy between the new breast and the remaining breast. Then you have to consider procedure options that will come closest to matching the remaining breast. And that has to do with the amount, quality, and thickness of the skin, and the size and shape of the other side. Based on these considerations, there is a menu of procedures to select from. Patients have different levels of goals. They are willing to go through different levels of hassle and discomfort to achieve certain standards. Some older patients don't want to do anything. Anything is too much trouble. In other patients, if they can just get an internal prosthesis, such as an implant so that they look normal in clothes, that's okay.

The first level is nothing and an external prosthesis in the bra; the second level is an internal prosthesis but not out-of-clothes symmetry or subtle symmetry in revealing clothes. The next level is an out-of-clothes natural-looking breast. I group them into those three categories. In different patients, the higher the standard, the more complicated the commitment.

Do you have a favorite procedure?

No. Anybody who does breast reconstruction well has to have all the colors on the palette to work with. The key to it is being able to select the right color for the right situation. You always try to use the simplest procedure to achieve the result you want. In the ideal situation, you have plenty of remaining skin and all the skin is healthy. Then you just put an implant in and you're

(continued)

through. When we're doing preventive mastectomies, where we are removing the breast tissue and leaving the skin, 91.5 percent of the time it's a one-stage procedure. Mastectomy, immediate implant, nipple graft, done. The patient has all her own skin and there are no flaps. But that requires that you have plenty of available, healthy skin to use. If that's not available, the next step is the expander. You can make up a difference of about 5 to 7 centimeters of size deficiency with an expander. The next step would be a flap, either from the abdomen or the back. The back flap advantage is that it's much simpler on the patient. The discomfort and risk factors for complication are much lower. On the other hand, it will get about 7 centimeters of surface dimension, 9 maximum, and it requires an implant. Finally, the last on the scale is tissue from another location, because it's the most complicated procedure. You can get an almost unlimited surface coverage of the breast by manipulating different blood supplies from the abdomen or hip.

You go from the simplest to the most complex in every patient. The next factor that comes into it is the shape of the remaining breast. Each of those operations might provide a normal-looking breast, but it might not have the same subtle characteristics as the other breast. So there's a second set of factors you have to consider. In general, a mature breast without an implant is best matched by no implant on the other side. An implant breast tends to be firmer and higher than a natural breast. You end up with better symmetry with either implants on two sides or no implants. It's very hard to match with an implant on one side and a natural breast on the other unless it's a very firm adolescent breast.

With all the experience you've had, going through this range with women, what is the biggest lack of understanding? What's your message to women about what they don't understand?
The most common misunderstanding is that women assume that all of the results are the same and they're only supposed to

(continued)

pick between which *method* they would prefer. That's a false assumption. Anyone would pick the simpler technique. But what they often misunderstand is that there would *be* no other techniques if the simplest ones got a good result all the time. The reason there are different techniques is because in general, the more complicated the technique, the more elegant the result.

With the future of implants undecided, do you see more women choosing the microsurgery options? And are there fewer plastic surgeons who can do them?

Yes to both. It is technically a very tricky procedure, so not as many people do it well. Secondly, the complication rate is high.

How can a women find a plastic surgeon who is expert at microsurgery?

From the standpoint of microsurgery, it is a part of every plastic surgeon's training. So someone would not offer you a microsurgical technique if they were not comfortable doing it. The answer is also not how many they have done, because proficiency can be achieved at a relatively small number under good training circumstances if you have the basic talent to do it. If you've done none, the answer is that it's not good to be the first one. But the key is the success rate.

Is pregnancy possible after the TRAM?

Nobody knows. That is listed as a contraindication to a TRAM. Because nobody's really sure—since abdominal weakness and potential weakness is one of the concerns, it's usually not considered wise to do that. The truth is that there have been very few patients who have tested that hypothesis.

What is the complication rate with microsurgical techniques?

Overall, a 10 percent significant complication rate around the world. Another 10 percent reoperation where you have to fiddle

(continued)

with it. The transplant died, or the vessels clot and you have to go back and reopen them. The problem is that the vessels that you go into in the chest around the mastectomy are not a good pattern.

So as you move down the echelons of complexity from simple implant to microsurgery, the complications follow?

Right. That's true. In terms of healing, the back procedure is by far and away the sturdiest, healthiest, least complicated of all. I'm not saying it doesn't hurt. I'm saying it's relative. If you do a back flap immediately, at the same time as the mastectomy, it doesn't feel any different than the mastectomy. It's the same dissection bed. The most important part of the back flap is that it's by far the sturdiest healer. The healing complication is less with latissimus than with any of the other procedures.

Explain the subcutaneous and total glandular mastectomy.

The blood supply to the skin comes through the breast. So if you do a complete mastectomy, where you take all the tissue but keep the skin, then the skin dies in a significant number of cases because there is not enough blood flow. It isn't that the surgery was done badly, it's that the breast is not designed for it. Not enough people's skin is strong enough for the blood supply.

So we developed the subcutaneous in the mid-sixties, with the idea that to reduce the complication rate, we'll just not take the flaps quite as thin and that way they'll be healthier. But it also reduced the thoroughness rate and has lost respect at major cancer centers because it is viewed as incomplete.

Now we have developed the total glandular mastectomy, which is a terrible name, but means we are taking it all out instead of part of it. The TGM is a mastectomy like what you would have for cancer surgery, but we don't take the skin because it's not involved. The problem, again, is that the complication rate is high because of the blood supply.

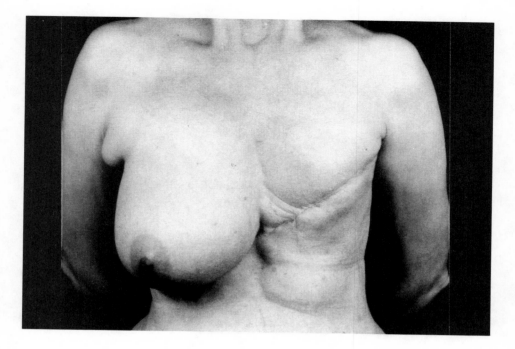

Expander Reconstruction

This fifty-five-year-old woman was reconstructed with an expander four years after a modified radical mastectomy on her left breast. Her right breast was reduced for symmetry.

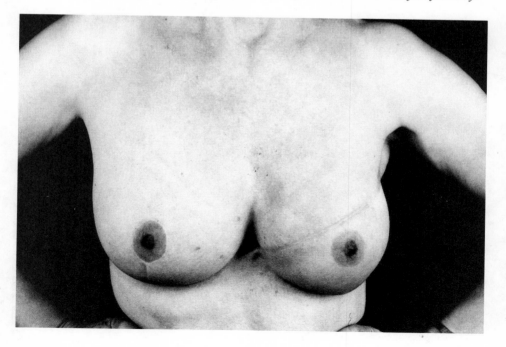

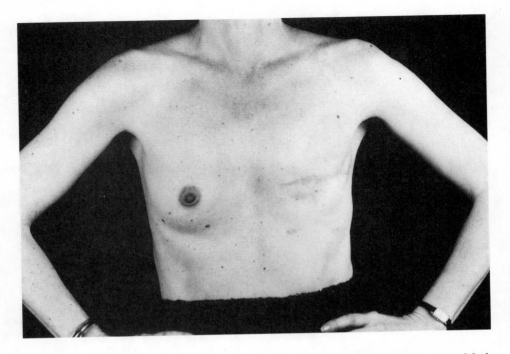

This forty-six-year-old woman was reconstructed with an expander one year after a modified radical mastectomy on her left breast. She chose a total glandular mastectomy on the right side because of a precancerous condition.

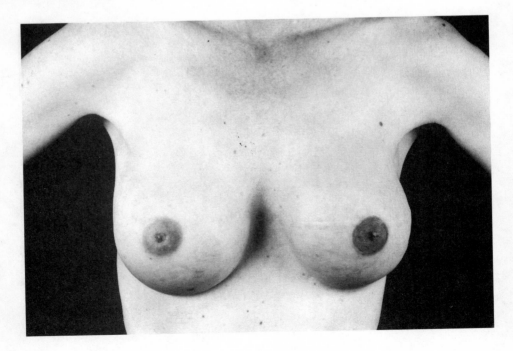

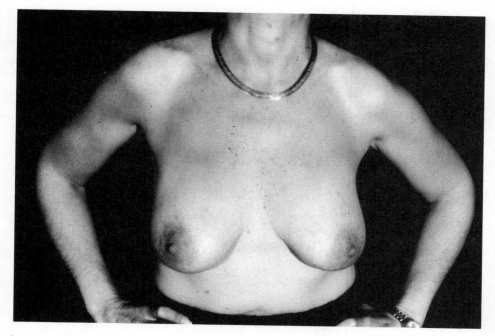

Latissimus Flap Reconstruction

This forty-one-year-old woman chose immediate reconstruction with the latissimus flap procedure at the time of the modified radical on her right breast. Four months later she chose to have a total glandular mastectomy on the left breast.

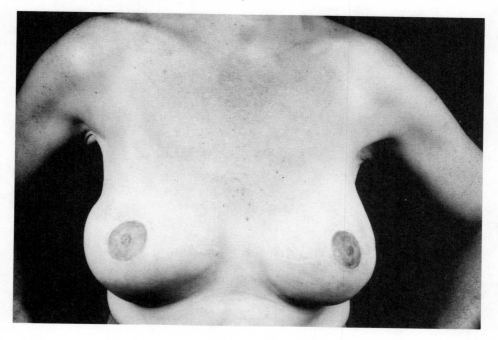

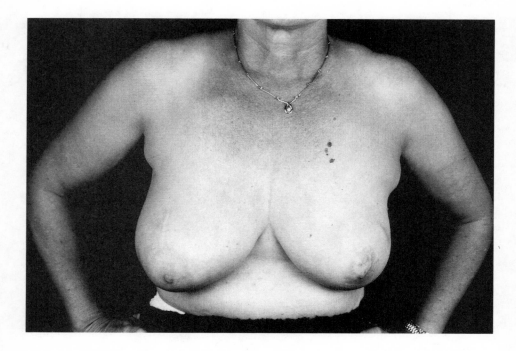

This forty-eight-year-old woman chose immediate reconstruction with the lastissimus flap procedure at the time of the modified radical on her right breast. She chose a total glandular mastectomy on the left breast because of her strong family history of cancer.

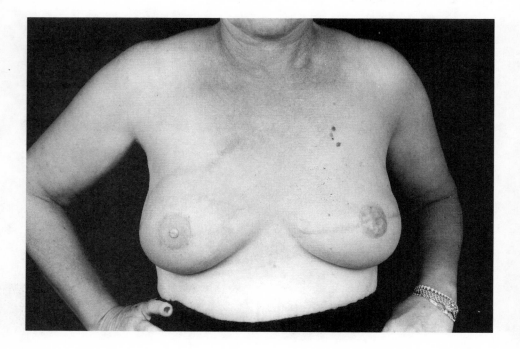

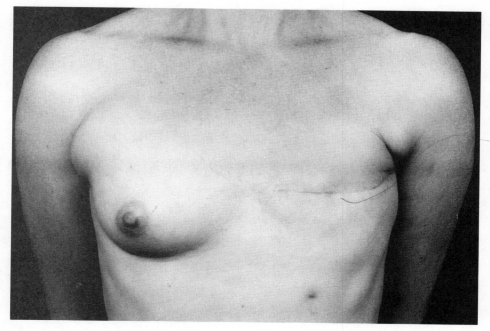

TRAM Reconstruction

This forty-one-year-old woman chose a TRAM reconstruction eighteen months after a modified radical mastectomy on her left breast. She chose to have her breasts enlarged with reconstruction and her right breast was augmented with an implant for symmetry.

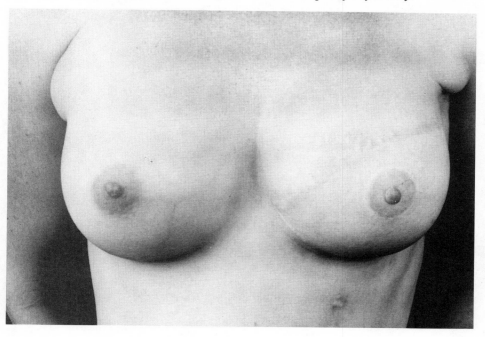

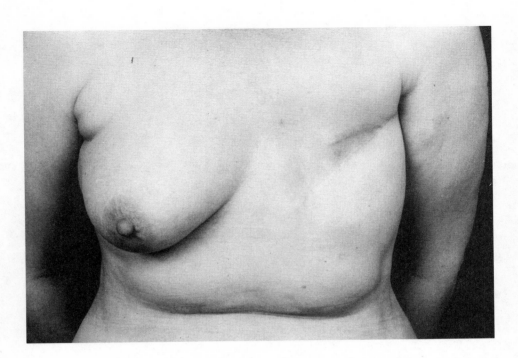

This forty-eight-year-old woman chose a TRAM reconstruction four years after a modified radical mastectomy on her left breast. She chose to have a total glandular mastectomy on her right breast at the same time because of precancerous indicators.

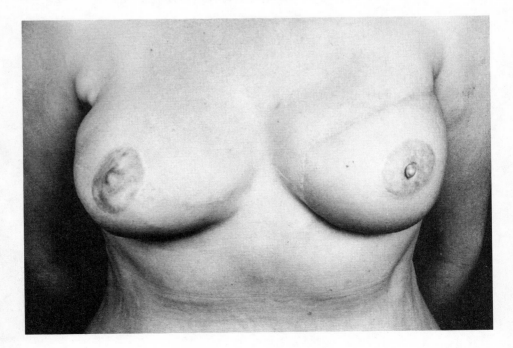

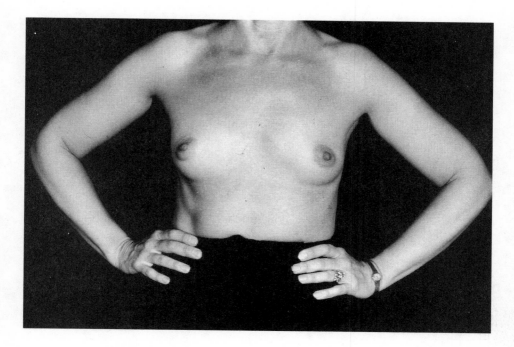

Total Glandular Mastectomy

This fifty-year-old woman chose a bilateral total glandular mastectomy for a precancerous condition.

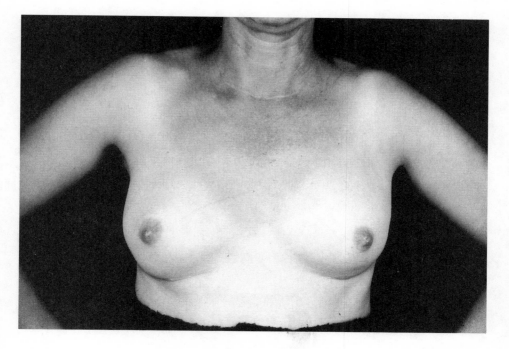

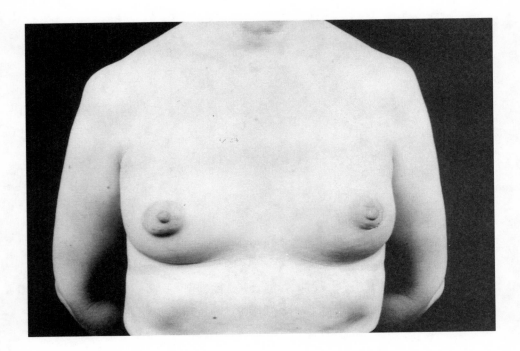

This forty-six-year-old woman chose bilateral total glandular mastectomy for a precancerous condition and because of her strong family history of cancer.

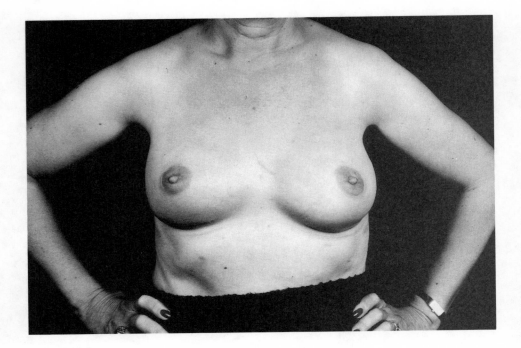

THE IMPLANT CONTROVERSY

"I would not have had surgery had silicone implants not been available, in which case I would not have known I had an invasive tumor under the calcifications. For me silicone implants were a lifesaver."
—Diana

"Let us make that decision about implants. For some women it's their sanity."—Teresa M

"Do I worry that I'm going to get cancer from the implants? I worry more about getting cancer from the substitute sugar I use. I've read so much about implants that to me it doesn't pose a threat. I'm not remotely concerned."—Joyce

"My surgeon said that the whole thing is really amazing. The same materials have been used for years for penis implants, but you would never hear a word about that, and in pacemakers. So he says it's a lot of crap. And as far as the attention, if as much press was given to breast cancer as there was to silicone implants, we'd be in a whole new ball game with early detection."—Bridie

To begin any discussion on silicone implants, you have to begin at the beginning, which in this instance was a network television show in 1990 in which women were interviewed who had had "problems" that they felt were linked to the fact that they had silicone breast implants. It was the beginning of a barrage of continuing media coverage that has exploited sick women while ignoring healthy women with implants and turned a complicated issue into a good guy/bad guy scenario that doesn't help anyone determine the real facts.

What followed during 1991 was an investigation by the Food and Drug Administration, which asked to see evidence from manufacturers that silicone implants were safe. The manufacturers of the silicone implants relied heavily on time as their proof, explaining that since silicone implants have been on the market for thirty years with few complaints, there was no specific research that followed women or any research to indicate that the problems being presented were scientifically linked to silicone leakage.

So the FDA heard from some sick women and many, many more

happy women. After a three-month moratorium in early 1992 on the use of silicone implants while evidence was collected, the FDA panel came back and recommended that silicone implants remain on the market for unlimited use by women who have had mastectomies and in a very limited study setting for women choosing augmentation. In April 1992, David Kessler, the head of the FDA, adopted the panel's recommendations but continued to warn women that they should think twice about using a silicone implant.

What we know, and what has been speculated about in the media and expanded on by the FDA and enhanced by litigation attorneys, provides little conclusive real evidence about the big question, which is whether silicone implants are safe **enough.** The FDA's job is to determine if the benefit of a product outweighs the risk. Yet after many of us traveled to Washington D.C. to testify before a Food and Drug Administration panel about silicone implants in fall 1991, it became clear that the voices of women who were happy and healthy and who had silicone implants were way down on the list of those being heard—with the loudest being the attorneys who stand to gain millions in settlements for cases that have been tried in the media.

It is clear now that the availability of silicone implants for women will be decided by lawsuits and the financial ramifications for the manufacturers, which have already seen one implant removed—not because it was proven that it caused problems, but because the manufacturer could not afford to fight. Indeed, since then two other manufacturers have pulled out, citing litigation fees. Dow Corning, the focus of most of the media attention during the controversy, left the market in March 1992, committing $10 million to research.

Part of the legitimate problem with the issue of silicone implants is the lack of follow-up on women who have them. It's not even clear exactly how many of us there are. Figures from 1 to 2 million have appeared. And because no one knows exactly how many women have silicone implants, no one knows how many women have had *any* kind of problem from silicone implants.

But there are a number of areas on which everyone agrees. Everyone agrees that the primary physical problem women have with silicone implants is not long-term immunological disease but capsular contracture. This condition occurs when the body forms a hard scar casing around the implant. It's uncomfortable, but not debilitating and certainly not deadly, and it is a condition that every woman is warned can happen.

I am a perfect example of this result. After getting my first smooth silicone implant in 1988, I developed severe capsular contracture. My breast was hard. It wasn't painful, but I could forget about ever sleeping on my stomach again. In 1989, my plastic surgeon replaced the implant with one that was covered by a thin coating of what looked like foam rubber. This "polyurethane" coating helped the body's tissue bond with the implant, keeping the hard scarring from forming again. It has been performing the same function on the exterior of heart valves and other medical devices for a number of years. It has been used on the breast implants since around 1985. I still have this implant and like it very much. My breast is soft and feels natural.

Mine is also the implant that I heard more than one expert testify **will** give me cancer—no ifs, ands, or buts. They theorize that the cover will break down into a carcinogenic substance. This was presented as fact, although no actual cases have been reported, except in manipulated experiments with lab animals and in experiments where the coating was heated well beyond a temperature it would ever experience in a live human being. But at the first hint of trouble, the maker of my implant, which plastic surgeons called the best product they had ever had, pulled its product from the market. It did not have the financial resources to fight this battle.

Fritz Barton, Jr., M.D., former head of plastic surgery at the University of Texas Southwestern Medical Center, says that this theory about the cover breaking down arose when silicone implants were removed and it appeared that the cover was gone. Barton says that it was a mistake on the part of the surgeons, who didn't recognize the shell as it had bonded with the scar tissue, which was exactly what it was supposed to do.

While capsular contracture is the primary physical problem with silicone implants, the lawsuits and the focus of true concern on everyone's part are on women who reported much more serious problems. Some had immune disorders that were debilitating and crippling. They said they suffered from joint pain and fatigue as a result of the immune-system response to the silicone, which had bled from their silicone implants.

Again, the evidence about who these women are and what is wrong with them is sketchy at best. No one knows how many women have had immune-disorder problems after getting silicone implants. Figures have appeared from anywhere from 200 to 2,000 women, and none to date have been identified as having a certifiable connection between their symptoms and the silicone, since no scientific link has ever been established. What has become apparent is that there are some women who have had physical symptoms that became better when the silicone implants were removed. What researchers don't know is why these women have had a reaction when others haven't and whether they are women who were predisposed to immune disorders and the silicone implants precipitated the onset of symptoms.

Statistically, 30,000 American women in any given year will contract immune disorders with or without implants. Since 100,000 women a year received silicone implants before they were banned, there could be a coincidental overlap. Even if there are 2,000 women who are reportedly suffering an immune problem as a result of their implant, and that's at the high end of the estimated statistics, this is still only a fraction of a percent of the number of women who have implants.

Remember that the FDA's job is to determine benefit in relation to risk. The risk we take every time we have general anesthesia that something will go wrong is 1 in 12,000. There is risk in everything we do— and certainly in every medical treatment we choose. We also have to remember that a significant part of the process of reconstruction is a woman's ability to heal. Some women just don't heal well. I have talked to women whose skin stretched far beyond expectation. I have talked to women whose incisions would not heal properly or whose bodies scarred more severely. We are each unique, and our response to surgery will be unique. It's the risk we take when we choose to be reconstructed.

In an April 1992 article in the *Wall Street Journal,* two plastic surgeons from the Mayo Clinic responded to the implant controversy on behalf of the 4,000 women who had received implants at their clinic. They said in the article:

"At the Mayo Clinic, we have never seen a patient with documented autoimmune disease. Our colleagues at Memorial-Sloan Kettering Cancer Center in New York and M.D. Anderson Cancer Center in Houston say the same thing. There is no question that those with implants may develop rheumatoid arthritis, scleroderma or breast cancer. There is no evidence, however, that they are more likely than the general population to have these problems. But because of the controversy surrounding implants, many of those with implants have been led to believe that every symptom they experience, from fatigue to joint pain to occasional fevers, are associated with implants. This is not grounded in fact."—Dr. John E. Woods, professor of plastic surgery and vice-chairman of the department of surgery, and Dr. Phillip G. Arnold, chief of plastic and reconstructive surgery at the Mayo Clinic, Rochester, Minnesota.

Indeed, where are the voices of the plastic surgeons during all this debate? They are the ones who insert the silicone implants and follow the patients. Plastic surgeons have thirty years of history with silicone implants. Plastic surgeons have not been consulted throughout the silicone controversy. Nor has any of the "scientific" evidence collected even been given to them for review. And there was not one present on the FDA panel that determined the scientific viability of silicone implants. Basically, plastic surgeons were treated as the enemy—a great medical conspiracy of doctors who were fighting this ban because it would mean a loss of money. They were painted as greedy purveyors of vanity, with no thought to women's health.

This couldn't be further from the truth for the thousands of legitimate, talented, concerned plastic surgeons who do this procedure. One of my surgeon's first concerns was the limited options for reconstruction and how much **more** expensive and complicated are the procedures that don't involve silicone implants. If making money were his first concern, he should be eager for a ban.

Women testifying before the FDA panel held up pictures of reconstructed and augmented breasts that looked like they had been done with a can opener and pen knife. Those of us who had shopped for a plastic surgeon and found board-certified, caring professionals were insulted that the work of those surgeons, whose patients came as a result of their advertising in the weekly shopping guide, was being held up as the norm. Bad surgeries were lumped in with silicone implants, and women who wanted a bargain-basement boob job to look better in sweaters got lumped in there with breast cancer patients—for whom the loss of silicone implants will mean more costly operations and more fear.

The Mayo Clinic authors ask the question at the end of their article: "Is it logical that because perhaps one out of 2,000 women with implants has significant problems, implants should be withdrawn from the market? To do so would be analogous to withdrawing aspirin, insulin, penicillin, digitalis and many other beneficial medications because of the potential problems."

The big losers in all this are breast cancer patients. I have talked to women who want reconstruction terribly and have been frightened into immobility at the thought of a silicone implant. And, according to Dr. Barton, it's beginning to look like the continuing debate will be ended not by the courts but by malpractice insurers, who are threatening physicians who insert silicone and by the one remaining silicone gel implant manufacturer, who is considering leaving the market because of financial considerations.

IF YOU HAVE SILICONE IMPLANTS

If you have silicone implants and have no physical problems, there is nothing immediate you should do until the studies on silicone are complete—and that may take years. The risk from surgery to remove the silicone implants is far greater than your risk of having a problem.

But you should be aware of your implant and contact your plastic surgeon at any sign of difficulty. If your surgeon is not keeping you informed about implants, ask that he or she do so. My plastic surgeon has sent out continuous updates on implants.

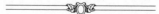

Tip—If you had your silicone implants put in by someone other than a board-certified plastic surgeon, you may want to consider changing surgeons. But be aware that the litigation craze surrounding this issue has made plastic surgeons cautious.

Specifically, watch for a lump or change in the shape of your breast, which may indicate breakage of the implant. Breakage does not mean that you are at risk for any of the problems listed. It means that there is silicone in the pocket around the implant that may cause disfigurement. Be aware of your breasts and note any changes. Chest pain, lumps under the arm, or anything else suspicious should be reported.

See your plastic surgeon at least once a year for a physical exam. Relate any kind of consistent body or joint pain. Keep records, and know what kind of implant you have.

Replacing implants is a personal decision. I have talked to women who have had the same ones for twenty plus years. Again, discuss this with your plastic surgeon.

RESOURCES

Be aware that the organizations that distribute information about breast implants do not appear to be objective. They are either for or against implants. A number of these organizations were waiting to assist in any studies that are begun on silicone implants. Medic Alert has begun a registry for women with implants, and for a $25 registry fee and $10 annual fee you will receive updates on recalls. Call (800) 344-3226.

The American Society of Plastic and Reconstructive Surgeons, 444 East Algonquin Avenue, Arlington Heights, IL 60005; (800) 635-0635. Will send a list of board-certified surgeons in your area and general brochure with pictures.

Implant Information Center (Dow Corning) P.O. Box 994, Midland, MI 48686; (800) 442-5442. Has a pocket of free information about silicone implants and current manufacturers.

Against silicone implants:

Command Trust Network, Breast Implant Information Service, South Linden Drive, Beverly Hills, CA 90212; (310) 556-1738. When I contacted Command Trust, I received a packet of information about implants that was fairly objective, considering the group's stance. It had a list of symptoms to look for and things to ask your surgeon.

BOOKS:

The Guide to Cosmetic Surgery, by Josleen Wilson, Simon & Schuster (April 1992), ISBN 0-671-76105-6. A whole chapter on reconstruction and good information on how to choose a doctor.

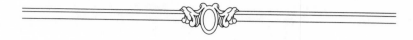

PART II

EMOTIONAL ISSUES and HEALING

THE BODY AND THE SPIRIT

Chapter 5

WHAT IS HAPPENING TO ME?

"In the English language there is no female equivalent of the term 'castrated' or 'eunuch.' In a span of two weeks I lost a breast and the ability to reproduce. I lost two very important vestiges of femininity. I had a hard time with that. I am not female anymore. What am I?"
—Mary H

"It was like a rollercoaster. We're sure it's not cancer; we're sure it's not; oh, yes it is. And then, Sure, you'll have a lumpectomy; No, you have to have a mastectomy. And then the next thing was, Well, we're sure it's not in your nodes, and then it was. And then, You won't have chemotherapy, but, Yes, you should. So I was just emotionally gone."—Sandy

"I was angry. I've taken good care of me. This is not fair. I've done my part. I've done all the things I'm supposed to do."—Gale

NOW WHAT?

The weeks surrounding my diagnosis and surgery were a confusion of emotions. I remember staring dumbly into space until Tom would recall me from my trance to ask what I was feeling. The sensation is hard to describe. Mostly, I lived with waves of an emotional syrup that mixed an angry determination to live with guilt and suffocating fear that resulted in a kind of physical paralysis.

I would finally shake off the omnipresent dread long enough to begin functioning again, only to be reminded of my dilemma by my infant daughter, who during this time was trying diligently to take her first steps. How many more of the firsts of her life would I be able to see, I wondered, feeling myself slip into that cold hard place in my gut called terror.

At the same time, I was trying to make peace with a body that I felt had betrayed me. After surgery I had to reclaim it from the doctors, this new body that was wrapped around my new, but altered, soul. Nothing fit anymore—my clothes, my personality, my life.

Ironically, I recall a friend at church calling me an "inspiration" during this time. My automatic pilot was taking me to the store, changing diapers, cooking dinner, finishing free-lance assignments, and moving on, while my soul was trying to unstick itself from a slow-motion morass of dread, fear, and anger.

I think our bodies protect us during this stage. We call it denial, but the selective hearing, the sense of unreality are the body's defense—to screen the world and allow only what we can handle at the moment. To try and get the big picture would be overwhelming both physically and emotionally.

"I think you're in a state of shock when it first hits. Thursday we had the biopsy, and Saturday night Tom and I went to a movie. We thought we should get out and do something. About halfway through the movie it hit me. This is me; this is happening to me; this is real; it's not somebody else. I held together pretty well until the end of the movie. Then the lights came up, and he said, 'Are you okay?' And I started crying hysterically."—Joan

As I look back now, I see how the emotional reaction to breast cancer had distinct stages. They may last for varying periods of time depending on the woman, her personal coping mechanism and support, and her prognosis, but the majority of the women I talked to agreed that they experienced many of the same sensations and feelings.

While the medical approach to breast cancer is relatively similar for most diagnoses, the emotional response is more complicated. Every woman brings to this experience a personality and a history of personal growth and relationships that may or may not lend themselves to a healthy assimilation.

This is not news you want to read at this point, perhaps. But the message from the majority of the women in this book clearly was a wish that someone had prepared them for what was to come emotionally and helped them realize that they were not alone in their feelings.

Lynne said that the emotional impact did not occur until months after the surgery. "*I wanted to immediately become a Reach to Recovery volunteer after surgery. I couldn't understand why they wanted me to wait. But three months later I understood. I know now that I was in denial. Breast cancer happens to other people. On the outside I looked good, but on the inside I was a basketcase. I hadn't dealt with a lot of the issues. My attitude was that as long as I stayed busy and didn't think about it, I would be okay. And then one day, it sneaks up and hits you on the head. I have had breast cancer, I have had CANCER. Then you begin dealing with a cancer diagnosis, death and dying, and your own mortality.*"

While Lynne's was a common reaction among younger women, the older women tended to be more accepting of a life-threatening illness and grateful that their diagnosis came when their children were grown.

A word here about age that is best stated by a member of my support group. Let me preface this by saying that Pat G is a vibrant, youthful woman who owned a figure at fifty-seven that I didn't have at twenty-five. When I began this book, the focus was on premenopausal women, who the National Cancer Institute classifies as under fifty at diagnosis. I explained this designation to my support group when looking for those who wanted to be interviewed. Well, I continued to receive good-natured ribbing about "older" women and came, as my editors did, to the conclusion that the issues surrounding breast cancer can be somewhat generalized to age, but that women with breast cancer are individuals. So this book became about women at all ages and soon included women twenty-three to seventy-three. I have found since then that the issue of disfigurement may be as severe for a sixty-five-year-old as for a twenty-five-year-old. Mortality may be somewhat more easily digested by a woman in her sixties than one in her thirties, but not necessarily so. It all depends on a personal vision and when a woman sees her life work as finished.

My group was delighted with the news that the "older" women would be included, since some were eager to tell their stories. Pat G responded in the form of a letter that I see as a better explanation than any I would write on the issue of age. She wrote:

"Dear Kathy, I still can't fathom why the fifty-plus women were excluded in the first place. Most of the women I know who are fifty plus have the same dreams and goals as you who are numerically younger, and a few I know are physically younger than a lot of women thirty-five to forty. Age, darlin', is only a number. I truly believe we all come into our own at fifty plus. Since I was fifty I have studied art at the Villa Maria Center for the Arts in Perugia, Italy. I am a dedicated swimmer who swims a mile a day during the summer. I am a five-mile runner. My paintings and ceramics, drawings and printmaking, which I do professionally, continue to grow. My gallery connections, thank God, still want me after a year and a half recovery following treatment.

"I am a fighter, Kathy, and I think I can speak for a lot of us who are fiftysomething. I plan to keep growing and enjoying life until I decide to check out. I'll fight to stay well and to be physically fit for the rest of my days. I find lots in common with friends from age six to ninety-six. That tip at the end of the branch keeps growing and growing. You have lots to look forward to. Love, Pat. Fiftysomething."

One of my favorite interviews for this book was with Ida Rose, who shattered yet another age stereotype. I asked her how her relationships had been affected by her diagnosis, expecting that she would say her women friends had been helpful or distant. Instead, she said that she did break off with the man she had been dating when she was diagnosed. *"But that was okay because it was just a sexual thing,"* she added. Ida Rose, by the way, was diagnosed when she was seventy-three!

THE REALITY OF CANCER AS GRIEF

"You cannot short-circuit the grief process. It's just not possible."—Dr. Michael Fitzpatrick

"The problem is, I don't know who or what to be angry at." —Andrea

"I've never gotten mad. Maybe I've internalized it and become depressed, I don't know. But I never got mad. I never said, 'Why me?' I just said, 'Blank. Now what are we going to do?' "—Elizabeth T

"I thought about committing suicide when he called me that day and said I had breast cancer. I keep a handgun beside my bed for personal protection. That afternoon, I pulled it out and looked at it and thought, Do you really want to do this? But I am such a chicken-shit, I really couldn't do it."—Mary H

No one can prepare you for the confusion of feelings that accompanies a breast cancer diagnosis. The cancer diagnosis and loss of a breast for a young woman is a physical loss of a body part as well as numerous less tangible losses—among them the loss of invincibility, femininity, control over our lives, relationships. For older women, it's the sense of being cheated out of the "golden" years of retirement when, their children grown, they finally have the time and resources to enjoy the fruits of their labors. In one sense we lose our entire personhood as we make the changes necessary to live with this disease. Even when we feel that we have licked the immediate tumor, the implications of breast cancer linger far into the future.

Many of you will read this with alarm, slam the book shut, and resist any notion that this is not going to be over and done with after surgery. Indeed, I have met a few women for whom this approach seems to have worked. Do I believe them? Somewhat. I suppose that there are those who are purely fatalistic about life. "What will be will be" really works for them. They can look at this as something to get through and then get back to their life. Breast cancer becomes more of a bump in the road than a detour. In some cases these women have already experienced incredible trauma in their lives. Breast cancer is serious, but for those women who have faced the loss of a child or, in Maureen's case, cope with a severely retarded child, it becomes another crisis instead of *the* crisis in their life. These women, some of them quite young, seemed to handle their diagnosis better emotionally. They had already been introduced to life's hurdles and in coping with them had begun the process of maturation earlier than their friends. I sense this is why counselors find that older women have an easier time with a cancer diagnosis. Most have lived long enough to have experienced both losses and acceptance. They are at an age where friends are more likely to have had health problems, and it seems more acceptable.

Other women express a resignation that comes from intense denial more than acceptance. My sense is that these women are going through the motions. They have stuffed their feelings so far down that they reject even the suggestion that there may be unresolved issues.

I am quite thankful that the nineties seem to have brought breast cancer out of the closet emotionally. Think of how many of us there are now. In 1992 an estimated 181,000 women were diagnosed with invasive breast cancer—around 50,000 of them premenopausal. Add to this the thousands more who lost a breast to an intraductal diagnoses. Add an average of 100,000 women for each of the past ten years, and there were 1.5 million survivors in early 1993. Unfortunately, the majority of women—particularly young women—diagnosed with this disease even as late as the early eighties got the message clearly that this was only a medical disease, leaving them to struggle alone through the grief process that accompanies a breast cancer diagnosis.

It seems there is a legion of women, their bras stuffed with cotton and their psyches filled with pain, who are living with this disease and never talking about it. While this may be simple denial for some—for the daughters of women who deny their disease, and who must understand their risk—it is both dangerous and debilitating as it adds to the fear of the unknown.

Doris went back to work after her mastectomy only to find herself crying in the lunchroom. Her boss asked if she wanted more time off. She said no. *"My attitude was that I'm stoic and I'm going to beat this thing. I wouldn't admit that I needed any emotional support or help. That night I went to a Reach to Recovery support group and was on the verge of tears. One of the women noticed and asked me about it. I said, 'I just can't handle this. I don't know what to do. Emotionally, I'm coming apart.'"*

Doris said her mother's breast cancer had *never* been addressed in the family, giving Doris no model for coping.

After my diagnosis, I had a few older women call me. They spoke in hushed tones, letting me know they had had "the operation" too. They patted my hand or hugged me and that was it.

I needed to stand on the roof and shout and scream about the injustice of what had been done to me, to my body, to my life. But this was 1986, and while I know now that there were other young women out there, they, like me, were feeling isolated. The much-needed emotional network to bring us together to deal with breast cancer was not yet in place.

Besides, with all the other work of a new mother that needed doing, it was easy to pretend. It was easy to stay busy enough to mask the emotions. Somehow, for me, beating this disease became synonymous with ignoring the emotional pain. Sadly, there is in our society more support for those who just get on with it and stuff their feelings than for those who let out the anger and pain associated with doing the kind of grief work necessary for assimilation.

I know now that I was guilty of what I so frequently accuse men of—being macho. I was proving I was tough enough to take it with a stiff upper lip. Of course, the rest of me was mush. Since I am a fairly strong person, I was able to keep the defenses up for almost two years. It was finally my resistance to intimacy that led me to believe that something else was going on. I was isolating myself from feelings. But why? I was, as my students often say, "clueless."

In 1983 I published my first book, *For Those Who Live: Helping Children Cope With the Death of a Brother or Sister*. The book, based on interviews in families in which a child had died, dealt with my resolution of my brother's death in a helicopter crash in 1972.

What I learned as I researched that book was that the suppression of grief can also suppress all strong emotions. The image I used to describe this phenomenon was a strongbox where all life's strong emotions are kept. In order to keep a lid on grief, you have to keep the lid on all the strong emotions, because they are all tied together. Passion and pain are closer than we think. I knew a lot about grief. But in 1988, I didn't know that I had succumbed to the stuffing I had written about earlier. No one told me that breast cancer was a *grief* experience.

A mention to my surgeon during an annual visit in 1989, almost three years after my surgery, that I was confused and upset led to her recommendation that I see Jan Pettigrew, a Ph.D. clinical nurse specialist in oncology and grief counseling, whom Dr. Knox had recently added to her staff after seeing a number of former patients six months to a year out who were doing well physically but remained confused, angry, and frightened.

I knew I was in deep emotional pain, but the source was truly elusive. I thought I had dealt with breast cancer well because I never talked about it. I had gotten on with life—or so I thought. I met with Jan and we talked, and as we talked, I became aware that the lock was being broken on that little black box. When the emotions came, I couldn't stop them. I basically had to start over and feel all the feelings again in order. Shortly after, I decided to write this book. I was ready to look at the new person after breast cancer.

In May 1991, my five-year-old daughter asked me, "Mom, why are you always talking about breast cancer?"

Because I have to. It is the primary factor that has shaped who I am today and who I will be. And politically I want to effect in any way I can a system that may find a cure for this heinous disease *before* my daughter has to face it as a possibility in her life.

Today women will find many more options for emotional as well as physical recovery. Doctors are beginning to understand that you cannot remove a woman's breast, demand that she face her own mortality, and then expect there to be no life changes. Support groups are blossoming across the country, many of them begun by nurses and counselors who saw the need for emotional support.

Gone, it seems, is the incredibly unhealthy stuff-something-in-your-bra-and-get-on-with-it expectation that our mothers' generation faced. The emotional healing needed in this disease is finally getting the attention it deserves. We want more than the physical answer to living with this disease. They can cut out the cancer and kill any remaining cells with chemo or radiation, but it takes something even stronger to eliminate the fear. For while the medical cure is in someone else's hands, we must find our own internal cure for the emotional pain of breast cancer.

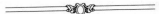

Tip—Those who counsel young women with breast cancer contend that the stages of shock and denial, bargaining, and anger must all be addressed before there is resolution and assimilation.

Michael Fitzpatrick, M.D., chief of Consultation-Liaison Psychiatry and associate professor at the University of Texas Southwestern Medical School, was instrumental in establishing the six-week program through the American Cancer Society that women can attend immediately after surgery. Fitzpatrick says that a woman can often be her own worst enemy in the resolution process as she tries to protect herself and those around her.

"Women often need to deny that having cancer has affected them. They want to make sure that their role-functioning is not diminished in any way. They want to reassure everybody that they are the same person. They want to protect their husbands or mates, children, and friends from fear associated with change and uncertainty by demonstrating that nothing is different, at least externally. That's an unhealthy process.

"To deny loss has occurred only postpones the time when grief will reemerge in one form or another. When delayed, it may later be experienced as physical exhaustion or perhaps as subtle changes in behavior or personality—for example, shutting people out, avoiding intimacy, indecisiveness, or general irritability. Sometimes complicated grief emerges as clinical depression. There are times when grief associated with earlier loss is experienced years later."

"A psychologist visited me in the hospital and said, 'There are steps to this and you can't skip around. You may think you are going to jump over all of them, but you're not. Remember this: You have to grieve. You have to feel like there's a death in your family.' I thought, No, I don't have to do that. Everything is going to be fine. I'm going to leave here and I will not even know this happened in six months. I found out I was wrong and he was right."—Joanne

Our losses from breast cancer are multiple; some are very tangible—our breasts, sometimes our hair—and some are less obvious. The list here from the women interviewed in this book is in no intended order. Indeed, you might want to number them according to **your** sense of specific losses. Then ask your husband or lover to do the same.

loss of health

loss of a body part

loss of femininity/ self-concept of being attractive

loss of self-concept that we are healthy people

loss of a significant relationship/ friendship

loss of innocence/ invincibility

loss of guarantees of the future

loss of family as we knew it

loss of the chance to bear a child

loss of financial stability/ insurance

loss of job

loss of control over life

loss of person we used to be

loss of goals and dreams that must be put aside

loss of mate or significant other

loss of ability to fulfill the parental role

How do we cope with such a laundry list? The best way we can. Accept the loss, feel the feelings associated with that loss.

"I got in a really bad place when we came home from the hospital. It's just so strange. Here's your life, you try to get back in it and everything's totally different."—Amy

"I never took the anger out on a specific person. I was just mad. I had a good marriage, three children, I was happy, and this wasn't supposed to happen to people like me. I started jogging after my mastectomy and that helped me deal with the anger. I put my shoes on and just ran and ran and ran."—Lynne

"I always had a systemically wonderful body. Everything was always on schedule and always felt the same way on the same day, and I could plan. I respected it so much. But now I'm thinking whenever I read about ovarian cancer or uterine cancer, Do I have this?"—Elizabeth T

"The diagnosis was just almost indescribable. When I first found out, my main concern was my kids. I remember thinking, My little boy

is two. If I die, he probably won't even remember me when he's ten other than a picture. My husband was swearing up and down—he'd never remarry, he'd never remarry. I said, Yeah. You're going to have to for the kids. You can't do this alone."—Madeline

THE EMOTIONAL STAGES OF BREAST CANCER

PHASE 1

"Dying was my first reaction. The word cancer *is so scary; it is just synonymous with death."*—Dot

"All I could think of was dying—leaving my family, what my family would have to go through, what I would have to go through, what my family would have to see me go through."—Sandy

Only a few women said they did not have an immediate vision of their own death when they heard the word *cancer* or *malignant.* "I am going to die—no ifs, ands, or buts." For the period right after diagnosis, we are like the rabbit caught in the headlights. Blinded by fear, we are frozen and can only stare at the destructive monster coming at us as we wait for the fatal blow. Then the surgeon or oncologist begins talking survival rates and sets the course for treatment, and we begin to understand that breast cancer is not a death sentence. Emotional denial sets in and we begin on the second phase, which focuses on the medical aspects of the diagnosis.

PHASE 2

"I think when you're actively participating in your treatment or you're going through the treatment, you really feel like things are going okay."—Linda H

This phase, which surrounds surgery and treatment, is the "I will live" stage—"we will fight this together and overcome it." The initial sense of immediate doom passes and we move into the fighting/bar-

thought about this I will die. I have to have positive thoughts and imagine the chemo doing its thing and always be positive and think that I am going to lick this thing and live."—Dana

"*I remember thinking, Now what did I do? I'm a good person. I go to church. I've never committed any crimes. I've never broken up a marriage. I don't strike children or dogs. It's like, I must be being paid back for something. I went through that for a while. I guess the thing that sort of took over for me was, Well, maybe God wants me to live my life differently. Maybe this is a message. Maybe it's not punishment. It is a message to get me to do something different.*"—Marsha

About three months after I finished chemo, a casual friend and former business associate called. She was distressed after learning that the twenty-six-year-old wife of a high school friend had just been diagnosed with terminal cancer and given only six months to live. She went on about the unfairness of it all and ended one sentence with, "And she isn't even the cancer type. She eats right and has always worked out."

It hit my guilt button hard. So what am I, I thought to myself as she kept prattling on, chopped liver? No, I guess I am *the cancer type*. It's a depressing reality that there are many people out there who believe that people who get cancer somehow caused it—and therefore deserve it. More depressing is the fact that some of those people are us.

What drivel—and yet how easy it is to buy the whole line about causing our cancer. I had barely moved from the fear-of-dying stage after my diagnosis when well-meaning friends began dropping off the plethora of books about cancer being about unresolved issues and high-fat food. Of course, it was the people who had not had cancer or dealt with it in their lives who were the first to tell me to buck up—a positive attitude is the answer.

I read the books intently then—and still read them, since I have found a road to health that for me includes many life-style issues. But I don't think I caused my cancer, nor do I think getting angry will cure it. I do know that expressing myself makes me feel better and that less stress will be better for my immune system to do its work. In the past five years I have come to understand that just as there are all kinds of cancer, there are all kinds of people. But more important, there are all kinds of women who get breast cancer. *We aren't a type.*

Yet I devoured all the books looking for the *WHY*. I needed answers to questions. What is this stuff called cancer? Why did I get it? What could I have done to prevent it? What can I do to keep from getting it again? Why me, God?

It didn't have much to do with getting through cancer, but I needed desperately to know why I got cancer. I know now that other women have the same need. I asked each woman I interviewed why she felt she had gotten cancer. The answers varied from standard environment issues, high-fat diet, genetics, stress, and the pill to drinking wine, eating grilled food, inhaling sculptured-nail solution and, my personal favorite, the woman who swore someone had put a curse on her.

As far as I am concerned, a curse makes as much sense as anything else.

And the answer is—there is no answer.

Everyone has cancer cells in his or her body. They are the cells gone berserk, in reaction to a lifetime of exposure to carcinogens triggered by chemicals, age, smoke, and who knows what other combinations of twentieth-century abuse. In most instances the body has its own methods for eliminating the little misfits. *When, how,* and *why* they decide to cluster into tumors in some people and not in others is probably the unanswered question of our time, and chances are we will know how to stop their division before we know what made them begin to divide in the first place. In one of those moments of anger when I wanted to pin my cancer on a specific, I asked my oncologist why no one had asked me life-style questions or quizzed me in any other way to find the link we all shared that caused our little berserk cells to settle in our breasts and begin to grow into tumors.

His response: "Because it is easier to find the cure than the cause."

Getting caught up in the *why,* and the ensuing guilt that question entails, does little to help us cope with the *hows* of breast cancer. Indeed, it infuriates me to meet with women who are bald from chemo and struggling to care for small children, who are beating themselves up about high-fat diets, anger, depression, or the latest cancer link described in the daily paper.

"I had guilt because I smoke and that is totally under my control, but I haven't stopped. So I thought, Well, I don't exercise and I don't eat properly and I am overweight. The guilt comes from not taking

care of myself. I joined the sports club and started swimming once a week. I am trying to cut out fatty stuff and I have stopped drinking. Now, if only I can stop smoking and eating."—Dana

"I pretty much think I gave it to myself. I went through a very difficult time, and I never was quite sure what caused it, but I was very severely depressed. At that time I was not really wanting to live, and I think I gave my body the opening."—Sherry

If the depression from being a new mother, or of having an unhappy marriage, or an unsatisfying job could cause breast cancer, we would have generations of documentation to that effect. But the bigger question is: Does the cancer patient really need some do-gooder sending her a book that is going to make her think that cancer is her punishment for depression?

I spent a good many months berating myself for a variety of things that may or may not have contributed to my cancer. I should have had a baby sooner; I should not be carrying around the thirty extra pounds that I constantly lose and regain. I regretted every animal-fat-soaked fast-food french fry I ever ate and seemed to get mad at my husband for every moment of anger I stuffed into our seven years of marriage.

Then I interviewed women who were thin, ate healthy diets, and had their children in their early twenties. Many of these women could be called fitness fanatics. They had none of the high-risk factors being touted today. Indeed, some would be called low-risk. They were happy, healthy women who did everything right, and they had breast cancer, too. Then I realized that I knew women who took birth control pills longer and earlier than I did, are fatter than I am, function under more stress than I do, and live at fast-food restaurants. They don't have breast cancer.

We hear the deceptive high-risk factors daily about family history, obesity, late childbearing. But the reality is that around 70 percent of the women who are being diagnosed with breast cancer right now HAVE NONE OF THE HIGH-RISK FACTORS.

All this concentration on life-style issues seems to ignore the exposure issues of these women. How do you document possible groundwater contamination? I look back at my life now and think of the DDT exposure while they sprayed for mosquitoes on every military base I ever lived on. Then there were the gallons of bug spray I used trying to keep the cockroaches under control in that apartment I lived in for ten years—not to mention the gallons of pesticides that filled the air from the manicured lawns of my childhood. There is no way to even begin to explore our food chain and possible carcinogens that come into our bodies through pesticides and additives. Then there is the evidence that women who begin menstruation early are at greater risk for breast cancer because of the increased estrogen.

My PBC (post–breast cancer) friends and I like to add to the list all the newly cataloged causes of cancer. We call each other with tidbits such as the friend who called this morning to say that women who eat a lot of soy sauce are at lower risk for breast cancer. Since my family was stationed in Japan for three years when I was five, I have used soy sauce as a condiment for years. It clearly didn't help. Besides, a recent article in *The New York Times* says that it's a defective gene we have to worry about. It seems that all the carcinogens have finally damaged the DNA and no matter what we eat or drink or how much we worry, there are those of us who are genetically at high risk.

Recently, the morning paper says that the stress of worrying about what causes cancer is what causes cancer.

Our bodies are complex, and what causes cancer is complex. Yes, there are a number of environmental issues that scientists and researchers say we can control to prevent cancer and prevent recurrence. But the specifics of the issues of diet and stress are hard to study. Each of these issues has a spectrum of internal issues that you must explore for your life and your situation.

A percentage of the women I talked to said stress was a major factor in their life the year before they were diagnosed. Others, like Kit, defied all the statistics. *"I had my children young and breast-fed all three. I was the one at school who got on all the other teachers for eating chips and drinking Coke for lunch. I never ate artificial sweeteners and grew my own food and baked my own bread. Now, I've said to heck with it. I eat junk food and never felt better."*

And before you say, "Aha, it must be that she is a repressed, angry person," I have never laughed as hard in my life as the two hours I spent with Kit. Her humor and zest for life were infectious. She remarried after her surgery and sees life as a new challenge every day in her work with children who have special needs. She is loved and feels fulfilled in her work. To my question about why she got breast cancer, Kit answered, "Just lucky, I guess."

The point is, stress does supress the immune system, and yes, there is statistical evidence that major illness occurs more frequently immediately following a major stressful life event. But right now all the whys in the world won't change the reality that you have breast cancer and must concentrate on getting well. The emotions of this time—fear, guilt, and anger—are stressful. But the goal should not be to pretend they aren't happening because you are supposed to be UP all the time. The goal should be to face them—lean into them. Let them be a part of this time—not the master.

I decided to decide why I got breast cancer. I have the right to do that just like you do. If you are fighting the guilt—pick something and let that be the why. Then work on getting well both physically and emotionally. Many women want to explore emotional issues as they relate to breast cancer because they want to feel that they are doing something toward healing. If you think you need to look at factors such as suppressed anger, do it. But find the style that works for you.

> *"All the books by Simonton, Siegel, and Louise Hay made me more depressed and feel more guilty. It's hard to channel the feelings, but you have to get as much as possible out of your body. If you let it sit there, it just drives you nuts. I've seen women in the groups who have just let it sit and you can see what it's doing to them. It's eating them up, so you have to find some way to get it out. Exercise or yelling and screaming in the bathroom or crying and talking to friends or whatever it takes. Channel it out."*—Andrea

Spend your energy from this moment forward concentrating on being and getting well.

Do I want to be well?

The answer to this one cannot be a "sort-of" answer. If you cannot stand on a chair and shout that you want to live and they will have to take you kicking and screaming from this earth, then stop reading this book and get yourself a good therapist quickly. Suicidal thoughts frequently accompany a cancer diagnosis and therapy is the only way to deal with that.

How can I best get well emotionally?

What issues do you think need resolving in your life? What stresses (and people) need to be eliminated who are hampering your wellness?

How can I take what research shows and best apply it to my life to stay well?

Not everything written applies to everyone. Filter, and decide what works for you. If the idea of seeing the good cells as Pac-Man eating the bad cells cracks you up, don't feel guilty—enjoy the laugh. If you cannot or will not face the anger you feel, but you know that you are angry, you are suppressing your feelings. Not a good idea.

Low-fat and high-fiber has been shown to be a healthy diet for all of us, and more and more information is being offered about the benefits of vitamins and a vegetarian approach to eating.

How can I own this experience as a part of my life and learn from it?

Breast cancer is a grief experience. Grief is hard work. There are many people and places to help you process this experience and learn to live with it. You must have someone to talk to.

How can I integrate my needs with those of my husband/lover, children, and family?

Our families need us to be whole, and that means processing this experience as it relates to the whole family.

> *"My friend Michael called, and I said, 'I don't have boobs anymore, I have these ugly scars now.' He said, 'Jo Anne, you are being petty; you are getting better.' The wisdom of that really struck me. Before I had the big question: Will I live or die? Now I was worried about the scars."*—Jo Anne

FINDING SUPPORT

> *"After I had my surgery, I started seeing a therapist because I'm a real planner. That's what I do in my career—plan for lots of things. So I thought, I think I need someone to help me through this, especially losing the breast, and even though the actual surgery was not that big*

a deal, I wanted to take care of that and also take care of some of the things that might have led up to my cancer."—Diane

"There were times when I could get real mad at myself. Why am I going through this all by myself? That was the worst part. I felt so lonely—especially during chemotherapy. And the friends I had, I lost most of them. They just kind of went by the wayside."—Sheila

You need a significant other in this with you for more than just moral support. You need his or her eyes and ears to help you listen and discern—whether it is in the form of someone who will take care of things totally or someone who is just a physical presence to go through the meetings and planning with you. If family is too far away, find a friend. If you don't have anyone you are comfortable with, tell your surgeon you need to talk with some of his or her former patients who have been there and who might be willing to touch base in the next two months, until you have a better grasp. The most helpful information will come from women who have been there, but be aware that your surgeon will be limited to referring you to the women who have voluntarily offered to be contacted. (Remember this later on and offer to talk to other patients of your surgeon.)

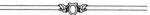

Tip—Don't forget to make time for emotions. During diagnosis and biopsy, things are moving fast. Set aside a specific time during the day to talk to someone about what you are feeling.

Although a number of breast surgeons around the country have established a support component for their patients, the majority still see emotional support as separate from treating the disease process. For this reason, you will probably receive little information on the emotional aspects of recovering from breast cancer from your medical doctors. Physicians, it seems, are trained to treat the body as a separate entity from the person—something that is impossible in breast cancer, in which women's very femaleness is being removed while they watch their future become doubtful. Laura Mae's surgeon actually told her to quit crying and get on with it. She was alive—he had saved her life.

Fortunately, a number of support groups connected with hospitals and particular surgeons have sprung up in the past few years. If you find one of these comprehensive centers, you're lucky, because in most cases you will be expected to seek these out on your own—something few of us are capable of initially. Have your friends research the emotional-support network available to you and your family in your city.

FRIENDS

"I have a couple of best friends who I have had for years and they are the ones who never tried to fix things for me. They never tried to tell me what to do; they just listened. If I cried, they sat and held my hand, and that is all I wanted. That helped more than anything else, and I treasure those friendships."—Lynne

Tell friends you need an accepting ear and heart for wherever you are, rational or not, in your healing. Keep close those friends who will allow you to be where you are at the moment, with all its inconsistencies and ambiguities. When they ask what you need, tell them: "I need you to ask me where I am and then listen without judging or trying to fix or offering solutions of your own. Just let me talk."

"Some friends rally to it better and more easily than others. In our last support-group meeting, one girl said, 'Well, you find out who your friends are real quickly, and those that can't rally around, I just discard them.' I was thinking people react differently to this kind of news, and that doesn't mean they don't care and that doesn't mean they don't love you and want to see you through it. Maybe they can't. And you need to give them a little break, too."—Diane

Although I have to concentrate to remember the specifics of what was said at that first meeting with Dr. Knox, what I can remember is a physical reaction. The adrenaline was pumping; I was ready to battle this beast in my breast. I wanted all those around me to be ready to fight with and for me.

I encouraged an attitude of determination from my friends and family and let them know that I wanted all of them to help me, whether it was through prayers, calls, practical needs, or just by sending good thoughts my way. It never occurred to me to be ashamed or embarrassed that I had cancer. I wanted all the good feelings and as much support as I could find. I wanted the troops on my side, as many as I could gather.

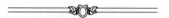

Tip—As hard as it is, ask for help. Much of what is happening right now is happening so fast that you don't have time to think about it or feel anything. But you have to remember to tell people what you want.

At this time, like at no other, you need positive, uplifting support. This is not to say you should put on a front of "fine, fine," when you aren't. You need friends in whom you can confide what you are feeling without fear of their judgment or your hearing of the latest cure they read about in a magazine.

One way to reduce stress is to accept and assimilate your feelings, not deny them because everyone is preaching about the importance of positive thinking. You can be positive and still accept that you are angry and afraid.

"Right after surgery, when I started feeling like I was going to die and it was going to come back, my friends' response was, 'Don't worry, today they cure breast cancer. You will be fine.' They kept telling me how good I looked. I stopped talking to them."—Mickey

"I would get real upset with people who started crawling out of the woodwork and calling me and telling me, 'Oh, don't worry about it.' Or, 'Be brave,' or 'Be strong.' I wanted to say, 'What in the hell are you talking about? I just had my breast cut off and have cancer.' It was really irritating. I've directed a lot of anger toward people like that. I think they need to say, 'I don't know what you're going through.

But if you just want to talk and want somebody to listen to, I'm here for you.' But they shouldn't try to say that they understand, because they can't."—Madeline

SUPPORT GROUPS AND THERAPY

"I have a friend who has had a bilateral and I tell her things we talk about in the support group. She's very concerned because she thinks it depresses me. I could not articulate an answer to her until it dawned on me that I gather strength from everybody in the group. I may cry and get depressed. I may be happy. But at the same time, I gather strength from each person there."—Judy D

"I just needed to talk to some women who had been through this and had survived it."—Joan

"I think she needs to go to a support group. Apparently, I'm not able to help her like she needs to be helped. And I want her to get over it, to feel better."—Cindy's fiancé, Larry

In the past few years, more than one study has confirmed that the women who do the best with a breast cancer diagnosis have someone to talk to.

Indeed, one of the most significant studies in the area of mind/body issues and cancer was conducted with breast cancer patients by David Spiegel, M.D., a professor of psychiatry and behavior sciences and director of the Psychosocial Treatment Laboratory at Stanford University School of Medicine. In his 1989 study, Dr. Spiegel decided to scientifically explore the issue of whether support would indeed have any impact on the lives of women who had metastatic breast cancer. Dr. Spiegel divided a number of women, all of whom had metastatic breast cancer, into two groups. One group met once a week in a group therapy setting with him; the other group received no therapy. What Dr. Spiegel found surprised even the most conservative researcher. The women in the group therapy, where they were encouraged to share their fears and feelings, lived, on average, twice as long as those in the group without therapy.

Those of us who have been there know that family and friends in our immediate support group may not be able to handle all the emotions we are experiencing. And even the most supportive husband or friend is soon exhausted.

> *"I realized that I needed something more than being able to talk to my husband about it. I can't tell you how much I have gotten out of the group. I've found out how differently people feel about their bodies."*—Pat H

> *"It was really helpful to talk to other women. It lost the hypothetical and theoretical when you could talk to people who had done it and been there and they were still walking around living their lives and it could all be dealt with and managed."*—Victoria

The women I talked to who had the most emotional difficulty with their cancer were isolated during their diagnosis and treatment. They were functioning under the "If I stay busy and get on with my life, it will go away" method. They didn't talk about what was happening and how they were feeling to anyone. Indeed, some spoke with pride that no one at the office even knew they had breast cancer. These were women who said they weren't sleeping, had withdrawn from society, and were sure they would die.

> *"At first I talked about the fear, and I could tell it really bothered my husband, that he didn't like me to talk about things like that. And I tried to talk to my mother. She didn't want to hear me talk that way, either. She would say, 'Everything is going to be fine.' So I just kept it all inside."*—Leanne

One of the most positive things to happen in the past five years is the proliferation of breast cancer support groups. There is literally something for everyone. Begin placing a few calls to find groups in your area, and then, if possible, talk to one of the women from the group to get a feel for how the group operates. This will also give you a friendly face who will be with you on your first visit. Nancy S became a support groupie after her diagnosis because she knew that the women who had been there had the best information for her. *"I am self-assured, but I wanted to learn as much as I could. I joined the support group with the surgeon; I joined the Cancer Society support group, which was six sessions, and my boyfriend went to those. I joined the support group that was starting in the suburb where I lived, with the American Cancer Society."*

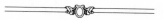

Tip for friends and husbands—Don't push when it comes to support groups for your friend or wife. Suggest that she might want to look into it. Offer to go with her the first time. Only someone who is ready to deal with the emotional issues will find support groups useful.

Support groups come in all shapes and sizes and have varying dynamics. They are not for everyone—but don't let one visit discourage you. Indeed, the idea of support groups has actually only taken root in the past five or six years, meaning they are blossoming at hospitals and in churches and private homes, initiated by one woman or a small group of women who want to talk. By early 1992 there must have been ten support groups in the Dallas area, and every one was different. The American Cancer Society, which has offered support groups for the longest time, generally has one for women who are newly diagnosed. These groups are generally information-oriented and have a beginning and end—say, six to nine weeks. They may include spouses or have a place for children. The ongoing support groups in Dallas offer women continued exploration as they move further and further away from surgery.

When I was newly diagnosed, I attended a group for young adults. The group included primarily women with breast cancer, but also a few with other forms of cancer. I was heartened to see other young women with breast cancer who were doing well. The ten or so people met at a church once a month. Each person introduced himself or herself at the beginning and then the floor was open for issues. At the time, this group was being facilitated by one of the women in the group who was a breast cancer survivor. She was compassionate and called me a number of times with information that was useful. Ultimately, what drove me from the group was one of the attractions. The women who had had breast cancer were farther out than I was. They were ready to talk about fear of recurrence—an issue I could not tolerate yet. I came away more fearful and frightened and stopped going. I have discovered since that I was not alone in this flight.

Marsha's first visit to a support group was on a night when an oncologist spoke. Since it was at a hospital, people were rolled in from their rooms. It frightened her to see such sick women, and she vowed never to go back. Marjorie B said she felt "inauthentic" at the group she visited, where persons with different kinds of cancer had gathered. *"I felt I was trespassing where I didn't belong. Like I was a healthy person trying to pass myself off as a sick person, because these people were so sick."*

Tip—You don't have to be dying to need to talk about your experience and what you are feeling. Your experience is valid no matter what happened to you.

I have begun to think that women really need different levels of information from the group encounter. First they need information; then they need a place to confirm that information as they absorb the disease; then they need somewhere to begin to understand how they feel about the disease. It's like they need a group for their head at the beginning and then one for their heart and soul.

I have been to groups where the women didn't talk, but listened to the facilitator talk about feelings and do assertiveness exercises. Joyce describes her group as a place where women can learn to have fun again after breast cancer. *"Our group teaches a woman how to be frivolous. And there are wonderful lessons about the child within."*

I have been to groups where the facilitator told the women how they should be feeling and what they were feeling. I have been to groups where there was always a professional whose goal was to increase the women's knowledge of the disease. I have been to large groups, of more than fifty women, and groups of only four or five. Some of the women interviewed for this book attend two or three different support groups, where different needs are met.

I ultimately found a home—a community of women—in the support group formed through my surgeon's office. The group, which meets twice a month for an hour and a half, is modeled more on traditional group therapy—with the difference that we all know why we are there from the outset. The group is facilitated by a Ph.D. nurse/oncology grief counselor. The group, which began meeting in August 1989, has evolved a number of times. At first we were all new to the experience—except for me. At the time I was the farthest out (and probably the most emotionally distraught, since I had entered the "what now?" stage and they were all into treatment and doctor bonding). Our standard at each meeting is to share our story quickly for anyone new in the group. Since we started, we have dealt with the death of five members and formed a truly tight-knit community of women who talk during the week and who have a newsletter (the *Mam-O-Gram*) that is a combination of news bits on breast cancer and gossip from more than one "raving" reporter. Every meeting is followed by a usually rowdy meal, when we do as much communicating as we did during group. (As the waitress was seating the ten of us one week, she asked if we were celebrating something. "Yeah, we're alive," Joanne shot back.) We love each other and have learned from each other how to grieve and how to feel the feelings of breast cancer. We are what I would call a serious group. We have become known among our doctors as "that group," which means to them that we are informed and demanding in our care—and at this point we are probably pretty scary to a newly diagnosed woman.

I joined my group in August 1989, when I was definitely in phase 3, accompanied by a lot of emotional pain. I have grown immeasurably in the past three years. I have also moved from a position where I "took" from the group to one where I now feel I "give" more. Joyce put it best: *"Six weeks in a support group is not enough. Twelve is not enough. An ongoing group is the only way to form bonds and actually become support for other women."*

I would wish for everyone the kind of group I have found, but it takes work. It takes a willingness to share your feelings and feel pain. It takes a professional who knows how to direct and keep people on track and doesn't project her own issues on the group (which is often the major pitfall of a group directed by an untrained facilitator who had breast cancer).

———— ❧⊙❧ ————

Tip—Look for a group facilitated by a professional such as a social worker, psychologist, or oncology nurse. If there is no trained individual, the group can get stuck on one issue or be dominated by one member.

"We had a woman facilitator who wanted to dominate the group. She had not had cancer and I don't know what her qualifications were, but I felt like screaming at her, 'Let these people talk.' "—Marjorie B

"The group was too big for good sharing. Just when I would get my courage up, the time was up. It wasn't as therapeutic as I would have liked. Then I found out about the young adult's group. It helped me realize how unresolved the personal relationship area was for me— sexuality and all the issues I have a need to talk through. That group opened all the doors again."—Jo Anne

"The support group is great to just compare things. You don't feel like you are the only one. You hear different stories and it makes you think. Sometimes I'm ashamed that I feel this way because I hear worse stories than mine and here I am complaining. It gives you courage a little bit at a time."—Mary C

Women sharing a cancer diagnosis, though quite dissimilar, can also find a fellowship and community unique to their experience. Sonja's husband had deserted her, and she knew no one in the city when she was diagnosed. She had two sons, ages three and seven, at the time.

"The week after radiation started I was a real screwball. The only thing that saved me was the support group. A woman asked how I was managing. She said, 'We all have husbands and none of us has small children. How are you coping?' I said, 'Well, I'm not doing very well.'

She asked what I needed, and I said, 'A nap.' She called her church, and every night a different couple brought me dinner and picked up the children. I went to bed and slept for two hours. I couldn't believe it. It really kept my job for me, and the kids were excited to get to go somewhere and be treated like guests. They had a great time."—Sonja

Marjorie S attends two different support groups, one through her surgeon's office and one facilitated by the Susan G. Komen Breast Cancer Foundation in Dallas. *"I have met some of the most fascinating people, and I'm getting a lot out of it, because it is an outreach I have been looking for. It gives me an opportunity to do something for others."*

Tip—Even if you feel you don't need it, seek out someone supportive to talk to and practice completing the following: "Right now I feel _____." If the word in the blank is "nothing," you may need to seek further help. You should be feeling something—if only confusion and fright.

For women who don't want a "cancer" setting for support, regular group therapy or one-on-one therapy are also options. A few sessions alone with the professional facilitator of the group—or with another professional, if your chosen group doesn't have one—may help clarify issues. Judy D says she has always been the giver, which made asking for support difficult. *"After a few visits with the therapist, it became very obvious that I needed support. I needed my family, my friends, and so I did an about-face emotionally and said, 'I've got to have help.' I called friends and asked them to listen and hear me cry, and they did. I feel fortunate. I learned for the first time in my life to ask."*

Judy describes her first meeting as a "two-tissue-box meeting" and the next as a "one-box meeting." After a few individual sessions, Judy joined the therapist's ongoing group.

Marjorie B visited a therapist after her mastectomy, which followed a lumpectomy two years earlier. *"When I went to see a therapist, I really felt it was a relationship issue, not breast cancer. The first day I walked in, she said, 'Why are you here? Why did you come?' And I said, 'Well, I divorced, I got married, I got cancer,' and then I cried for an hour."*

A therapy setting will require a more serious commitment on your part to explore the issues in your life, with breast cancer as the focal point or the crisis that leads to exploration of underlying problems. Dana recalls the day she decided to get help. *"I began to wonder why the diagnosis wasn't bothering me as much as it should. I had met this guy and we had been dating a few weeks when he broke it off, and I remember thinking, God, Dana, you have had breast cancer and you are going through chemo and this guy has broken off with you and yet you are kind of bumbling along each day, getting up and going to work and coming home. I knew I was home alone, drinking two or three glasses of wine a day, and it hit me that something wasn't quite right. I should be crying or mad or going out and learning to hang-glide or something. That was when I contacted a psychologist."*

> *"I got into a support group and that didn't help. That was what was scary for me—it was helping other women, and it didn't help me. After I was hospitalized for depression, I kept going to a psychiatrist, where I dealt with a number of major life issues that had nothing to do with breast cancer—except they were keeping me from feeling what had happened to me."*—Mickey

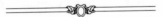

Tip—Choosing a therapist should involve the same procedure as choosing any other doctor. Find one who is recommended, check credentials, and be sure there is an emotional fit.

> *"I had met with the therapist after my parents died, and she was the first therapist who was able to get me to confront my feelings and my anger and my fears. With the breast cancer, I returned to her and found that just confronting the feelings and talking them out helps me be able to solve them myself."*—Melissa

Amy visited a few cancer groups but felt totally out of place because of her extremely young age at diagnosis. She was twenty-five and looked about seventeen. She chose instead to go back to a therapist she had seen in high school for individual counseling and then joined the therapist's group. *"In some ways it's gotten worse, because therapy really stirs it up. But I think I will also work it out sooner because of that. Like I said, they really don't let you get by with much in there. They really keep you coming."*

"I didn't like groups and didn't want to have anything to do with them, because I felt like I didn't want to be like one of them. I didn't want to be one of those people who had cancer and sat around and cried and boo-hooed and didn't have any hair, and I didn't want to be depressed. I just refused. The one-on-one therapy helped a lot, because I could talk to her and she is also a good friend. She could give me good advice, but I didn't have to be reminded about cancer because she was wearing a turban. I just didn't want to be reminded. I wanted it to go away."—Angela

Be aware that support groups are just that. They are not designed for those who clearly need more significant therapy. All kinds of women get breast cancer. Some were diagnosed when there were other unresolved issues in their lives that had nothing to do with the cancer. But if there are other unresolved issues, a woman may find her emotional recovery from breast cancer has to get in line behind other more basic issues.

"The support group leader who was a nurse counselor said she didn't have much to offer me. She said her job was to help me deal with the grief of the cancer loss, but she said, 'I don't sense that you are grieving.' She said it could be that I was not going to grieve over it, which she said was a little unusual, but she said that more than likely, I had not begun to grieve over it because I had never grieved over anything. I wasn't in touch at all. That was when she sent me to a psychiatrist, who agreed that there was a lot of co-dependent stuff."—Dana

Many women who have been through breast cancer see support groups and volunteering as a way to give as well as get. Kim decided to join the hospital's cancer-volunteer program after her bilateral. *"I remember sitting there and looking out the window at the hospital the night before my surgery, and I felt so alone. It would have been so nice for someone to have walked in, whether they be thirty-one, forty-one, fifty-one, sixty-one—and just say, 'I don't know what I can say to you that would help, but there is life after breast cancer. After your surgery you'll be okay.' "*

"Joining Reach to Recovery has been a very good thing for me. Some people feel like they don't want to go see people—they don't want to deal with it on a regular basis. It's better for me to go see somebody and have them ask me how long it's been. I can say now it's been three years, and watch them say, 'Oh, three years! That's good.' It's good for them to hear that, and it's good for me to say it. And I've met some great people, women."—Harriett

GRIEF VS. MAJOR DEPRESSION

Women and their significant others should also watch for signs when a woman clearly needs immediate therapeutic intervention. While the normal processing of grief can lead to strong emotions as a woman moves through the process, it is a healthy movement that happens in its own time. When anger persists for months and there are other indicators that recovery has been replaced by strong stagnant emotions, it's time to get help.

"I always blamed myself for things. I think I blamed myself for the cancer, too. I was depressed and it got worse and then all of a sudden I was thinking about killing myself and starting to plan it. When I started talking about it, my husband took me to a hospital. They helped me see I was co-dependent on taking care of everyone else instead of myself. I thought that someday there would be time for me and then I realized that there might not be. I was very angry."—Mickey

"After surgery I was on a high, and I felt wonderful and everybody was so wonderful to me and I just felt like everything was going to be fine. Then after a month or so I began to get depressed. I just felt like nothing was right and never would be again and I was sort of paralyzed.

I felt helpless. I couldn't walk down the hall without crying over nothing. It was a terrible feeling."—Betty L

Pat F said her depression began when her mother died after Pat's first mastectomy. When her cancer recurred in the other breast, Pat said her depression worsened and she began taking a mood elevator. *"It was frightening, because I thought of death a lot. I still do sometimes think of death, not my dying, but doing it to myself to ease myself."*

Depression is a side effect of many crises, and while it is easier than feeling the pain, resist the urge to medicate your depression. If you do choose one of the mood normalizers on the market, do it in conjunction with psychotherapy to help resolve the root cause. While some depression is chemical, most is life-based.

Dr. Michael Fitzpatrick warns against a quick fix of medication for grief.

MICHAEL FITZPATRICK, M.D.:

"There are women who will develop the illness of clinical depression, which is both qualitatively and quantitatively different from grief. These are women who are not just experiencing the sadness associated with loss; they are persistently and pervasively down in the dumps. They often are unable to respond positively to those people and activities that had been sustaining for them in the past. They may have insomnia and weight changes. They feel anemic and are easily fatigued. Concentration is difficult to maintain. Perhaps they may feel either that life has lost all meaning and that they would be better off dead, or they have actively contemplated suicide. Clinical depression is a syndrome with many symptoms occurring simultaneously. The lack of a reactive mood, apathy, and the inability to both experience and anticipate pleasure are especially key symptoms. These women need an evaluation and further medical treatment. Once treated, the grief work still must be addressed.

"On the other hand, sadness and some depressive symptoms are certainly to be expected. Many physicians will prescribe medications if their patient is spontaneously tearful or is just having a bad day at the time of routine examination. Without a thorough inquiry and an active investigation over time, a patient is often treated inappropriately for depression with antidepressants and tranquilizers. These medications are not benign. They have complications. They are often sedating and may actually inhibit the cognitive clarity that's essential for good recovery. Secondly, the implicit message given is that if you take this pill, then everything will be okay. So in many instances, the medications are not only inappropriate but also harmful.

"There are times early on in the grief process when some symptomatic treatment is appropriate. If one is having trouble with insomnia, then some mild sedative is appropriate for a time-limited period—perhaps two to three weeks. After that, one begins to develop rebound insomnia that occurs as the drug is being withdrawn. Persistent insomnia is worrisome. It ought to be evaluated by a competent professional rather than just medicated away, and may be a sign of complicated grief.

"There are no magic pills here. Many physicians want to be helpful and, as a result, prescribe inappropriately. Patients want simple solutions as well.

"You cannot short-circuit the grief process. It's just not possible."

HUSBANDS AND LOVERS AND BREAST CANCER

To generalize about how men will respond to cancer is to generalize how women will respond—and that can't be done. Add to this equation how the couple responds as a team. As with the women interviewed, the men had a number of reactions to the diagnosis: shock, denial, and fear. But again and again I heard the words *helpless, frustrated,* and *out of control* as the men struggled to explain their inability to fix what threatened their family.

For those of us who were part of a couple when diagnosed, our husbands and significant others shared the pain of diagnosis and were usually the primary source of support. Some women felt their partners took the diagnosis harder than they did. Few said they resumed the same relationship with their partner as before the diagnosis.

"You're talking about a fundamentally important body change. It's just as simple as that, and you're not going to snap your fingers and

say, Okay, are you better now? Can we get everything back to the way it used to be? I think the thing is that you've got to sign on for the long haul. It is not the three weeks in the hospital or the six months after that. That is the easy part, because you know your enemy is right there and you are rising to the occasion. Two years later, it's not immediate anymore. You have a tendency to get back in your own life and forget about it—it's over. But it's not over."—Marjorie's husband, Chuck

"It makes me so mad to hear that women think men are going to leave. I bet for every man who leaves his wife there are 10,000 like me, who were desperate to help and wanted to do it for her."—Dot's husband, Jack

"I felt helpless; I felt inadequate. I felt like there should be more that I should be giving her. I did not have the answers. Always before, I had answers; I could always figure out what to do."—Mary-T's husband, Leonard

"I think that men need sort of a caveat to be ready for this changing every aspect of your life, possibly in a big way, a significant way. It's not something that you can sweep under the rug or try to ignore. It is scary. The feelings that I was aware of were anger and being afraid— anger at this intrusion into our life, this potential loss, this disruption."—Elizabeth T's husband, Hugh

"I didn't know what was expected of me—what I could do or should do."—Dot's husband, Jack

"I remember you were throwing up from chemo, and I had to take Kirtley to the doctor. She had a respiratory problem and was clearly in distress with her breathing. So I left you and remember sitting in the doctor's office with her and wishing I was at home with you, thinking, It doesn't get any worse than this. Now I look back on it as positive because we got through it."—my husband, Tom

The accepted differences in the ways men handle a crisis situation are often highlighted by a cancer diagnosis. Most of the men said they tried to understand as many of the facts as possible and functioned on a purely analytical level—assessing information and making decisions, getting done what had to be done.

"I don't think I experienced anger as much as I experienced frustration at watching her go through the hell that she was going through, and there wasn't anything I could do to help her. I honestly think that at that time we probably did a terrible job of communicating, verbally, but I think it was because I was simply trying to do everything that I could think of to make it easier for her."—Dot's husband, Jack

"I know many times we would lie side by side in bed and I would start crying and say, 'I want to say something, but I don't know what to say. I want to tell you something. I want to try to comfort you, and I don't know how to do it.' Or, 'I'm hurting and I know you don't know how to comfort me in this situation.' Men tend to respond in a way that we mask these feelings, and you just can't do it. You can't do it for your wife. You can't do it for yourself."—Mary-T's husband, Leonard

"It was the first time in my life I've really had to face something that I couldn't do anything about. I've always been able to get my hands on something. It was very frustrating. I started reading, trying to find out everything I could."—Cindy's fiancé, Larry

"I think men are expected to be able to control all situations. And it's quite a shock to realize you're out of control and have to depend on somebody else. All of a sudden I realize that no matter what I did, I wasn't going to change things. That's what I had the most difficulty with and it still haunts me. I talked about that with the counselor a lot."—Sherry's husband, Kerry

Most men said they approached the emotional aspects of the diagnosis like Cindy's fiancé, Larry, who felt he had to put up a strong front and act like everything was going to be fine—and then grieve in his office alone. In the two plus years since Cindy's diagnosis, his approach has been to try and protect her from his feelings of fear. He recognizes that they need to communicate. *"It's something I've got to get used to—talking about it. I guess most of the time I just block it out and work. I don't want to think about anything happening. I don't want to acknowledge that it can. I refused to. I guess that's a weakness on my part. I found out Cindy is extremely strong. Probably stronger than me. There were a lot of times that I felt guilty because I felt like she was probably helping me get through it more than I was helping her."*

Pat F's husband, John, said that the hardest thing was trying to be the strong and brave one. While he accepted that as his role, it was sometimes tiresome. When asked what he did when he got tired of it, he said: *"I sucked it up and was strong and brave."*

Craig, Leanne's husband, said he learned about dealing with his own emotions and how important that was to help his wife. *"Once the time is right, when you've got the opportunity, make sure you consider yourself. Because in an indirect way, that's supporting her too. You have to have your head in the right place to give her the support she needs. I know now that that may be why she is having trouble now, almost four years out, because I've put it away as much as I can instead of dealing with it. So don't just shelve it."*

Marjorie's husband, Chuck, said that his approach was to be himself and not try to guess what Marjorie needed. *"What my wife needs from me is me. She doesn't need me acting one way or another. You can only be what you are and try to understand that it's real life; it's really a horror that someone is going through this and there's no answer for it."*

With the American divorce rate hovering at 50 percent, it is clear that breast cancer occurs in many families where there are already problems. A breast cancer diagnosis may add to existing barriers, particularly when communication is a key issue and neither party has sorted out exactly what he or she is feeling.

Some of the women said their husbands or partners were all they needed to help cope with the emotional aspects of breast cancer. Others—both men and women—accepted that they needed outside support, sensing that their primary relationship could not sustain the level of intensity. This is not a condemnation of the primary relationship. Nor does it seem to be linked to the woman's prognosis. Women need to tell their story repeatedly in an environment where it is acceptable. They need to express emotions that they may not be able to express at home if they have been protecting their partner. This need may become particularly pressing when the woman begins to cope with her fears of recurrence. Larry says he struggled to understand Cindy's depression, which set in more than eighteen months after diagnosis. *"That's been frustrating to me because, jeez, we've got all the crap behind us now! Now we ought to be feeling good and moving on and getting back in the swing of things. And I find her going the other way, and I don't know what to do about it. And of course, I tried to get her to go to support groups. I've tried for over a year because I felt like she needed it. I said, 'You know, there's something that I'm not providing. I don't know how, or can't, or something— I don't know.' "*

Norm said that it took him a couple years and some retrospection before he realized that he had been insensitive to the emotional aspects of Lynne's diagnosis. At the time of her diagnosis, Norm and Lynne had been married for fourteen years and had already faced a major crisis when their first son was born with a heart defect. A former navy pilot, Norm said he approached the cancer the way he was trained to handle all crises: Dissect the problem, remedy the problem with the goal being to preserve life—very systematically. *"For me it was fixed. We have cancer. We went in. We fixed it. We're going to live a long and healthy life. Thank you very much. Now we just go forward. I didn't have the emotional sense of loss. To me the deal breaker was survival. Don't get me wrong, I love my wife's body, but the answer was, You don't look back and wish things weren't as they are. You march forward and make the best of what you've got. That's my type-A personality."*

Lynne described Norm as a tremendous support during this time, but Norm recalled becoming aware during the year after her surgery that Lynne was troubled. At one point she made a comment to him about never wanting another woman to sleep in her bed. *"I said, No problem. If you die on me, I'll just get rid of this bed and get a new one. So you have two choices. If you don't want me to sleep with another woman, you better not die. She laughed, and it was black humor, but again that's how pilots are trained to cope."*

In the months that followed, Norm began to understand that his perception that the cancer was in their past was not how Lynne felt. *"I really didn't focus on the emotional aspects of the cancer. I think I was sympathetic, sure. I mean, I listened, but I didn't understand."*

Norm says his advice to men is to be aware that the grief and fear last much longer than the treatment. It is interesting to note Lynne's feelings more than seven years after diagnosis. *"I just sent my oldest child back to college yesterday. I sobbed and cried. And my family doesn't understand that I am not crying because I am sorry to see him go but because I am still here. I can remember thinking in the hospital and wondering if I would see the twelve-year-old graduate from junior high, let alone go off to college."*

There must be an acceptance between husband and wife that, even in loving, caring relationships, there may be a chasm between partners in coping with the unknowns presented by breast cancer.

My husband, Tom, thanks to his own therapy in years past, was able to really listen to me and deal with my fear at diagnosis. When I would shut down, he would encourage me to talk about my feelings. And then he would do the active listening and ask what seems to be every therapist's favorite question, "What does that feel like?"

It was when my treatment was over and the waiting began that we seemed unable to communicate. The feelings were no longer easily verbalized, so I couldn't figure out what was wrong, which made it impossible for me to communicate what was happening with Tom. We have also discussed at length the difference between men and women and how the sexes cope with the unknowns presented by a breast cancer diagnosis. While I will fantasize endless scenarios about what might happen **if . . .** Tom does not comprehend the void, the unknown, the "what ifs." His male cognitive mind must have something concrete with which to cope. My mind seems much more willing to contemplate the unknown.

Marjorie's husband, Chuck, describes it as the difference between a strategic response and a tactical response. *"Strategically would be, 'Oh Christ, you're going to die. What am I going to do? And it's going to be terrible for you.' Tactically is, 'How are we going to get through this situation? How are we going to keep your spirits up? How are you going to deal with the changes in your body?' Things that you can deal with. The other stuff you can't deal with."*

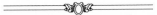

Tip—In general, men act and women feel.

While Norm and Larry concede that they could not comprehend the fear, they were open to the feelings being expressed, and both Lynne and Cindy described their partners as completely supportive. Their memory of how their partners reacted often didn't mesh with the men's. Indeed, it is important to remember that both the woman and her partner are in shock initially and may move through the stages to acceptance at different stages.

> "I decided that before surgery we should talk to a friend who was a counselor and this was the first time I actually sought help. He called to get some information about the situation, and I told him I was concerned about Sherry. She seemed to be handling it well, in fact to a degree that I wanted to make sure before surgery that she was comfortable with it all. After the first session, he said that she was handling it well and I was the one having the problem."—Sherry's husband, Kerry

> "Well, I'm not sure how to articulate this, but I think there's some denial that goes on at first. I just think I didn't want to deal with it, so I found myself holding back, trying to distance myself a little bit from the hard reality. You're doing the best you can, but you're shaky. There was certainly recognition of that. I remember trying to bolster her up the best I could. It's a real feeling of helplessness, though, on the patient's part and on the family's part. Nothing you can do."—Elizabeth T's husband, Hugh

---

Tip—Talk about what kind of help he is going to need while you are in the hospital and recuperating at home. If women are bad at asking for help, men are terrible.

As I said, I went into surgery the perfect candidate for a lumpectomy: small tumor, good location for clean removal, and large enough breasts that the loss of breast tissue would leave a fine cosmetic result. The lumpectomy would be followed by six weeks of radiation.

When Dr. Knox walked out of the operating room to tell Tom that we were now talking about plan C for chemotherapy, Tom read the frustration on her face and immediately assumed that I was dying. All of a sudden, my "I can handle it" husband needed emotional support worse than I did. I was out of it. Luckily, our assistant pastor was with

Tom when the word arrived. I asked Tom later how he reacted.

"I cried," he said.

I received phenomenal support immediately following surgery. I wish more friends had called Tom and asked how *he* was doing. He was dealing with reality and the subsequent depression. Remember also that the man must take on the daily family responsibilities for children and home in addition to his job while his wife is incapacitated, often leaving him no time for his own reflection or time to grieve, adding to the stress of the situation. Leonard took over the day-to-day responsibilities for the house and two children and learned to cook while Mary-T underwent chemotherapy. He was also facing additional stress at the office. *"I think the hardest thing was there was never a time just for me, because I had excessive demands at work and obviously excessive demands at home and there was no in-between."*

Ray and Evelyn had been married fifty-two years in a very traditional marriage when she was diagnosed. They laugh now at Ray's cooking for himself during her hospital stay. *"I said, 'Ray, just go to the store and get something that's easy to fix and you can do.' He said, 'I don't know what to get. You make a list for me.' I said, 'Ray, I've been cooking for fifty-three years,' and he said, 'Well, I've been cooking for a week. Aren't we even?' We laughed about that."*

Madeline was furious at how friends and family reinforced the macho approach that the man should be strong for his wife. *"My poor husband. People kept coming up to him, saying, 'Be brave. Don't worry.' This kind of crap. And he said he just wanted to shake them: 'What do you mean be brave? My wife's going to die and I've got two little kids.'"*

Luckily, I have a husband who knows the value of therapy. The day after my surgery, Tom paid a visit to his former therapist, Harold, whose wife had undergone a mastectomy twenty-five years ago. Because of their established relationship, Tom had no trouble expressing his fear of my death. I really appreciated Harold's response to Tom's query of "Why?"

"It is clear that God made a mistake," Harold answered simply. I like that.

Men, as a rule, have fewer outlets where they can express their feelings in such a situation. Men just don't have the same permission as women to call each other and get upset and display fear and anger. This doesn't mean their need is less; they just have not had the socialization in which our communities accept that men can need support. They are supposed to be supportive but somehow not need their own support.

Lise's husband, Bill, sought a support group for men but didn't find a match. *"One was a group of men who were in their sixties, which I totally couldn't relate to. And the other was a group that was younger than me, and their attitudes were totally different. One young guy married this girl and she had her breast removed and he was really bitter about it. Here, he just got married and now he has this deformed wife. And I guess if you've been married six months or a year, your attitude might be different than if you've been married sixteen years or something. But I still couldn't relate to it. If you really love someone, does that really make that much difference? And he didn't want her to have chemotherapy because he didn't want her to lose her hair. It was a very strange attitude."*

With few exceptions, both the men and women interviewed for this book agreed that the physical aspects of the breast cancer were not as big an issue for the men as what the women perceived they would be. They overwhelmingly agreed that the sense that the loss of the breast would impact the relationship was a much more significant problem for the women than for their partners.

> *"The one thing I probably resent was that she thought I was going to love her less because she only had one breast. And I don't give a damn if she doesn't have any. That's not what I married her for. It's the person—the person, and that's all."*—Dot's husband, Jack

One of the greatest misconceptions about couples and breast cancer is that men immediately abandon women—either literally or emotionally—when their wife or lover has breast cancer. I met only a few women who felt that their cancer had contributed to the end of their relationships. And in all those cases the women said there were problems prior to the cancer.

Amy and Chris both divorced after breast cancer. Amy was twenty-five at diagnosis and her husband was twenty-four. They had been married a year. When they separated a year after the diagnosis, Amy said she felt sure it was due to the cancer. *"I think I took a lot of it out on my husband, which I've dealt with now. I've had a lot of guilt about it. I was just crazy. I think I became very abusive towards him, because he was*

the anger and to verbalize it so that, cognitively, one can set limits on the anger and can begin to diffuse it.

Where is the anger projected?

Frequently, at physicians—and sometimes it's deserved. At times it is projected toward God. It may be projected toward one's spouse.

So what is the healthy way to resolve it?

It's important to look at what has helped in the past. The best way is to try to get the couple to do things together rather than to have the anger separate them. Another way is to be in a support group where they hear other men say, "I felt the same thing. I know exactly how you're feeling. This is what worked for me." At times the couple may need more intensive work with a couples therapist when recovery is more complicated and not going well.

CHILDREN'S ISSUES AND BREAST CANCER

"Each of the four children reacted differently. Number one said, 'Are you going to die?' Number two said, 'You must be eating too much fat.' Number three said, 'How is Dad going to handle this?' And number four said, 'Why couldn't it have been Mrs. Findley?' "—Lola

Nothing seems more a focal point for the emotional pain we are suffering than our children. They are the pinnacle of our fear as we contemplate their lives should we die. Yet they consume our energy at a time when we have none to give.

Children of all ages need *information* and *participation* in any family crisis. They need to know what is happening and be given the option of being part of the process. The level of information and participation will depend, of course, on your child's age and ability to comprehend what is happening. Yet even an infant may react to the tension in the house and the disruption of his or her schedule.

"The kids lost control. The little one was three and took a pair of scissors and sliced up the new sofa. I spanked him, and I never would have done that. He had never had a spanking before. This was a week after radiation started."—Sonja

The best a family can do is keep communication open, encourage questions even when you don't have the answers, and keep in touch with teachers and significant others in the child's life. If there are clear problems, get help. Parents of older children must remember to include their grown children and tell them what they need.

"From the first day we had made the decision not to hide anything from each other, such as feelings and emotions and the very real problems, and also not to hide it from the boys, who were teenagers. She was still up in bed, groggy from anesthesia, when the kids came in that afternoon and I sat down with both of them and told them exactly what was happening."—Mary-T's husband, Leonard

Their need for information will also depend on where they are developmentally. Young children and teenagers may be very self-centered about the disruption to their lives. The best advice is to ask what they want to know, then let them tell you. Answer their questions simply, and don't supply more information than they want. Prepare children with honesty. Listen to their questions and respond. Don't be afraid of tears.

Madeline's daughter was five. *"I'd just been home maybe a week, and I was taking a bath, and I went to get out. And just as I was getting out, she walked in, and she saw me, and she kind of jumped back a little bit, because I still had the stitches in. And she said, 'Oh, Mom. Is that what they did?' very matter-of-fact. And I said, 'Yeah. This is what they did.' And I said, 'But I'm going to look better as time goes on.' And she seemed to accept that."*

Nancy W saw clear signs of distress in her five-year-old son immediately after her diagnosis. Her mother had had ovarian cancer for a number of years, and she knew that her diagnosis would be taken to heart by her sensitive son. *"Because we recognized some problems, we wanted to get some help for him. We asked about it, but the insurance company wouldn't refer us. We asked about it again because the problems* were getting worse at school. He was out of control. So we were able to finally get a referral. But then, they wanted to talk to him, and I had to say, 'Look, I'm not taking a child in to be assessed. That's not how one does it with a five-year-old.' The idea is to try to find a play therapist or someone who's competent at dealing with these issues."*

Children, like everyone else, go through their own adjustment issues when a parent has cancer. They too may be fine during the surgery and treatment, as they are "strong" for mom, and then begin to show signs of fear and anger as time progresses and the constant stress of cancer builds on the family dynamic. Add to this the complication of development issues for children and you may see a wide variety of reactions from your children for years.

Teresa M said that initially her six-year-old son handled her diagnosis very well. She took him to radiation with her, and he seemed to be coping. *"Then a year post-op he started having a really bad time. He was a very bright child and all of a sudden he stopped learning. And the teacher sent him for tests and did all the logical things. Finally, I took him to a therapist and it turned out he was having nightmares his mommy was going to die. He was concerned that Daddy wouldn't be able to take care of him as well as Mommy did. Then he was feeling guilty about that. That was the hardest thing I went through."* Teresa said that later, when her son was a teenager, she talked with him about this time and the decision for him to see a therapist. *"I said, 'You know, it was hard to put you into therapy. It was hard for me because I thought I had failed. And then I worried about friends who would know you were in therapy—would they tease you? Or would you regret it? Or when you got older, would you look at me and say, 'Why did you do that?' He said, 'Mom, it's one of the best things you've ever done for me.'"*

Very young children may be fearful of being left alone and be consumed with issues of their care should you die. Young children are also very much magical thinkers: If they wish it, then it will come true. It's possible that your child may feel responsible for your cancer, that he or she caused it because of anger at you.

Also be aware that a child's imagination will usually supply the details if you don't. Leanne's daughter was four when Leanne was diagnosed. *"At first I think she was concerned that she was going to get it too when she got breasts. I said no. She was very concerned and asked what they were going to do and how I was going to wear my clothes. I tried to keep her involved in everything. When we went to get the prosthesis, she was with me. She knew about everything so that nothing was scary to her."*

> *"One night after I came home from the hospital, I was taking a bath and all the children, who were eight, ten, and twelve, found some excuse to come into the bathroom to see. My son wanted to see it, and then the little one came around the door. She was smiling when she came in, but I thought when she saw it she was going to throw up. I just told her it looked bad now but it wouldn't always look that bad."*—Kit

We often forget that our children can feel very deeply even as young as three or four and have the distinct ability to absorb our fears and reflect them. If you are fearful, your children will know it.

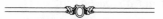

Tip—Don't forget to tell the children what is happening. If you are having treatment, prepare them. When you are depressed, tell them.

My daughter was six when my mother was diagnosed in October 1991. Because I had already been in the process of writing this book for more than two years, Kirtley knew very well that her mother had had breast cancer and it was what she did for her "work." At lunch after church on a Sunday shortly after my mother was diagnosed, I was discussing breast cancer with a friend. In mid-sentence, I looked at my daughter, who seemed troubled. She looked up and said, "Mom, I wish you would stop talking about breast cancer because I think I am going to get it." That, of course, is my worst fear and a very real concern. We talk about it often and Kirtley knows more than most adults about breast cancer, knowledge that is her comfort *and* protection.

Older children generally understand the process a little more fully and, depending on their personalities, will be present in the moment and able to share their fears of death. Children will generally ask you what they want to know. Allow them the time and place to do this. If it is clear your child is troubled, but he or she is unable to share feelings, gently suggest that this is a scary time for you and see if the child agrees that he or she is scared also. Watch for signs of trouble at school or in patterns of sleeping and eating.

"The older boy was seven and scared, and when I started chemotherapy, he was afraid that I would lose all my hair. He took out his frustration and his fear by throwing screaming fits, saying that he did not want me to come to school if I came up with a wig on, that the wig might blow off and everybody would make fun of his old mother, and he cried and cried."—Lise

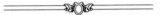

Tip—The greatest gift you can give your children is to share how you feel. Remember to tell them how you feel. Don't press them to talk, but make time together that will allow them to talk.

Teenagers are in a category all their own. They may even be angry at you or disappear entirely during your illness, for a variety of reasons: Teenagers generally turn to peers to express themselves. They may be in denial or unable to handle their own emotions about your illness. Developmentally, teenagers want to separate from the family and may have begun the process when Mom's illness brings home the reality that parents aren't forever. They may feel guilty for those very normal adolescent rejection-of-parent feelings. One mother called her teen a "total schizo" about the whole thing, alternately offering support like an adult and then regressing into childlike behavior and being very difficult. Remember that this is where teens are—one foot in adulthood and one in childhood.

Mary-T's husband, Len, found that his fifteen-year-old son was turning to a neighbor for support. *"He became more or less a surrogate father, because my son could relate to him, could express himself. I remember telling the neighbor that I didn't have any problem with that and I knew that my son has got to get through this and I feel very fortunate having him here. I didn't feel threatened, so that worked out real nicely. He had someone he could express those fears, frustrations, anger and anxieties to."*

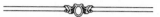

Tip—Resist the urge to rely on your children too much for emotional support. They are still children, even into adolescence, and should not shoulder the entire responsibility of being your support network.

My stepson, who was sixteen at the time of my diagnosis, did not visit me in the hospital after surgery. Indeed, he avoided me as much as possible. We had just begun communicating again when he caught a glimpse of me without my wig, and off he went again. He was twenty-two when my mother was diagnosed, and he was very concerned and wrote and called. At one point he said, "I know I wasn't there for you." It was just not something he could handle.

What's normal behavior for teens and what signals trouble with them is often very difficult to distinguish. In families where everyone is healthy, the teenage years can be frustrating and angry as the child works to separate and become independent. Often the place where issues are expressed the most fully is school. A drop in grades during your illness may be a reflection of difficulty, but normal nonetheless. We can't concentrate, yet we expect that our children will be able to. They need permission to have their lives interrupted also. So what if their grades drop a little? This is life. We are having a major crisis in our family. It's okay to be a little crazy.

I had a student in journalism once whose mother was diagnosed with cancer during the semester. I had seen enough of her skills to know she was an A student, but class assignments became a real struggle for her. She was confused and frightened by what was happening to her, and although she knew at one level that what was happening at home was affecting her, she didn't understand that it could have such an impact on her ability to concentrate. I told her to keep a journal of her feelings for the rest of the semester instead of doing the class assignments. She did, and I gave her an A.

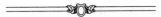

Tip—Be sure to call the teachers yourself and let them know that it's okay with you if the children need down time at school.

Signals that normal grief and anger need more significant intervention may be indicated by the extremes. Instead of just a drop in grades, your child refuses to go to school. Drugs and alcohol have been the opiate of adults for decades; they are also available for children now. One interview I did for my first book was with a single mother whose sixteen-year-old daughter had been killed in a car accident. She was concerned about her surviving son, only fifteen months younger than his sister and her best friend. She was concerned he was taking drugs to alleviate the grief, and she knew he was skipping school. When I suggested counseling, she said she couldn't handle it because she was on so much Valium herself that she had trouble getting to work. Somehow she didn't see her dysfunction and drug-taking as a model for her son's.

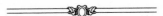

Tip—Children model on their parents for coping. If you are open with them, they are more likely to be open with you.

Talk of suicide and hopelessness should be taken very seriously and professional help should be sought. Because of the high number of family issues being brought into the schools, many have begun counseling programs. Call the school and alert them to the situation.

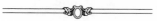

Tip—Just be sure your teens are talking to someone. Call the parents of your teen's close friends and alert them.

Getting teenagers to talk about feelings can be the most frustrating effort a parent faces. So don't. But make time to just **be together.** Don't set it up as "our time to talk." If your teenagers are taking a stab at expressing themselves, just try to reflect back what you hear. "I hear a lot of anger and that's okay. I am angry, too."

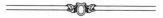

Tip—Call your local American Cancer Society and ask for a copy of 'Helping Children Understand: A Guide for a Parent with Cancer.'

Parents should remember to include their older children also. When Sandy was diagnosed, her five children were eighteen to twenty-five. On the day of our interview, her twenty-one-year-old, Melissa, who had just graduated from college in another state, was home and joined us for the interview. When I asked Melissa about her feelings when her mother was diagnosed, she immediately teared up. Because Melissa was at school and had an important interview for graduate school, Sandy and her husband decided not to call Melissa at college and tell her what had happened. This was the first time Sandy had seen such emotion from her daughter about the cancer. Melissa stated emphatically that she wished her mother had told her about the diagnosis. As it was, an older brother told her and got the information wrong. "It was like everybody knew but me," Melissa told her mother.

Melissa ended up doing her senior thesis on the importance of support groups and breast cancer. She came home after graduation to be closer to her family.

Older children who may be in college or on their own should not be excluded from the information and participation process. Let them decide if taking the final or coming home to be with you is more important. But also be sure to be honest. Do you want the child home? Try to discuss your feelings openly and honestly.

When an older woman gets a breast cancer diagnosis, a whole other set of dynamics can take place, depending on the woman and her relationship with her grown children. At best this is repay time, when the children can be there for the parents who have been there for them. At worst it is an emotional tug-of-war as the children resist the idea that their parent is ill while the parent is demanding time and attention.

It may also represent the point at which the children become responsible for their parents. This is what happened in my family when my mother, Mary, was diagnosed in October 1991 at seventy-two.

Because my mother had been in good health, she was caring for my father, who has Parkinson's disease, at home. She had insisted on caring for him alone at home for more than three years, despite me, my sister, and my brother admonishing her to find good nursing-home care. My father required constant attention and had to be assisted with eating and dressing and was diapered at night. My sister-in-law came in during the days, and my father went to adult day care three days a week. But it was clear that the burden was become overwhelming for my mother. Indeed, the morning of the biopsy, before we knew she had cancer, my sister and I had a frank discussion with my mother in which she finally admitted that she was emotionally and physically spent. We decided to begin the process of finding a good nursing home for my father. Little did we know that the next two hours would necessitate the immediate move of my father from the family home and an activation of the family to care for both him and my mother during her surgery and chemotherapy.

While my brother, sister, and I sat in the hospital room during surgery, we made plans to move my father to my sister's home while we began looking for a nursing home. We divided responsibility for Mother and Dad's care. We explained to Mother when she woke what we had done and asked her permission to take over. I think there was a visible sigh of relief as my mother gratefully handed over her life and that of my father to us.

When you as the patient decide you want your adult children involved, you may or may not find that they are willing participants. It is painful for children to realize their mother is aging and can no longer be the caretaker but instead must be cared for. Dealing with adult children can be painful if they decide to pull away from what they see as the possibility of your death.

Joanne says she felt abandoned by her thirtysomething daughter. *"I would get up three mornings a week and there would be the sweetest card under the front door from Sherry. She would call, but she wouldn't come by. I got my feelings hurt because I wanted to see her. I didn't want little messages from her here and there."*

Mary C was a widow when she was diagnosed at seventy-one, and her forty-year-old daughter had always been there for her. Mary says that her daughter became a different person after the cancer, and despite Mary's repeated attempts to identify the problem, her daughter remains aloof. *"She is just too busy to come over or be with me. She says there is no point in listening to me feel sorry for myself. It really hurts me. She went out of town for Christmas, and I really wanted her here. I really don't know what to do next."*

Ida Rose talks about her cancer as if it were a common cold, but when she began talking about her children's reactions to her illness, her pain was visible. Ida Rose had four grown children, two sons and two daughters, when she was diagnosed. The sons both lived close; the daughters were both out of state. *"They're accustomed to me just coping and doing for myself. I had built up a lot of resentment over them not saying, 'Is there anything I can do? Do you need any help or anything?' They're so used to me just doing it on my own."* Ida Rose says her oldest daughter told her that her needs were too great, that she would have no energy left for her own family. Ida Rose says she wanted a call and a card occasionally.

The complications of the child-parent relationship are legion, and resolution is never easy. A lifetime of dynamics make up these relationships, and nothing tests them like a crisis or illness such as breast cancer.

PEDIATRIC ONCOLOGY NURSE CLINICIAN JULIE STEELE,
R.N., CHILDREN'S MEDICAL CENTER, TALKS ABOUT
CHILDREN AND CRISIS AND SUPPORT GROUPS

Julie Steele, a pediatric nurse clinician at Children's Medical Center in Dallas, since 1982 has worked with children who have cancer and in 1989 started A Time for Me, a support group for children whose parents have cancer.

Tell me about what's happening with different age groups.
Children under five are not likely to have been exposed to the word *cancer*. If they have, they're probably not real sure what it is. I think children who are less than five are basically feeling just the chaos of what's going on. Something is wrong. Mommy's sick, and I'm being shipped off to Grandma's house and I'm not real sure why.

What age are the children in your group?
It begins with eight-year-olds. Not that there is something magical about an eight-year-old, but there is something about how much they will talk and how much they are able to communicate ideas.

How do you begin your work with children?
The children are given a pre-test of questions like:

What is chemotherapy?

What happened in the first place that made your mom or dad have cancer?

Did you do anything to cause their cancer?

Did they do anything to cause their cancer?

What is a blood transfusion?

(continued)

Then we give them a test at the end of five weeks to see if we have accomplished anything. Almost always there has been a vast improvement.

How are the groups structured?

In the first group setting, we usually start off by taking a seat and then I ask questions like "What is cancer?" Most of them have a pretty good idea about what it is. We'll talk about if you can catch cancer and I let them know you can't. We talk about what causes cancer.

One child's mother had had a baby not too long before she discovered her breast cancer. She was nursing and I think the baby bit the nipple and it got infected and from that they discovered the cancer. Well, the child thought that the baby had caused it. So we went through the process of explaining that no, he didn't, and maybe it was a good thing he bit her because they discovered the cancer. He said, "Oh, yeah, yeah, I knew that."

Is it all medical—helping them understand?

About half is educational and half is support. We just talk to them about whatever they want to talk about. We do art therapy, where they make a "need book," and there are different pages that say things like "I don't like cancer because . . . " Then they draw a picture.

Or sometimes they will just write something. One girl wrote, "I don't like cancer because it makes my dad angry." Anger is a picture that comes up a lot. I'll ask what the biggest thing that's different now that your mom has cancer. Half of them will say their parents are mad all the time.

What should parents tell the kids about the hospital?

It depends on what is going on. If it's just an IV, then I think it's okay for the kids to see the hospital. If it's a more serious situation, where there are tubes or whatever, someone has to ex-

(continued)

plain to them what all those tubes are for. "That's scary. But it doesn't hurt—there are all these tubes, but Mom and Dad really can't feel any of them"—that kind of thing.

If you are a woman with breast cancer, what can you do to help your children in this eight- to eleven-year-old age range?

First of all, encourage children to communicate; encourage them to ask questions and let them know that it is okay to ask questions—and that sometimes you may not know the answers. I think one of the reasons parents don't encourage their children to ask questions is that they are afraid they won't have the answer. And one of these questions is, "Are you going to die?" Be ready with an answer. And what that answer is needs to be left up to you, but you shouldn't lie about it. I think that parents need to know that it's okay to cry in front of their kids, because crying in front of the children gives the children permission to cry and be upset. Let the children help. Have the child hold something for you.

What is the single most important thing for a parent who has cancer in dealing with children?

The main one would be to keep the lines of communication open.

Chapter 6

===≫〇≪===

COMPLEMENTARY THERAPIES

THE MIND-BODY CONNECTION

"He gave me a relaxation tape and he told me, 'This is medicine. You listen to this three times a day like you would take a prescription for an antibiotic.'"—Nancy W

"I was a tough customer for my oncologist because I was doing the visualization and all that good stuff, and he really wasn't into that. He never told me, 'It's bullshit,' but he never would really talk to me about it. I was taking vitamin therapy-type things, and I had them in my hospital room. The doctor picked it up and kind of looked at it and had this kind of smirk on his face, and I said, 'What? It can't hurt.' And he said, 'Yeah, but it doesn't help.' And I said, 'Yeah, but you don't necessarily know that.' Then before surgery, he told me I was in the top ten patients he had seen as far as tumor shrinkage for preoperative chemotherapy in that fast a period of time. He was really pleased with how I reacted. I said, 'Well, I'm helping you as much as you're helping me.' So that doesn't surprise me that it's going along that well."
—Diane

The plethora of information on self-healing has brought the issue national attention but, unfortunately, has provided little real guidance or clarity on the subject.

Even the terminology is open to discussion. For my purposes **orthodox** therapies are those offered by mainstream medical science, which for breast cancer are surgery, chemotherapy, radiation, and hormone therapies. **Complementary** therapies are those used **in ad-**

304

dition to orthodox medicine that do not interrupt or change treatment. They include visualization, nutrition, and other mind/body techniques. **Alternative** therapies are those used instead of orthodox medicine.

This chapter focuses primarily on complementary issues—those things you can do while undergoing regular treatment that will

- enhance the immune system naturally through diet or stress reduction.
- give you a sense of control over what is happening to your body.
- make you feel better about yourself as a person in the midst of the disease process.

Complementary approaches to healing are often seen as black and white—you are either for the idea or against it, when in reality many people don't know what *it* is.

> *"Nothing seems outrageous when you're talking about a serious illness. Things that you might not normally consider—all of a sudden you really want to consider. It wasn't that I would go away from traditional medicine, but I wanted to find out about other alternatives. I took a whole regimen of vitamins and lots of raw vegetables."*—Anne

Actually, there is a broad spectrum of practitioners and approaches in complementary healing. It ranges from the zealots, who protest that their diet is the one true way, and who will chastise patients for exploring any other approach, to mainstream clinicians, who seek to work with patients to explore whatever is the best way for them—often in areas that until recently were ignored or criticized by mainstream medicine.

Unfortunately, the sensational side of "alternative" healing is what gets the most press, and those who are the most vocal about it are the fringe "healers," who offer miracle cures as they attack traditional medical science. As a result, many cancer patients totally dismiss the "new age" mumbo-jumbo and stop their own exploration into what may actually benefit them—or go to the other extreme and abandon their orthodox treatment regimen when someone offers a miracle cure.

To add to the confusion is the increasing number of mainstream medical studies that show effective links in complementary healing issues but do little to show patients how to locate practitioners or apply such findings in a concrete way in their own lives. Medical doctors are getting the message from their own community that many of the complementary healing methods work, but because there are no standards nor integration of practitioners, most M.D.s don't have a frame of reference from which to discuss the treatment possibilities or practitioners they can recommend.

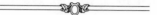

Tip—If you do research on your own, share it with your M.D. Take this opportunity to teach him or her.

While there are literally hundreds of books on complementary healing, there was no one good overview that offered an objective look at complementary healing until Bill Moyers, *Healing and the Mind* (Doubleday, 1993). This book appeals to me as an excellent place to start researching the issue for two primary reasons. It is written by a highly respected journalist whose goal is to explore and present information, not judge its value; and it looks at primarily mainstream medical practitioners who have moved into a more holistic approach through question-and-answer format. You can read the question and the answer. It explores meditation, diet, exercise, stress reduction, and cultural differences in healing between the United States and China. It is a good balanced place to begin your exploration without the emotionality and fanaticism that shapes so many complementary healing approaches. It is also proof positive that healing in this country is changing and expanding to encompass the individual's participation.

What, then, are the facts and how does a patient sort out the right course for herself?

The basic premise behind complementary therapies is a holistic approach to healing. The cancer cannot be separated from the body in which it grows—and that body has a mind and spirit that should not be ignored in the healing process.

The recent medical findings that support this premise are simple.

1. The immune system is the body's first front against disease of all kinds, and scientists are only beginning to understand its vast capabilities. When it is strong, the immune system can assist in fighting the cancer cells. A healthy spirit and well-fed body help the immune system.
2. Specific things can suppress the immune system—and build it. Certain kinds of stress have been shown in studies to suppress the immune system. Conversely, studies show that people who discuss life issues are sick less often.
3. Nutrition is important in building the immune system. Certain nutrients and vitamins have been shown to build those blood cells that are most effective against cancer. In 1990 new dietary guidelines were released that showed a diet high in fiber and lower in fat was better for a healthy life. Studies have shown that while Americans eat a lot, they often do not get the minimum daily requirements of many vitamins and minerals.

So far this is common sense. A healthy, happy person is going to be better able to cope with and fight cancer than someone who is depressed and malnourished.

The confusion and controversy come in the myriad approaches and applications of each of these areas, and practitioners range from emotional profiteers to those who have developed one theory after years of working with cancer patients to those who have moved into the mystical.

Cancer patients, who need balance and support in exploring the psychological and health issues relating to cancer in their lives, often find instead theorists who are ready to categorize them as "cancer personalities"—repressed individuals who never show their feelings or their anger.

Dottee, who had been involved in holistic medicine for more than twenty-five years, kept a detailed journal of her journey through the breast cancer experience. She offers parts of it here for you.

When she was diagnosed with cancer, Dottee recalled sitting tearfully in her surgeon's office. " 'But I don't have a cancer personality,' I recall *saying while simultaneously blinking back tears wanting to spill. 'I'm an artist and I enjoy expressing and creating. How could I develop a terminal illness?' "* Dottee, who admitted that a prior involvement with a doctor had left her leery of the medical profession in general, contacted the director of the cancer research center at the university near her home. *"Accepting conventional medical treatment to destroy the cancerous lesion was my first decision for therapy, and surgery if necessary. Simultaneously, I commenced an exhaustive search into my mind for clues to any condition that had permitted some type of stress to cause my body to create abnormal cells. But my first priority was to get the awful growth out and away from my body."*

After surgery, Dottee wrote out her plan in her journal. She chose a combination of medical and complementary healing, beginning with a lumpectomy and radiation:

"I opted not to do chemotherapy, for I felt my body would heal the best with one medical therapy at a time. Instead, I made my third choice, that of accepting my own personal therapy options. I wanted to call forth creative powers for healing. Feeling my own needs, as well as being truthful to myself, was important to me. These were my summaries:

1. *It was okay to react to shocking news concerning my body.*
2. *I was not going to die tomorrow, so I could take plenty of time to make my choices on my personal treatment.*
3. *I would receive as much education as possible concerning any planned treatment—doctors had readily admitted that they didn't have all the answers (particularly as to why a person contracted an illness that might be terminal).*
4. *The science of medicine has advanced enough to aid in the destruction of an abnormal growth, yet it is up to me to begin to recognize how my body created the imbalance. I would look into my experiences and into my mind to find the answers.*
5. *My life-style habits would be important, so I would open my mind to begin to tap my own creative power to help me heal by adding more art of living immediately into my life.*

In addition to surgery and radiation, Dottee used visualization, color work, personal body work, exercise, nutrition, and laughter.

PSYCHOLOGIST CHARLES KLUGE, PH.D., TALKS ABOUT EXCEPTIONAL CANCER PATIENTS

Dallas psychologist Charles Kluge, Ph.D., has been working with cancer patients since 1974. He became interested in the topic as a graduate student, when he was introduced to the mind/body concepts by the chairman of his department, a clinical psychologist who had worked with cancer patients at MD Anderson in Houston as early as the late 1950s. He has since adapted a California study, completed in the early seventies, which he uses with clients in his clinical practice.

When did you begin working with cancer patients?

In 1974 I was in New York finishing my clinical residency and got a call that Southwestern Medical School was looking for psychologists for a cancer rehabilitation project. It was a multidisciplinary approach. We explored a number of things with patients, and among them was the mind/body connection.

What were you looking for?

We wanted to know what the patient could do to impede the disease. Out of that work grew my perspective on working with patients in terms of fighting the disease mentally and emotionally in addition to medically.

Why? What happened there?

What I remember in particular was one young man we were working with who had testicular cancer. We were doing imagery and group work and seeing him frequently. The physicians kept saying, 'We don't know what you are doing with Johnny, but he has gotten much farther than we thought." He lived out his prognostic clock several times over. Then one time he came in and said, "I am tired." He died six weeks later. Once he gave up mentally and emotionally, the disease consumed him. That experience

(continued)

burned in my memory that you don't give up. From that point forward, I've encouraged every patient I work with not to give up.

Then you do believe there is a connection between mental issues and wellness?

We are seeing a body of research today that supports a connection between what happens in your mind and what happens in your body and that, properly channeled, you have some power there that you probably don't use.

Tell me about the program you use with your cancer patients?

I use a six-point plan that is modified from a California study done in the early seventies. This study was conducted on patients who had experienced the "miracle cure." This group of people had undergone all the medical therapeutics and were not responding and were told to go home and enjoy the time they had left; there was nothing else medical science could do. But they didn't die. They went home, but didn't sit under a tree and wait for death to arrive. They changed their lives in fundamental ways. And the study was done to correlate what the factors were that this group of people had in common. The six factors are what they found.

What were they?

First, they changed their diet. They stripped out the red meat, or greatly reduced it, and cut out a lot of fat. They ate more fruits and vegetables—not necessarily something radical: They just ate a healthy colorful plate. Lots of fruit and vegetables and less meat and fat.

Second, they all began to exercise more and exercise every day. Not necessarily anything strenuous like jogging, but something that was significant for them at their physical level, for a half hour a day.

Third, they began to do some kind of introspective reflection. Something as formal as biofeedback or as informal as praying. It was a deep meditative process and it was highly individualized. I

(continued)

always ask patients to do imagery work. I am looking for a specific focus of mental imagery. Each patient individualizes the imagery to his or her own needs. I start by asking them to get into themselves and visualize attacking the cancer cells at a cellular level. Each person will do that in a unique way that means something to them. Some use soldiers; others flush the cells out of their body—whatever imagery works for them. I also add to that something called mirror work. Bernie Siegel likes to have people talk to themselves in front of a mirror. I tell them to stand in front of the mirror without clothes on and have a conversation. Talk to yourself and say, "I love you and I am going to take care of you." Make that contract to yourself out loud every day. I call that mirror work.

Fourth, they all became more religious. Not necessarily in an orthodox way, where they were in church whenever the doors were open. But all of them began to believe that something bigger, stronger, and more powerful than themselves was helping.

Fifth, they began to order their personal schedule in life so they did things that gave them pleasure. All of us have a busy schedule. We are active, dynamic, and involved. That can range from being a CEO to a mom taxi. But all of these people, regardless of their station in life, began to restructure their priorities so that they did things on a daily basis that gave them pleasure.

Sixth, they each began to do something where they involved themselves in a community outreach. They began to give something back to the community—some sort of selfless outreach.

How do your clients respond to these changes?

It requires basic life-style changes and those are hard to do, so there can be some resistance.

What is the resistance on the part of medical doctors who treat cancer to advising psychological help for cancer patients?

I don't know. That has mystified me for a long time. This is a team approach and everybody needs to be seen by someone. The

(continued)

psychological aspect is a very clear part of this and should be part of the overall plan. It should not be *instead* of anything. Surgery is necessary and chemo is necessary and radiation is necessary. But in the same way, your personal and internal coping need to be looked at. The cancer is one issue. If you are married, that is another issue. If you have children, that is another dynamic. All of these issues need to be addressed in coping. Now that you know you have cancer, you need to add the dynamics of the care and feeding of this issue. This doesn't mean every day has to be a battle. It means you should do certain things to care for your body. If you think about it, it is all very logical.

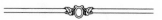

Tip—In looking for a psychologist or therapist, follow the same procedure as you would in choosing any doctor. Get recommendations. The first visit should be your interview of him or her. Ask about his or her theories, training and background. If you feel pressure or coercion of any kind, this is the wrong person. Yet be aware that emotional healing requires work.

HEALING IDEAS (Writing, Art, Music, Pet Therapy, Humor)

There is no magic pill or thought to make your cancer go away. And if it comes back, it's not because you were not good enough or didn't work hard enough. But for many women interviewed for this book it was personal work on the complementary therapies that brought them the gifts of insight into who they are as people who had cancer.

Because of the reluctance of medical science to offer research or any other introduction to complementary healing issues, you will have to do this exploration on your own. Begin with Bill Moyers's *Healing and the Mind* and the list of books at the end of this chapter. Then make a plan of those areas that work for you in your personal plan as a partner in your own care. Look at it as your surgeon's job to remove the cancer, your oncologist's job to kill the remaining cells, and your job to add as many factors as possible to aid in self-healing.

Lawrence LeShan, Ph.D., and author of *Cancer as a Turning Point,* says this exploration should begin with making a commitment to finding out who you are and what gives you joy in life. LeShan, whose pioneering research in mind/body issues began more than forty years ago, addressed the 1992 assembly of the National Coalition for Cancer Survivorship, where he presented a number of personal anecdotes about former patients who had survived cancer by reexamining who they were and why they were alive. LeShan said that this determination to discover one's own uniqueness and to live toward that potential sends a message to the immune system that the body wants to live, thereby assisting the outer healing with inner healing.

It's a great place to start.

Amy read Bernie Siegel's well-known book *Love, Medicine and Miracles* before going into the hospital for surgery. She took tapes with her to listen to during surgery and chose a hospital room that had a view. She entered therapy before surgery and remained in therapy afterward. *"A lot of it didn't fit. A lot of it did. Going to therapy and doing certain things like that. The outdoors helps me a tremendous amount. I really have started camping more and just trying to get outdoors at least one time a day and just be quiet and be there. But the typical things about visualization . . . it just wasn't working for me. I was becoming more stressed trying to do it and thinking I wasn't doing it right, or I was trying to close my eyes and I'd start thinking about something else, or start thinking about work, and I was like, 'This is stressing me more.'"*

"Massage therapy began as a curiosity. I thought it was interesting and I responded to the massage therapy physically. My philosophy was that massage increased the amount of oxygen to the tumor, which provides healing. Very few doctors felt like it was worthwhile. I asked for a prescription so insurance would pay, and they laughed."
—Elizabeth P

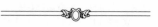

Tip—Massage therapy must be approached cautiously for women with metastatic disease. Discuss it with your doctor.

"I felt more at peace with myself after reading Siegel's books. I felt first of all that I wasn't quite as alone, that I got more of a feeling from other people after dealing with the same thing. It's sort of like Dr. Siegel is trying to give you the message that it's okay if you have cancer; you shouldn't feel guilty about it. You shouldn't feel like it's something you've done wrong, or because you didn't do this or whatever. You've got it and you deal with it and go on from there. And I like that attitude."—Theresa

WRITING

Some found that writing their thoughts and feelings down in a journal helped clarify and express their emotions. Clinical studies done by James Pennebaker, Ph.D., described in his book *Opening Up,* indicate that writing and talking about crises has a direct impact on the immune system. Pennebaker's research followed college freshmen through their first year, an experience that everyone would agree is one of the most stressful of our lives. Those freshmen who kept a journal in which they wrote about issues that made them anxious, adjusted better, and more of them stayed in school. Pennebaker's research also indicted that the tears we cry from emotion are chemically different than those we cry from an irritant.

Dottee kept a journal of healing, and in its introduction she says, *"It is not intended to be even remotely a sad tale, but rather an offering of hope to many who face similar situations. Most importantly, I intend to cover the many choices that I made concerning my right to control my own life and how I created a personal road back to health."*

ART

Drawing, painting, sculpture, and photography became outlets for others who worked best with a visual symbol to release their feelings. A number of cities have groups of artists who meet to explore illness and healing and art.

In addition, those with a creative bent will find time for relaxation as they practice their art. Hobbies and making time for yourself are critical for self-love and healing.

Don't dismiss the idea of art because you have never had a class. I spent hours in my bedroom gluing antique jewelry on hairclips and bracelets during the years after my diagnosis. I enjoyed the hunt for unusual pieces, the bargaining for bags of old mismatched jewelry that I would turn into clips and combs. Now I string old beads on fishing wire to make colorful necklaces. I have even sold a few of my creations—and I have never had an art class in my life.

Dottee, who was an artist and color therapist when she was diagnosed, found a therapist's request that she draw her cancer cells an intriguing assignment. *"Without so much as an analytical thought, my hands flew over the paper to form a large jellyfish shape, with tentacles and a long tail. (Later I realized that my tumor, too, had a long root.) I colored it 'yuk' (yellow-green, like yellow pea soup) and made the tail more distinctive, with accents of mustard yellow. The surrounding picture space of my drawing I shaded the softest of violet. I was amazed that the total painting of a cancer cell had come so easily, without effort. Then, putting the drawing up on the wall, I sat back to analyze its color and form as I had critiqued hundreds of artists' paintings when teaching art classes."*

In visualizations that followed, Dottee was able to bring rich carpets of emerald green and brilliant purple pouring out of a huge space that were forced to crush the hundreds of little yellow-green jellyfish below them. *"This was the power, the source that I had been searching for. My visionary rocket fuel meant power, my inner power of spirit, healing from the supraconscious of the mind."*

MUSIC

Some felt drawn to a particular kind of music for relaxation and reflection. Amy and Nancy W took music into surgery. Others kept healing soft music playing in their hospital room. The right music for you is the music that makes you feel good. Bernie Siegel recommends Gregorian chants, and there are actually a number of cassettes that are sold at bookstores as soothing, healing music.

I find that Native American flute music has a very calming effect on me, and since my diagnosis, I have begun identifying physical reactions to music that I may rely upon.

One of the most wonderful workshops at the 1992 National Coalition for Cancer Survivorship Assembly was presented by a music therapist named Deforia Lane, a Ph.D. in music therapy and a stunning woman with a voice that was meant for opera—until it became clear that hers was to be a much needier audience at the Ireland Cancer Center in Cleveland, Ohio, where for a number of years she has been singing to and with cancer patients.

Dr. Lane, who is also a breast cancer survivor, has been involved for a number of years in the study of music's impact on the immune system. The study's significant results are now gaining acceptance at an increasing number of hospitals. It was found that music can help the body release endorphins to bolster the immune system. At the workshop, Dr. Lane gave examples of comatose patients speaking in response to music and other cancer patients being calmed and having less pain as a result of music.

PET THERAPY

The distraction and nurturing required to take care of a pet can be a positive for healing. Kim went out and bought a dog. *"I thought, Well, I want something warm and fuzzy that wags its tail when I walk in the door. I got a dog, I need some life in my house."*

HUMOR

Lola was a humor therapist at the time of her diagnosis, so she said her immediate reaction was to find the humor where possible—and encouraged her friends to do the same. One instance stayed with her. *"I'm Catholic, but go to church anonymously because I don't want to get involved. I just like to go. Someone gave me some holy water from Lourdes back before the cancer, and I was in the habit of blessing my husband before he left for work. For fun, you know, 'Wait, you haven't been blessed.' Well, I ran out of water and wanted some and didn't want to ask the priest. So I took my little bottle and filled it from the fount after everyone left the church. I told my friend I felt bad about stealing holy water. Anyway, after the biopsy she said it was because I had gotten hold of some bad holy water, and when I woke up after surgery there was a big poinsettia from her and a juice jug of holy water. I still have some in my closet. It's got algae growing on the bottom, but I can't bear to get rid of it."*

VISUALIZATION

"I try to practice stress reduction, deep breathing, detaching. When your positive self-talk becomes negative, I intervene and say, 'Wait. I am okay.' I am a recovering type-A behavior."—Jo Anne

Visualization is a process of relaxation and mental imagery that can be used for stress reduction, simple relaxation and, some say, healing. In the healing visualizations, the person imagines the cancer cells and then creates something that will destroy them.

Because I have always loved horses, I formed a visualization that saw hundreds of snow-white wild horses galloping across the prairie of my blood supply. For the most part I just enjoyed watching their powerful muscles ripple and their manes blow in the breeze, but occasionally some nasty little black lumps would appear in my mind's eye. My horses at this point would rear majestically and stomp these unwanted invaders to dust, leaving the prairie a lush unbroken green once again. Does it work? It can't hurt if it gives you a sense that you are actively participating.

Visualization has helped a number of women not only with healing issues but also with treatment issues. Lise visualized conversations with healthy women who had survived breast cancer while undergoing radiation to help battle her claustrophobia. Cindy used visualization for pain after her biopsy and surgery. *"On the way home from the biopsy I was in a lot of pain. He only gave me Extra-Strength Tylenol. I closed my eyes and in my mind I visualized my hand reaching over and pulling the pain out of my chest and putting it in front of me. Every time I did it, the pain was less and it scared me, because I didn't know how much control I had over my body. On the way home from chemo I would start the same*

.process, pulling the pain out. I listened to the ocean on a tape during chemo and it totally relaxed me. You must distract yourself."

Dottee integrated color into her visualizations. *"Color meditation is a mind practice where a person visualizes a color, sees it all around them, and then breathes the color into themselves, filling their being with the essence of the hue. I would begin my breathing exercises by seeing a certain color in my mind, then imagine it surrounding me in a powerful mist, breathe it in, and mentally direct its energy to every cell in my body to assist my overall healing. My color meditations became as important to me as any of my cancer treatments."*

Dottee, who is the author of *The Language of Color* (Warner Books, 1988), chose the colors from her meditations based on their effects. *"Pink soothed and rescued my tumbling feelings. Green offered calmness, while the color blue offered me more control, red energized, and orange and yellow expanded my thoughts; violet felt good and quieted my mind. Each color left me with a different sensation."*

Dottee also did mind-painting, in which she visualized a peaceful landscape and added colors that felt pleasing.

More and more psychotherapists are trained in stress reduction techniques that include self-hypnosis, visualization and other relaxation exercises. There are also a number of relaxation and guided meditation tapes available.

NUTRITION

A magazine proclaimed on its fall 1991 cover: "Absolutely, Positively, the Last Word on What to Eat."

I doubt it.

In the past decade Americans have been besieged with information on nutrition. It has gotten to the point that we are told everything and anything we put in our mouths has the potential to harm or heal us. Sometimes I feel like everything should be labeled: *Warning—eating may be hazardous to your health.*

At first the attacks were on what we ate—and what we ate too much of. The American diet, high in animal fat, red meat, and sugar, was clearly linked to heart disease. We were admonished to cut down and cut out. Then we began to hear about what we weren't eating and the effects of that. According to some, the lack of basic vitamins and trace minerals leaves our diet and our immune system severely lacking in the needed elements to keep us healthy—and, some say, cancer-free.

Much of the emphasis on food has resulted in better food and an increased awareness of what is put into the food we eat. Those who produce our food have responded with variations that are lower in fat and calories, claims that some consumers take with a grain of salt. The hue and cry now is that the food chain has become so complex and complicated that even if we are told what is or isn't in our food, those divulging the ingredients may be lying or unaware of exposure to carcinogens in the food chain. Even so-called organic food has come under attack. Who says it's organic? Unless you live in a state that has begun regulating organic labels and farmers, there is no proof that the higher-priced lettuce from the health-food store is indeed healthier for you.

To complicate matters, the information relayed to the consumer via the media often turns a molehill into a mountain. Reports of studies that show *some evidence* that there *may be* a link between something and something else is reported as though it is indisputable fact.

> "I take a lot of vitamins now. I do a mega and separate mineral and beta carotene and separate E and fish oil and a booster of zinc. I took a low-fat-cooking course. I love chocolate, and the farther out I get from diagnosis the less attention I pay to that. We eat very little red meat and I don't do caffeine. But there are days when I buy a bag of chips and bean dip and sit down in front of the TV and eat it in one fell swoop."—Joanne

> "I take mega doses of vitamin C now. I think it helps me not get so tired. You know how it is when you work and have young children. I am exhausted. I have always believed in a lot of fresh fruit, and I continue doing that."—Lise

> "I visited a friend who started a feed company in Oklahoma and he gave me a list of vitamins and minerals, trace minerals, and something called Korean white ginseng root, which he said would detoxify my body. I was on chemotherapy and I started multivitamins and mega-doses of C, some A and E. Very specific vitamins and minerals and a

way to take them. In thirty days there was no comparison—how I looked, how I felt, my skin tone, everything. I am convinced the ginseng root was one of the things that helped me get through the cancer. I was never sick from chemotherapy. He was actually a horse-food manufacturer, but he got into that by studying nutrition and did lots and lots of researching. He said, 'When science tells me one thing and the horse tells me something else, I believe the horse'."—Gale

While all this confusion about nutrition is irritating to the general public, for cancer patients the headlines about cancer cures and nutrition can lead to a frenzy of fad foods or vitamins that might even be unhealthy.

As with other issues in complementary healing, we need to find a balance and it is often left to the consumer to sort out what works and what doesn't. Even the basics become complicated, since it seems every proven food-related issue has a study that says it isn't so. Even the seemingly accepted high-fat link to breast cancer has come under attack by those who have their own studies to show that fat is *not* linked to cancer. The truth about food and cancer is elusive at best.

For these reasons, I have endeavored to offer you the basics, reluctant as I am to add to the confusion. Indeed, as a cancer survivor, you must explore and become educated beyond the headlines and the latest fad.

If you want to become knowledgeable about what you eat, resist getting your information from health-food-store clerks. Visit your local library or university bookstore and find a good up-to-date textbook on nutrition. In the back of the book you will see food tables that break down food into every possible component. Then find a licensed dietitian through your local hospital. Sit and talk about diet. Begin subscribing to magazines that focus on nutrition. Then decide on what you think would work for you and your life-style.

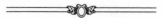

Tip—Many of the fad cancer-cure diets can actually be harmful, such as mega doses of certain vitamins.

**Be sure you have consulted with your doctor before
beginning anything extreme.**

At this point I would like to offer an overview of what we do know
about the nutrition/cancer link—the facts and the myths.

It is a fact that nutritionists have known for years that our diet and
our immune system are linked. Poor nutrition can significantly decrease
immune function, and certain dietary modifications can enhance the
immune system.

How it is suppressed and why and what will enhance it become more
complicated.

It is a fact that by 1991 the Four Basic Food Group approach to
eating in this country had been replaced by "Five a Day," a new approach that encourages consuming less fat and more fruits and vegetables. Recommended are a high-fiber, low-fat diet and:

1. Five servings of a *variety* of fruits and vegetables a day, particularly
   those high in vitamin A and C and fiber, and several servings a
   week from the family of cruciferous vegetables. (A serving is equal
   to about a half-cup of a vegetable, a medium piece of fruit, or 6
   ounces of juice.)

2. For fiber it may turn out the old saw "An apple a day keeps the
   doctor away," may have some truth in it. Apples provide vitamins
   and are an excellent source of dietary fiber.

3. Learn to read package nutritional information. The number of fat
   grams should be less than 30 percent of the total calories per serving. To determine this, multiply the fat grams by 9 (the number of
   calories per fat gram). Is the total less than 30 percent of the number of calories for a serving?

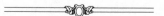

**Tips for low-fat diet—Use butter or margarine spar-
ingly. Avoid bacon, sausage, ribs, snack foods like
potato chips, cheeses, cream, ice cream. Also, bake**

or broil or steam foods. Remove skin from chicken, which cuts the fat in half. Use water-packed tuna instead of oil-packed. Eat more meals comprised of pasta or vegetables.

The search for high fiber provides an example of just how conscious Americans—and those who sell to them—have become of catchwords. A few years ago, a study suggested that bran had special nutritional qualities. Before we knew it, every item on the grocery shelves—from cereal to beer—proclaimed to be "high in bran." It took government intervention to get manufacturers to be more honest about what was and what was not in their products.

Instead of looking for high fiber in all the wrong places, go to the sources: whole-wheat, rye, oatmeal, and corn breads; whole-wheat English muffins and bagels. Breakfast-cereal labels should be checked to be sure that the "whole-grain goodness" is not being overwhelmed by the other, unhealthy, ingredients. When possible, stay away from products made with refined and enriched flour and add whole-grain products and fruits such as apples, pears, apricots, bananas, oranges, prunes, raisins. Vegetables are also a great source of fiber as are many beans and peas, which also offer good nonanimal protein.

While there are those who suggest high-dose vitamins for cancer cure and prevention, be aware that it is possible to overdose with some vitamins and this can cause serious problems and organ damage. Number one on that list is vitamin A. Yet beta carotene, a substance found in yellow and green fruits and vegetables, allows the body to make vitamin A naturally, guarding against overdose. Beta carotene is also one of those substances that has been touted as a natural cancer killer and an immune-system booster.

Getting beta carotene is as simple as eating a plate of green and yellow vegetables a day, particularly spinach and carrots, the two top vegetables on the list. Others are sweet potatoes, kale, winter squash, broccoli, cantaloupe, brussels sprouts, and apricots.

Beyond these issues, the entire issue of nutrition and cancer becomes much more complicated.

NUTRITIONIST GEORGE LIEPA, PH.D., TEXAS WOMAN'S UNIVERSITY, TALKS ABOUT THE FOOD CONNECTION IN HEALING

George Liepa, a Ph.D. nutritionist, former NIH research fellow, and faculty member at Texas Woman's University, has been studying nutrition and its impact on disease for more than twenty years. His emphasis changed from kidney and heart research to breast cancer in 1990, when his wife, Candy, was diagnosed with the disease. Since then he has begun an exploration of how different fats affect cancer and this year will oversee a study of the effect of fish oil on breast cancer.

When we talked in late 1991, Liepa had just returned from a breast cancer conference in San Antonio that was sponsored by the University of Texas Health Science Center in San Antonio. More than 700 oncologists and other cancer professionals from around the country were present to discuss a variety of aspects of treatment of breast cancer. Liepa found that physicians were more accepting than ever of looking at nutrition and its impact on health.

How do you see nutrition as a part of breast cancer treatment?

For one thing, oncologists have historically had problems getting cancer patients to eat at all because of the problems they've had with chemotherapy and vomiting and nausea. Now we have new drugs on the market that prevent side effects like that. I think we'll now be able to get cancer patients, for the first time, to eat foods that we think might enhance immune function. In the past we were always told, "Hey, we're lucky if we get them to eat anything."

What's the balanced approach, as far as nutrition is concerned, if you want to build your immune system?

We've got good data now about certain things in the diet that tend to be immune-enhancing and certain things that tend not to

(continued)

be immune-enhancing, and good information about what kinds of things will bind the carcinogens and estrogen metabolites in the bowel and help remove them from your system.

Like what specifically?

There are no absolutes, but there are epidemiological trends and many laboratory animal studies; you can pull all of this together and synthesize something that approaches reasonable advice. The basic information that we can present, with some confidence, is what the American Cancer Society has been saying to you—we should cut down on total fat. For the time being we advise an increase in the total consumption of fruits and vegetables. We should eat a variety of fiber, not just one kind of fiber. We should not drink a lot of alcohol, and we should not eat a lot of spicy or pickled foods. That's the classic approach right there.

Could you talk a little about fat?

There are people who eat a lot of fat who have very little breast cancer. Rural Eskimos, for example. According to their diet, these people should be dead when they're twenty-two. They don't have banana plantations on the North Pole and they don't have pineapples and they don't have anything but lots of fatty food—lots of walrus and whales and fatty fish to eat. They don't eat fiber, so they should be constipated, and their kidneys should be failing due to excess protein intake, and they all ought to be overweight and have hypertension and they all ought to have cancer coming out their ears. The truth is, they have hardly any breast cancer. They don't have kidney disease. They don't even have a word for diabetes. They're fat people who eat a lot of fat and who are quite healthy. Many researchers feel that fish oil is probably a type of fat that is of some benefit and may be helping this population avoid all these dietary problems. Many of us feel—meaning the people in the nutrition community who do research—that we ought to be studying that particular type of fat vigorously, and

(continued)

one of the directions that a lot of people are looking at is what fish oil does to immune function. We know that some fats, and some seed oils, tend to depress immune function.

What are the seed oils?

Most of the oils you find in a jar are seed oils: corn, soybean, safflower, cottonseed, sunflower.

These suppress the immune system?

Studies have formed a tendency to think in that direction. I prefer being conservative because I don't want to overstate. But also, we are finding that there are exceptions. Certain seeds, like rapeseed and linseed, tend to do better than others. We're just now starting to look at specific immunological factors and see if there's improvement in people when they eat certain oils. As that body of data accumulates I think we'll find that certain foods are very immuno-stimulatory and others are very immuno-depressing. I tell people now that they can basically eat the kind of oils they want to eat, but I think for the time being there's some wisdom in eating more ocean fish. I don't recommend fish-oil capsules. Eat more cold-water ocean fish.

Which are?

Albacore tuna. Not oil-packed—water-packed, because you want the fish oil, not the oils that they've added. Salmon is a wonderful source of fish oil. We are beginning a study soon that we hope will help us confirm some of these proposals.

Why can't women just take fish-oil capsules?

They could work. I believe people need to eat right. I think cancer patients need to take time during the day to sit down with friends, family, or somebody—their dog or whatever—and relax. And I think people need to get back to eating a meal instead of something they take out of the freezer and just microwave. The

(continued)

answer, in my view, is not popping another capsule. If we see real strong trends that could warrant that, I'd say go for it. In the meantime, I'd rather do it with diet. There could be something wrong with fish-oil capsules. There could be something wrong with fish oil. People who eat cold-water ocean fish have less breast cancer. A lot less. Is it the fish? I don't know. Japanese women have far less breast cancer until they come to America. Once they've been here one generation, their incidence of breast cancer is one in nine, like ours.

You have two daughters who were seven and five when your wife was diagnosed. Are you concerned at all about their diet? About hormones in chicken and beef? Do you buy only organic?

When you put a hormone in beef—first of all, it's in super-small amounts. Second, it goes through your GI tract. These hormones are often made of amino acids and proteins, and they should be digested and they should go into your body as normal amino acids. There's no reason to think otherwise. Now, Europeans are quite concerned, but I don't understand that. I've talked to American scientists and here, very little concern exists. I am not down on meat. I am big on fiber. I think there's good data on that. So by pushing fiber and cutting back on fat, you're going to naturally cut down on meat consumption. There are populations, some Mormons as an example, that eat higher than the national average of meat. They also eat a lot of beans, but they eat more meat than the average American and yet they have a much lower cancer incidence. So there's something wrong with that whole meat hypothesis. I won't tell you that down the road we won't find that meat might cause a higher incidence of *something*.

We're really just at the beginning of understanding what all this is, aren't we?

Yes, but we're finding new things all the time. We're finding that certain amino acids tend to enhance immune function. Ar-

(continued)

ginine is one of them. Arginine is found in higher amounts in plant products generally than in animal products. Does that make an animal product bad? No. Does that mean you have to stop eating animal products? No. Does that mean that if you have a family history of cancer, you might eat more plant products? Yes, I think you could consider that. Does that mean you should go out to the public school and make everybody stop having hamburgers? No.

Was your shift to breast cancer research totally because of Candy's diagnosis?
Overnight what became a labor to make a living became a labor of love. I'm a good nutritionist and I know that there's nobody who'll do as good of a job researching literature as I will. I went into computer banks to pull out breast cancer information and I've got tons and tons and tons. I thought, Well, if I'm doing this, I should also be looking at setting up a study. I've got a number of students whose mothers or sisters or relatives had died of breast cancer. So I just pulled it together—research literature, students, and breast cancer patients who wanted to help.

How do you deal with it emotionally now that breast cancer is your work and home issue?
The thing that is interesting is that there are times when I feel like walking away from a talk on breast cancer, not from the field, but from a talk, because I feel like I need to hear something good, and the data I'm hearing is bad. I badly wanted to hear something really, really good at the breast cancer conference in San Antonio, and I heard some very promising things, but I heard more things that confirm that we're not as far as we want to be. I left that meeting feeling like our nutrition work is even more important. And it's even more important that I turn doctors around and make them start having some respect for nutrition as a part of the patients' therapy. Instead of feeling that everything will be answered

(continued)

via chemotherapy, they should view *nutrition* as a type of chemotherapy. It can act as a type of hormonal therapy. There's a potential that through diet, we can get your body to turn around and improve itself and hopefully kill off a stray tumor cell that got away when surgery and chemotherapy were used as treatment.

But can you do that with nutrition?

I think so, but the research is slower, because we're not sure of the combinations of food which give ideal results. If we bring up your natural killer cells with diet, the next question is are there four other types of tumor-killing agents that we've decreased but we haven't measured yet? But the point I want to make is nutritionists and oncologists are trying to find innovative ways to let your body heal itself—we're heading in the same direction. Instead of killing healthy cells while we kill bad cells, we want to find a way to let you selectively kill the bad cells. It takes painful, tedious research that needs to be done with various foods to find out what the magic combination is going to be. And I can tell you with good conscience that the more people we have out there looking from different directions—chemotherapy being direction one, diet being direction two, genetic engineering being direction three—the more likely a cure will be found in your lifetime. I feel that when people look at nutritional research support for cancer patients with disdain, they are being foolish.

Where does a woman find a nutritionist?

I think it's important for the public to be aware that the people who are certified, who are trained, and who have been examined nationally are dietitians, not nutritionists. There are a variety of people who call themselves nutritionists who come out of non-accredited schools or who have taken a series of correspondence courses. And I think one has to be very careful of that.

(continued)

Where can I get a list of foods and what they have in them?

Any nutrition textbook has it in the back of the book. Health-food stores generally take a little bit of stuff out of the research and then blow it way out. They push zinc supplements, they push selenium, whatever. I think they do much more damage than good. People get into all kinds of trouble trying to treat themselves without going to a dietitian.

What about vitamin C?

I don't recommend supplements, but I think vitamin C is very important. Orange juice and apples are just two good sources. If you eat the fruit with the vitamin C, you get the fiber also. If you just take a vitamin C pill, you don't get the fiber. The vitamin C is a good anti-oxidant. It's of no doubt that it's good for cancer patients. We also know that some fiber tends to bind to estrogen and estrogen metabolites, which is good. It's so much more pleasurable to sit and eat a good juicy orange than it is to swallow one more pill.

SPIRITUAL LIFE AND CANCER

"I was very angry at God. I had had all these friends who had nice lives. It didn't seem fair. It wasn't fair. I am still working on that."
—Mickey

"I choose to think God had his hand in it. I don't think he caused it, but I think he used it. My philosophy comes from the Scriptures. 'Where I live or die, it is thee.' I have turned it over."
—Elizabeth P

"I had a religious experience in the hospital. I felt the presence of God comforting me. I'm not religious. He was just there for me in my crisis."—Debra

"I used to ask God why and how. I feel like there has to be a reason. Maybe we don't know it yet. Maybe I can help somebody else."
—Angela

"I have no relationship with God right now. I really went through a tremendous crisis about that and I'm to the point right now . . . I just . . . there's nothing there for me right now. I hope eventually that will change."—Amy

I don't know how as human beings we cope with cancer unless we sense that there is meaning to it and to our lives in a spiritual sense. I don't mean necessarily an orthodox sense, but the sense that as a result of this chaos will be something sane and reasonable that we can look at and say, "Oh, now I understand."

With cancer we are stripped of the future and of our daily ritual for living. We must in a sense begin again, as if babies, to see the world. And when we have trusted that God will take care of us, it is often difficult to reconcile our vulnerability with our faith.

Everyone handles his or her relationship with a higher power differently. Some women went into the cancer experience with little spiritual sense and emerged renewed. Others had defined themselves as strong believers and came out shaken and bewildered. Personally, I chose to rely on God's promise that we are never given more than we can bear, hoping all along that I could somehow bargain that I have indeed learned my lesson and this is quite enough, thank you.

Mary-T and her husband, Len, relied on Romans: "For the good who trust the Lord and live according to his purpose. *It helped us tremendously in realizing what we had to do was seek the purpose."*

Soon after Mary-T was diagnosed, her husband lost his job. Consequently, they were forced to sell their home in the midst of her treatment. *"I would run into people in the strangest places and I would introduce myself, and they would know me or say, 'I remember hearing about you. I prayed for you.'"*

Mary-T said she remembers the moment that was the turning point for herself and Len. In the midst of losing her home and being in chemotherapy, she and Len received an IRS audit letter. *"When that happened it was kind of like Len flipped a page and said, 'I can handle anything that you lay on me because I have got all the help I need. Just bring it on now.' That did not mean that it stopped coming; the problems did not stop, but all of a sudden my whole response to problems was that I can handle anything. I have got the love of people. I have got the love of God. I can handle anything."*

Joanne said God's presence was very real for her. *"The day I went in for surgery, I was waiting for X ray in the hall and I just said, 'God, we can't play games anymore. Because I can't go through this if you don't let me know for sure that there's something there besides me. I have to know.' Then they took me into X ray and I was up against the wall and I felt a hand on my shoulder. And with every chemo treatment that I had, I put my hand on my shoulder. And that's how I made it."*

I have often equated my experience with breast cancer to ten years of instant therapy sessions. In a flash we have been taken to the very core of our existence. Sometimes what we find there is not what we expect, and if our faith is something we wrap around us instead of inviting inside, we soon find ourselves on shaky ground.

Dr. Charles Kluge's list of the six things cancer survivors can do to help themselves heal included daily contemplation or introspection—it seems another word for that in the Christian context would be prayer.

Song was another great release for me, and I sing songs while I drive, most of which I learned in church. These songs move me and help me feel the presence of the Lord. Some days when I am driving and feeling sorry for myself, a hymn will begin to get me out of myself and I look at the world outside the window and see the people who have so much less than I in terms of comfort and community. It never fails to get me back on track. As my daughter has gotten older, we have begun to sing in the car together.

Whatever works on your spirit and soul is healing.

Those women I feel have gone way beyond me in their faith journeys immediately began looking for the gifts in their cancer.

Gifts? How can that be? Yet so many women listed those ways that their life was enriched and healed and helped by cancer. The gifts equation made some sense to me after I heard a sermon in which the minister was talking about church and what it meant and that it went beyond the walls of the building with the stained glass to the very real Scripture that says when two or more are gathered in God's name. In that sense, I have had a lot of church with my cancer.

Identify your gifts and surrender to them with passion—because your gifts are from God, and in surrendering to them you are doing God's work. And if you are doing God's work, you cannot help but make the world a better place.

Could it not be that cancer helps people find or engage their gifts and the power of this experience certainly makes us surrender no matter how strong we are. Are we not, therefore, by finding the gifts in this experience, doing God's work?

ALTERNATIVE "CURES"?

"I had a friend whose aunt had breast cancer and she was curing it herself with mind therapy. She was diagnosed six months before me and wouldn't have a mastectomy or any treatment. So she did nothing but mind control. But at the time this friend was telling me her aunt was fine and she was doing macrobiotic diet and mind control. Well, I talked to her about a year ago and her aunt died."—Mickey

When I began looking for women to interview for this book, I placed an ad in a local quasi-alternative paper that has a large personals section. Sandwiched between the men-looking-for-women section and men-looking-for-men section was a section for miscellaneous searches, where I placed my "writer looking for breast cancer patients" ad. The first answer I received was from a woman who began by saying she would talk to me if I was going to "tell the truth" about cancer.

Since I was still looking for "the truth," I eagerly sent her a survey form.

Her completed survey indicated she had refused all orthodox treatment for what she said had shown up on a mammogram to be a large cancerous tumor. Her survey was peppered with phrases about medical science such as "quackery in the most evil sense"; it said that we must be "deprogrammed from lifelong medical misbeliefs" and that the surgery suggested was "unnecessary mutilation." She chose instead "detoxification, enzyme therapies, electromagnetic therapy, castor-oil packs, vitamin C IVs, colonic therapy, spiritual de-stressing, biofeedback, wheatgrass therapy," and more.

I have to admit that at that time it threw me. As a journalist, I have been trained to look at things objectively. She was still alive; I had no reason to distrust her information any more than what was presented by any other woman. When I called her for an interview, I began asking more specifics about her diagnosis and biopsy. I am still not clear about whether there was a biopsy nor its outcome. She would not—or could not—answer my specific questions about her regimen. Neither could she give me any kind of statistics on a cure rate for her alternative cocktail. She would discuss these issues only in person with me at the location of her choice, where she planned to have other converts to talk to me. This was all presented in the best John Le Carré secret formula kind of presentation. I refused. My objective sense screamed "setup," and there was no doubt in my mind that had she produced a football stadium full of women who had chosen alternative therapies, I would still have been skeptical. I needed a balanced look, and I knew from the outset that the issues and the direction of this book would, like my own treatment choices, remain accepted medical procedures combined with complementary healing.

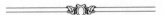

Tip—Anything that is a great secret is not a cure.

But assuming all she said was true, that she did have a large malignant tumor and was now fine—indeed, that she had become a professional alternative healer—why wasn't she dead? Had I been wrong? Was I not as good and smart as this woman? I never considered including alternative healing in this book because I never took it seriously. I kept thinking I would never find someone who had actually been cured. Now I was talking to her on the phone. She was emotional and committed and had not lost a breast; it was easy to get sucked in.

And then, as I began to talk about this woman and my second thoughts, everyone knew someone who knew someone who had chosen something other than orthodox medicine and had had a miraculous healing. One old friend even said, "I have a friend who cured his brain cancer with nutrition," a statement that leaves hanging in the air the unsaid second sentence, "Why didn't you do that? I guess you aren't as in touch or smart enough to cure yourself. You have to use *doctors.*"

Approaching the issue like a journalist, albeit one whose objectivity was greatly compromised, I visited the local health-food store, where the bookshelves were filled with the "truth" about nutrition, herbs, attitude, and the medical profession. I wrote to the addresses they offered and got thousands of photocopied colored pages of names of alternative "doctors" both in and out of the country who offered a mix of regimens that appeared to range from witchcraft to perfectly reasonable-sounding regimens for a healthy life-style. Along with these came the lists of names of those people whom I could contact for testimonials, and flyers of beautiful below-the-border clinics that showed pictures of the grounds and the rooms and gave detailed arrival instructions. Some offered medical regimens not significantly different than what I had encountered, but also blended complementary healing issues.

After laughing with my husband about drinking "juiced grass" to cure cancer, I began taking wheatgrass and felt a real surge of energy. I also found books by those who claimed to be healed by macrobiotic cooking. Bernie Siegel's books about his work with exceptional cancer patients pointed to incredible untapped sources in the human body that can heal if we know how to use them.

I read one book that documented spontaneous remissions in cancer patients who were doing nothing exceptional. Then I read accounts of the dangers of some herbs that told how for some people the limited "miraculous cure" diets can be very dangerous. I read case histories of those who had done all the right alternatives and died. I dug up the government's controversy about Laetrile, a drug that is still used today in alternative circles and that the government tested extensively and found useless. Then I read the other side, which said the government fixed the study, using only people who were too sick to gain any help because Laetrile was too cheap to produce and would ruin the medical establishment.

My oncologist would not comment on any of it, saying simply that if he couldn't see a study on it, it didn't exist. When I asked if he had seen any patients "will" themselves to health, he said no, but he has certainly seen people "will" themselves to a premature death.

I can see why people are drawn to charismatic healers who promise health. Our medical profession deals in numbers and studies, often without looking up at the terrified human being sitting naked before them. I had been fortunate to have doctors who were sensitive and humane. But I knew women who didn't, and I could see in much of the alternative writings a desire for more humane holistic treatment that was *driving* cancer patients from orthodox treatments. Indeed, the line blurred for me about whether it was the coffee enemas, the gallons of juiced vegetables, or the *faith* in the healer or the cure that brought about the heralded results.

It's exciting to think that it is possible to cure cancer through means independent of medical intervention. However, when faced with a cancer diagnosis, you must be aware of the temptation to embrace undocumented cures presented by people who are quick to point out the failure rates of standard medicine. Their success stories will be given to you in testimonial after testimonial; you'll never hear the grueling statistics from them that you have heard from your oncologist.

Where then is the unbiased, logical, rational look at all of this? Is there a middle ground? I found only black-and-white voices—either you were a pawn of the AMA or you refused to set foot in a doctor's office.

I finally found a voice of reason in the person of Michael Lerner. He is a Ph.D., former Yale professor, recipient of the MacArthur Foundation Fellowship, and consultant to the government on a study of alternative and unproven cancer cures. Lerner operates the Commonweal Cancer Help Program in Bolinas, California, a residence program where cancer patients are offered a variety of workshops in physical, mental, emotional, and spiritual healing. The workshops offer a wide range of *complementary* healing therapies to be used in addition to orthodox medical treatment.

Lerner's forays into alternative healing began in 1982, when his father was diagnosed with cancer. At that time he began a scientific exploration of alternative therapies, visiting thirty clinics. He published his findings in *The Cancer Report, a work in progress on Alternative and Adjunctive Cancer Therapies with a Primary Emphasis on Intelligent and Informed Personal Choice in the Integration of Conventional, Adjunctive and Alternative Treatment Systems.*

His conclusions:

1) "I have seen no cure for cancer among unconventional cancer therapies, in the sense of a documented intervention that reliably cures any form of cancer;

2) There are very few scientific studies of these therapies;

3) There is reliable case evidence and anecdotal evidence that some cancer patients have recovered from life-threatening cancer while using these therapies.

4) While there are unethical quack practitioners and desperate credulous patients, these old stereotypes are very unrepresentative of the field as a whole, in which many ethical physicians are treating patients who are making informed personal choices, and in a very large majority of cases, continuing conventional therapies as part of a combined program;

5) There is a movement toward convergence among some thoughtful practitioners and researchers in conventional and complementary cancer therapies, and a growing consensus that a higher level of constructive dialogue is possible about the benefits of psychological, behavioral, nutritional, and other complementary approaches to the cancer problem."

In his continuing analysis of unconventional cancer treatments, Lerner explores in detail a number of clinics and approaches, trying to provide balance where possible. There is one conclusion from *The Cancer Report* that comes after a discussion of the persons involved in offering treatments:

"Having said that there are certainly impaired physicians and inhumane practices in the field of unconventional cancer therapies, and that the unregulated nature of the field in North America contributes to this state of affairs, I wish to emphasize that the study of unconventional cancer therapies demonstrates the existence of many interventions and approaches to the treatment of cancer that could, today, immeasurably improve the lot of cancer patients. Let us not be distracted by the bizarre, the eccentric, and the esoteric elements in unconventional therapies and ignore the constructive side of the field."

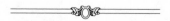

Tip—Remember that those who offer alternatives are saying what you want to hear. Be rational.

Admittedly, there is growing evidence that attests to the importance of complementary healing in areas such as nutrition and mind/body issues, and their acceptance as part of an overall approach to wellness and healing. And the distinction in the past few years between accepted complementary healing issues and alternative therapies has blurred.

But the results of complementary healing are not conclusive and present an impossible array of aspects that defy control-group analysis to determine their potential in *healing cancer.* Clearly, the cause and effect that many alternative healers present has no basis in science. But those trained to believe in and administer only what they can see verified in studies are coming around as nutrition and mind/body issues are being shown as clinically beneficial to their patients. And while few are inviting nutritionists to join their staff, others are, perhaps begrudgingly, listening and learning from patients who are demanding a more holistic approach to their care.

Indeed, even the government has sanctioned the existence of alternative approaches with the announcement in early 1993 that National Institutes of Health would open a new Office of Alternative Medicine. According to an article in *The New York Times,* the new office has begun accepting proposals for grant funds to explore the entire range of alternative healing: from homeopathy and the use of herbs to mind/body techniques such as visualization and guided imagery. The office is headed by a pediatrician whose upbringing included exposure to Native American healing. Typically, the reactions from the medical community to the new office have ranged from enthusiastic support (from researchers eager for the financial backing that would allow legitimate, scientific studies on their approaches) to criticism from those who think only their own approach is valid to blanket rejection from those who just holler, "Hogwash."

For the near future this still leaves each of us to address the issue of personal healing individually, with the understanding that medical science is not perfect and tends to discount those things it cannot "study." We must address with knowledge and skepticism all treatment options until convinced of their worth—and then be willing to look not only to others for answers to our lives, but also within ourselves. Perhaps in the next decade we will find a middle ground where finding the cause of cancer will become as important as finding a cure.

RESOURCES

If you are considering an alternative therapy, move with caution. An excellent resource is *Third Opinion, An International Directory to Alternative Therapy Centers for the Treatment and Prevention of Cancer*, by John Fink (Avery Publishing Group, 1988). This book offers some objective guidelines on alternative therapies as well as a listing of clinics, who operates them, a description of their services and the illness treated. It does not give any assessment of the quality of the treatment or if the treatment works. *Third Opinion* also offers an excellent resource section that lists educational centers and support centers across the country. Many of the organizations listed offer complementary as well as alternative healing.

At the same time I would recommend reviewing a copy of *Unconventional Cancer Treatments*. This document, which was published in 1990 by the United States government, has a summary that can be purchased through the government or your local Government Printing Office (GPO) for about $2. The actual document was out of print by November 1991. Unfortunately, when the government sells out of something, it's just no longer available. The clerk at the GPO in Washington told me that the Office of Technology Assessment would reprint something if there was enough interest, but it wasn't clear how that would happen. So call first to see if you can get the original document. If not, copies are available in major libraries. The GPO stock numbers are 052-003-01207-3 for *Unconventional Cancer Treatments* and GPO stock number 052-003-0128-1 for the Summary. Call the GPO (202) 783-3238 for information, or try your local GPO. Dallas had copies of the summary available locally.

The 312-page document explores both complementary and alternative healing approaches in the usual bureaucratic style, but with a balanced approach that is easy to read and extremely informative. The advisory panel that compiled this information included people from mainstream organizations and well as from what would be called complementary and alternative organizations, including the Gerson Institute, the Mayo Clinic, the Institute of Transpersonal Psychology, the Institute of Noetic Sciences, and George Washington University School of Medicine. The document explores behavioral and psychological approaches, dietary treatments, herbal treatments, pharmacologic and biologic treatments, immuno-augmentative therapy. It also addresses the questions of who uses unconventional cancer treatments and the laws governing such treatments. The bibliography alone is an excellent resource.

Varieties of Integral Cancer Therapy, by Michael Lerner, Ph.D., $26.00, Commonweal, P.O. Box 316, Bolinas, CA 94924; (415) 868-0970. Lerner's descriptions of each of the thirty cancer clinics he visited while exploring complementary and alternative healing practices is an excellent resource if you are considering alternative and complementary healing. It is updated with reprints of articles and gives the most balanced view of these issues, with a short explanation of the best-known alternative clinics.

Other Books on Complementary Healing:
There are probably hundreds of books that explore complementary healing issues. The ones that follow are only a few that were offered as helpful by the women I interviewed.

Dr. Bernie Siegel offers a catalog of books and tapes through his program for exceptional cancer patients. Write to 1302 Chapel Street, New Haven, CT 06511 or call (203) 865-8392.

Healing and the Mind, by Bill Moyers (Doubleday, 1993)

Cancer as a Turning Point, by Lawrence LeShan, Ph.D. (Dutton, 1989)

Triumph, Getting Back to Normal When You Have Cancer, by Marion Morra and Eve Potts (Avon, 1990)

Recovering the Soul, by Larry Dossey, M.D. (Bantam, 1989)

Medicine and Meaning, by Larry Dossey, M.D. (Bantam, 1991)

The Cancer Conqueror, by Greg Anderson (Word, 1988)

Quantum Healing, by Depak Chopra (Bantam, 1989)

Love, Medicine & Miracles and *Peace, Love & Healing,* by Bernie Siegel, M.D. (Harper & Row, 1986, 1989)

I Will Live Today, by Judith Garrett Garrison, M.Ed. LSW, and Scott Sheperd, Ph.D. (CompCare Publishers, 1990)

The Road Back to Health, by Neil A. Fiore, Ph.D. (Bantam, 1984)

Getting Well Again, by Stephanie Matthews-Simonton and Carl Simonton, M.D. (Bantam, 1978)

Help Yourself Heal, by Bill L. Little, Ph.D. (CompCare Publishers, 1990)

Choice in Cancer, by Michael Lerner, Ph.D. (available from Commonweal at $29)

Books on Nutrition:
Diet, Nutrition and Cancer Prevention: a Guide to Food Choices, the U.S. Department of Health and Human Services. NIH publication number 87-2878; available from 1-800-4-cancer.
Eating Hints: Recipes for Better Nutrition During Cancer Treatment, NIH publication No 87-2079. These are both free.
Nutrition Action provides research and recipes from the Center for Science in Public Interest, Suite 300, 1875 Connecticut Avenue NW, Washington, DC 20009. It costs $20.00 a year for ten issues.

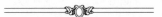

Tip—Call the U.S. government's Nutrition Hotline for more information. It is staffed by a dietitian. (301) 344–3719.

Information on Music Therapy:
To find a music therapist close to you, call 1-800-765-CBMT, or the National Association for Music Therapy, (301) 589-3300.

PART III

LIFE AFTER
BREAST CANCER

EMOTIONAL AND PHYSICAL ISSUES

Chapter 7

LIFE AFTER BREAST CANCER: THE EMOTIONAL ISSUES

"It's a chronic stressor. I did my dissertation on psycho-social stress on major life events versus the little daily hassles. And it's the chronic stuff that you can't really do anything about, that wears away, eats away on you. And this is just one more chronic stressor." —Elizabeth T's husband, Hugh

"When you have had cancer, you can't ever really throw it over your shoulder. I hate the thought that it's still on my mind." —Pat H

It has been a year or so since the diagnosis and surgery or treatment. Externally, we look great. Treatment is over, and our hair is long enough to wear without the wig. The prosthesis or reconstruction trivializes our losses as well-meaning friends comment on how good we look and make such statements as, "Aren't you glad that's over? Now you can put that behind you and get on with your life."

While our loss is hidden to the outside world, we may feel isolated and sense that our doctors have abandoned us. We feel that our family is as tired of hearing about breast cancer as we are of going through it. It should be over, but it isn't.

"Who is watching me now?" said one woman.

We are set adrift at the time when we are at last accepting that our bodies and souls and relationships have been altered forever.

Our friends and family have moved on to other issues. Our husbands

343

and children are back in the routine, eager to put this behind them. *We* want life to be as it was. We try to pretend it is behind us. But we are caught by our children's faces as they change, or an annual trip to a friend or relative brings sadness as a little voice says, "What about next year. Will you be here?" We brush these thoughts away, hoping no one saw. Our husbands or boyfriends look at us quizzically. If we can voice these feelings to them, they give us reassurance: It is over. It is time to move forward.

We are ready, yet with each step we know that life is different. Our bodies are different; our priorities are different; our relationships are different.

For those of us who haven't begun the emotional work of coping with breast cancer, we may do what my support group likes to call "crash and burn," when the intellectualizing and "get on with it" attitude have developed a crack. All of a sudden the fear of recurrence rears its ugly head. All of a sudden we just can't keep it together. All of a sudden we are back at *day one*.

> *"My first year was not that hard. I went through chemo for the first seven months after diagnosis. Then, at a year out, I got depressed. I went to see my surgeon and got up on the table and just wept. I just wept. I said, 'I don't understand this. I have been so strong and every-thing's gone right and the prognosis was good and I think I'm okay, that it's all right. But I'm not.' She made an appointment with a ther-apist, and I went to see her and wept for a solid hour."*—Joanne

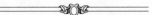

Tip—Many of the women interviewed for this book said the true emotional devastation of this disease did not begin for them until a year to eighteen months after the diagnosis.

A breast cancer diagnosis changes the woman and her family and their relationships. If the emotional adjustments are on track, there are family adjustments that relate to a critical illness in a family. These may mean dreams cancelled or lives rearranged.

Larry and Cindy loved to skin-dive, and shortly before Cindy's diagnosis they decided to sell everything and move to the Caribbean, but the cancer changed their dreams.

> *"We just figured we'd postpone everything five years. We just altered the timetable. And that's when I went ahead and opened the dive shop here. I thought, Well, that will keep me busy and keep me involved in the business while we're going through the remission period, and once we get to a certain point, we'll go ahead and do what we planned on doing. But now I figure we'll keep this shop here and keep the house here so we can come back. Because I don't feel like we could ever just pick up and move down there now."*—Cindy's fiancé, Larry

Nancy W had made a career change from computers to nursing school just before she was diagnosed. With three small children and the life changes she made during the cancer, Nancy ultimately put nursing school on hold to home-school one of her children, who had had difficulty during her diagnosis and needed to make up for lost time.

For some women the loss of professional time during surgery and treatment may mean lost credentials or professional standing. Teresa M, a Reach to Recovery volunteer, recalls meeting a young woman doctor. *"She was thirty years old. She had lost both breasts, and she and I were sitting there talking and she said, 'I really put my life on hold for this. I don't have any medical practice left. What am I going to do? I'm going to be in chemotherapy for the next six months to a year. I'll have to start all over again.'"*

Mortality issues strip us, and as we heal both physically and emotionally, we must accept that everything and everyone has changed. Change—some like it and others hate it, and how you feel about it will determine the ease with which you (and your loved ones) face this transition into the future after breast cancer.

SEX AFTER BREAST CANCER

"I have a nurse who asks the patients if they have returned to sexual intercourse in the same way they used to. The wife is waiting for the

husband to make some overture, and the husband wants to, but he says, 'I don't want to act like an animal. The lady just went through a big operation. She must be in terrible pain. And I don't want to jump on her body.' And then the wife says, 'Oh my God. I'm so ugly, he doesn't even want to—he doesn't even bring up the issue.' Whereas the husband is only trying to be polite. So then what you have is that frequently the two of them are not discussing it."—breast surgeon Jeanne Petrek, M.D.

Intimacy is the ultimate act of trust and acceptance, which means that in those first few intimate encounters, many other emotions may be intermingled with the passion as the woman begins to let down her guard and feel not only the good feelings of passion but the variety of other emotions connected to what has happened to her.

This new dimension of sex will invariably change our intimate encounters—at least for a while—and perhaps put a new spotlight on an act that in the past was mystical and magical. As Marjorie's husband, Chuck, says, *"I don't know how you put it, but it's like you change the deal. Whatever you had, you can't say, Look, we were this way and we're gonna find these methodologies and I'm gonna get back to exactly that. I think you adapt. You're going to change in ways and hope the sum total is going to be positive. But if you think you're going to go back the way you were before it happened in every respect, you're wrong. It doesn't happen."*

One of the most treasured moments of my life will always be the first time my husband kissed the scar where my breast used to be. I cried, but remember trying to hide the emotion from him, assuming he wouldn't understand. But then I recall crying, or stifling tears, frequently during those first few intimate moments, so thrilled was I to be alive and to be feeling so loved and accepted. Passion was secondary in those early months to the pockets of grief that tended to surface during lovemaking.

"For a while there he was into my sickness and feelings—holding hands doing the chemotherapy treatments, and he even volunteered to go with me into the radiation room because I suffer from claustrophobia. But afterwards when it was all over and done, it was like we were the same person, and I had a hard time relating to him sexually as a woman again. It was like he knew me so well that he was me. It took

us some time there to get over that. That we were separate sexual individuals again; we had some problems there for a while."—Lise

"Norm wouldn't let intimacy be a problem. We have very good communication in our marriage. I think men need to encourage their wives that they are the same person as they were before. Their personality does not change just because they have lost a breast."
—Lynne

"The sex part remains tough. I don't think I will ever feel like I was before physically. With the nipple done it will be better, but I just don't think we'll ever do it the same way. Specifically, I wear my nightgown all the time when we make love. Before, I wouldn't. I think it will be that way for a while. I don't see that changing. That is hard for me. I don't think Bill really even cares."—Ann

"It was so wonderful; it really was. After I came home from the hospital the intimacy was there and I don't know how he knew to, how he did it so well. I'm sure that many men try, but they are afraid they are going to hurt their wives after they have surgery, so they are not sure what to do. They don't mean to reject them but I'm sure a lot of women take it as rejection."—Dot

"She says that we're not as intimate, our sex life is not the same, and she's right to some extent. But the why is wrong. We have been so busy trying to fight this situation. I've been so busy trying to get this new business off the ground, that I come home at night after sixteen hours a day, seven days a week during the season. And there's sixteen years difference in age. And I keep telling her that, too. I said it doesn't have anything to do with the fact that you've had a mastectomy and all that. So we've had those kinds of talks. But I'm not sure she really accepts my explanation."—Cindy's fiancé, Larry

"I was sitting at the dressing table with my robe sort of open, and he whistled at me. I said, 'From there you can't see the other side, can you?' He said no, and then he came over and opened my robe and kissed me about four times on that side and said, 'This does not bother me.' The first time he held me, I probably cried for a couple of hours and he just held me. There was nothing to say to make that pain go away. We joke about it now, but there's still a deep pain."—Joanne

"The first time we had sex, all I could think was that I felt whole again. He was so gentle. I cried. I'm crying because this man loves me for who I am and not what I look like."—Diana

Conversely, the new tension in those intimate moments may come from one or both of you trying not to let go, for fear the feelings will be overwhelming. Marjorie said that she and her husband, Chuck, talked after it was clear that sex was not as it used to be. *"I don't re-member who initiated it, but at one point I said, 'Tell me what you're feeling. It can't be all me. Part of it is you. So tell me what you're feeling.' He said he was afraid of letting it affect him, and just his fear of letting it affect him, affected him."*

Marjorie said he told her that letting it affect him made him feel like he had failed her. *"I thought, Well, how natural. And it was really won-derful. But he expected me to get upset and sulk and be hurt that he had actually admitted to me, 'Yes, the changes in your body have affected me.' I didn't. I just said, 'Of course it has affected you. I'm not surprised.' "*

Chuck agrees that they have not dealt with the issue well, due to the confusion of issues surrounding sex. *"Part of the problem is that you can't look at a situation and say, Well, this percentage of the problem is due to this factor—cancer—and this percentage is due to my inadequacies emo-tionally or your self-image, which may or may not be positive. So it's very hard, because you have a tendency to overemphasize the effect of the thing that's easy to talk about. But it may or may not be accurate. There's no way to tell."*

For couples who have successfully experienced sex for many years at a purely emotional level, the analyzing and discussion may be as detrimental to the passion as any more concrete issue. As Chuck says, *"There is a consciousness of intimacy that there was not before this happened."*

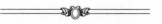

Tip—Work on getting your emotions to the surface. Sit naked on the floor in front of a full-length mirror with your partner behind you. Let him hold and caress your new body as you watch.

In my research on the grief experience, I came to the conclusion that stifling a strong feeling—no matter what it is—tends to stifle all strong feelings. It's like they are all in the same bag, and when we let one out, they all come out. So when we use our energy to keep our fear and anger suppressed, it also keeps passion and trust and love suppressed with it.

Communicating with your partner about sex and having sex during and after breast cancer can be a complicated, scary, emotional issue as each partner tries to sort out new feelings. As Mary-T's husband, Len, said, *"Everyone just has to work a little harder at it."*

"When Chuck touches my real breast, I can feel his indecision. Like, Do I ignore the other one? Do I touch that one? He makes the decision to touch it, to act like it's real, and I always want to say, Just ignore it, because it makes me aware that I can't feel it. It just feels weird. But I've never told him that because the only time I think about it is when he's doing it and that's just not the right time."—Marjorie B

Joyce's breasts were important to her sense of sensuality. *"I loved my breasts. They were very erotic. It was part of sex. It was part of orgasm. It was a big part of my sexual, sensual life. And frankly, for a long while I thought I would never orgasm again in my life. I thought sex was gone."*

Joyce sought a therapist who was experienced in sexual issues as they related to illness. The therapist recommended a book called *Great Sex.* *"We talked about technique, about dealing with my problem. What do I need? Am I able to communicate what it is I need? Well, hell no. I need a natural, normal body. I just want my boobs to be boobs! You know? Well, you work through all of that. And if you have a loving, caring husband, then you really work through it. And I have to say, sex is better than it's ever been."*

Joyce says that to her, the issue of sexuality is empowerment and women understanding that they have the right to enjoy sex and not just submit. She says the therapist encouraged her to explore her body, to experiment and discover what felt good. *"Does it feel good to be kissed on the neck? The biggest sex organ on the body is the skin. Nothing is more sensual than touch. What feels good? If he kisses your thigh? If he kisses your neck? If he touches, down the center, through the cleavage? Is there feeling there, close to the breasts? Do you worry about not feeling in your breasts? Eighty-five percent of sex is in your head. Once you know that, then what you think about as he touches your reconstructed breast mound—then all you're doing now is just focusing. Not on whether it feels, but on what DOES feel."*

The exercise that proved to be most valuable helped Joyce refocus during arousal or clitoral stimulation. *"The therapist said to breathe through the vagina. You took deep breaths. Your breath was coming in. It helped you focus. That was the purpose of that exercise. To breathe in and out. Your whole focus. It was easy for me to do that because when I meditate I focus on breathing. It still is a wonderful technique for focusing. For getting your attention off not having breasts anymore and on restoring the sweetness between you and your partner."*

Joyce also consulted with her gynecologist some weeks after her mastectomy, when she felt that her libido had diminished. She felt that she couldn't heal unless her sex life was healed also. *"I didn't want to be touched, and I knew that I really enjoyed sex years ago—in another life. I had a new body. I had to learn new things. I had done some research that said testosterone will sometimes bring the libido back to life. You don't take much—just a couple of milligrams a week. I still take it three years out and my libido is better than ever. It's not for everyone—if you are on tamoxifen, you can't take it. It took two years to put myself back in sync sexually."*

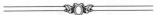

Tip—A low testosterone level can result in reduced sexual drive. Ask your ob/gyn to test your level if you suspect this may be a problem.

Intimacy can be complicated by the physical changes brought on by the treatment for breast cancer, such as tamoxifen and chemotherapy, which many women say affect their sex life dramatically. Also, there are changes in birth control for women who can no longer take the pill and must now become comfortable with condoms or other forms of birth control. It's one more obstacle to spontaneous sex.

"It never stopped the lovemaking. The only time we did stop was when I was in pain or was physically not able. It was difficult at first because he was trying to figure out how to hold me so he wouldn't hurt me. The hardest thing has been using rubbers."—Cindy

"We no longer have intercourse, because of the vagina shrinking and the tissue being so thin. It is too painful. But it has been better. He is more affectionate. Now it isn't just sex, it's the real thing. That's more important to me and a positive. On the other hand, some people might have a problem with that."—Elizabeth P

"I think of our relationship changing in terms of sexuality. After the surgery I wanted to keep my gown on, and he would get frustrated with me. Why is this thing on? It was a subtle thing. He didn't push me to take it off; he just made a statement. I remember he wouldn't touch me around the scars. I told him it didn't hurt and I had a real need to be touched there. Bless his heart, when he did touch me there my nerves were sensitive and then I would say, 'That is enough.' It was damned if you do and damned if you don't and you give off some real mixed messages."—Jo Anne

"If he had shown any reluctance or standoffishness toward me, it would have affected me. I would have been very depressed. But he didn't. The first thing home out of the hospital, we made love. It was the most important thing that happened to me. I don't think he was thinking, She needs to know I want her. He said, 'Does it bother you that I want you now?' So he wasn't thinking that. He was thinking I want her, and he had no idea what a boost he gave my morale right then."—Kit

"I was really worried that he was going to want to stay with me more out of sympathy than out of true love, and that was the thing that was a real kind of concern with me at first. It was strange because I got real timid. I felt like I had to prove myself all over again."
—Theresa

NURSE COUNSELOR AND BREAST CANCER SURVIVOR LOIS GREEN, R.N., FORMER PRESIDENT OF THE NASHVILLE COUNCIL ON HUMAN SEXUALITY, TALKS ABOUT SEX AND BREAST CANCER

Lois Green, a nurse counselor in Nashville, Tennessee, offers a unique perspective: She is a breast cancer survivor, a single woman, and the former president of the Council on Human Sexuality in Nashville. Since her diagnosis and modified radical in 1985 at age forty-four, Green has begun a breast-concerns support group for presurgery women and survivors. In addition, she counsels women and men about sexual issues prior to and after breast cancer.

What are the issues in resuming sexuality after surgery?

What I talk about from the beginning is the openness and communication and sharing about what each other needs. And I tell the partner that at the beginning, the woman is not going to be able to deal with his feelings until she is stronger and has recovered somewhat from the surgical procedures. He has to be the strong one and may need some help in dealing with it because she is often so confused she cannot give him clear messages about what is going on. She is overwhelmed. I tell her to include him as much as she can. Take him to the doctor; let him be with you.

How do you begin discussing sexuality with the women and men you counsel?

First, we explore a woman's three developmental periods surrounding the breast. From the time we begin to develop as preteens, we focus on the breast whether we want to or not. It is the rare woman who is not aware of the development of her breasts. For many of us it is a time of anxiety and happy anticipation. What are they going to be like and how big will I be and what

(continued)

will they feel like? There are those parts of us that say, What if they are too big, or too small? Are we going to be made fun of? So much goes into that developmental time that men are not aware of because women don't share that with brothers or fathers.

The second developmental issue is when women become intimate as teens—the first fondling, when someone feels your breast, and then full intimacy. Then the breasts take on a new meaning of sexuality. Many women are able to achieve orgasm just from having their breasts stimulated. For those women, the loss of a breast would be worse than for those of us who enjoy the feelings but don't reach orgasm.

So you have intimacy, and then when she enters the period of motherhood, even if she is not a mother, there is the sense of nurturing. It is human nature for women to bring men, women, and children to their breast to console and nurture them, and it is more profound if they breast-feed. Although I did not breast-feed, I remember so exquisitely holding my son in my arms and having him rest against my breast.

Most women identify strongly with those three things. When you add what society thinks and the *Playboy* attitude about breasts, we begin to think that our breasts are how men see us. When I talk with men, that is not how they see us. That is why it is important for me to meet with the man and woman and have her confirm that this is what she thinks and then have him say how he feels about her breasts. So often what the guys say is, "I love her breasts, but she isn't her breasts. *She* is the important thing." Women need to hear that.

What can you do to help the woman see that?
I ask if the woman holds her husband's testicles during intimacy. If she recoils, then I stay away. But if she agrees, then I ask if she enjoys the feeling. If she agrees, then I say, "If something were to happen to one, I am assuming that you would be sad, for yourself and for him, because this is an important part of his

(continued)

maleness. However, would you consider leaving him for a man who had two?"

And they say, "Well, of course not." Then I say it is the same thing with your breast. That is the closest analogy there is. The testicles are the closest comparable body part for a man.

How do you see the woman coping in reality?

There is withdrawal from the husband sexually. She doesn't want him to see the scar site. What I hear most often from women is the closed-door syndrome. The lights are off and the poor man doesn't know what to do. If he reaches for her, she sees it as horny, and he isn't thinking about her emotional needs. If he doesn't touch, she thinks he feels repulsed by her. It is a no-win situation for a while. If they both talk about it, they can work through it.

When is it reasonable to resume sex?

As soon as they feel like it. I tell him to listen to what she is saying but not to allow the closed door between them. When that starts happening, when she starts pulling away, he has to say, "How can I help?" and pursue that. I try to tell them both that when he does reach out to touch her, she may begin to cry and it's not because it hurts or it's wrong, but it's that all of a sudden you are missing a breast and it brings that all back. This becomes critically important because therapists know that for many couples, how it goes the first time they make love is going to set the stage for how healthy they are going to be sexually in the years to come after surgery. So it is extremely important that sexual issues are addressed and that women feel comfortable dealing with this from the very beginning. If they wait and things don't go well, then the wall begins to build. And in this society, sexuality is often not a healthy issue for most people already, so if you add any negative to that picture, you may have some real problems that may be hard to get rid of.

(continued)

Do you have suggestions for making that easier?

What I do is talk about the husband or partner touching the body again. Letting her lead in that and putting his hand where she wants it to be. Getting to know the body again. That is also true with reconstruction and the need to bond with a new body part. I say, "You got to know your breasts for years by touch and this is a new body part and you owe it to yourself to get to know this one." She should explore to find what feeling is left, with the understanding that for women who had a sexual focus on the breast and nipple and may have had a bilateral, they now have lost that connection between the nipple and the clitoris. It is sad that my reconstructed left nipple, as pretty as it is, has no connection with my clitoris. I miss that. And I miss the flexibility of my left breast. I miss that they don't match. One is soft and the other is firm. That doesn't put down the reconstruction. I am enormously grateful for what I have and what medical science could do for me. But I don't feel that reconstruction kept me from the loss.

What are the other issues you address?

Women must be given permission for self-pleasure, both those who don't have a partner and those who do. Men have this permission, but women don't. Men know their bodies and know what feels good, and most sex educators agree that if the woman doesn't know what feels good to her, she is not going to be able to convey that to her partner. We lose a lot by not knowing ourselves.

I do talk with the men about the loss of sensation in the breast and point out to them that if she was very sensitive, then the remaining breast, of course, is there, but he may want to find other places and other body areas to see what brings pleasure. For women who have had bilateral, I recommend they explore around the cleavage and up to the neck to see what sensation is left and what feels good. Explore that area. And I point out that we focus on one area where there may be many others that bring pleasure.

(continued)

Do you discuss other sexual techniques for those women who cannot have vaginal intercourse?

I don't generally in group, but I have had one woman who had some other problems and had very thin membrane and vaginal dryness, and I counseled with her individually. She did not have a partner at the time and was concerned about how she would be perceived as a partner for anyone. I said I didn't want her to hear that I was recommending that she be a receptacle for a man, but there are other parts of your body that can be brought into play and the mouth is not the only one. I have to be sensitive to those who are open to anal intercourse and those who aren't and help those women see that they can derive pleasure from this if they are receptive to it.

What does a support group offer in these discussions?

Women learn so much from other women. In one instance one woman in her fifties was talking about having sexual desire but being dry when one of the younger women in her thirties said, "Honey, let me tell you about Astroglide."

What about vaginal lubricants?

Doctors are recommending them. The advantage of Replens is that it isn't something just for when you are going to have sex. Replens is inserted three times a week and keeps you lubricated all the time. It is more like your natural body fluids and keeps you ready for action at all times.

As a single woman after breast cancer, how did you handle sex?

I had been married twenty-three years and was involved with several men when I was diagnosed. One had lost a mother to breast cancer, and I was aware of his departure and why. The others were very supportive, and one of those, I am still with. Before the breast was removed, I was thinking, How are these or

(continued)

any other guys going to react to this? I had been very sensual and sexual and open, and now I was wondering how they would deal with this maimed woman. Even with reconstruction, I knew there would be a time when it was not complete. It was a very scary time.

I remember the first time I showed a man, thinking I would watch his reaction closely. I don't remember how much preparation I gave him. I got into bed with clothes on, and as I was getting ready to remove the top, he said, "Are you okay with this." I said, I have to get this done. It was crucial. If he had looked displeased, I would have been crushed. I felt very, very vulnerable. He looked and there wasn't a change in expression and he said, "That's not bad."

SEX AND THE SINGLE WOMAN AFTER BREAST CANCER

"When my hair was falling out, a friend was setting me up with a guy, but I just couldn't go. I thought, What if my wig falls off or he hugs me and feels my prosthesis? I just wasn't ready to explain it to some guy I didn't know."—Karen

"I've thought about dating, but I just don't have a clue yet as to how it's going to go. I think, probably, I will not say anything unless somewhere down the line somebody seems like they're serious or something. But I don't think I'm going to mention it in just dating. But it's part of who you are. A big part of who you are. It is. It's weird to skip it."
—Amy

There is no easy way to be a cancer survivor, but when you are a young woman trying to establish and maintain relationships, you are caught in the "who am I" bind. Cancer has played a major role in your life, one that has changed your body, your body image, and your self-perception. To try and form new relationships and leave that part of you hidden is difficult. You may have become a stronger person, but there is still that fear of getting close and suffering rejection from those who cannot reconcile themselves to your cancer diagnosis.

Amy explored the idea of dating in a therapy situation with men in her group. She asked each what they would truly think when they heard the news and was generally dissatisfied with the "it would make no difference" responses she received. *"I told them, 'That's what everybody is supposed to say. But you're going to have feelings about that.' There was one man in group I felt was really honest. He said, 'I think you're really attractive, and it didn't change the way I think about you. But when I heard that, I just thought, Oh, she's probably really scarred.' And he felt bad about saying that to me, but it was so refreshing to hear somebody just say it. It was the first honest thing I've heard from a man. Instead of all this, 'Oh, it really wouldn't make a difference'."*

We say constantly that if a person cares for us, cancer should make no difference. But will the disfigurement and fear make a difference? Will the more serious outlook make a difference? Perhaps. Some women are not even willing to risk dating for fear of rejection when they break the news. Others have and were rejected. Others have met and married in spite of, or perhaps because of, the cancer and the person who emerged from that experience.

"How did it come up? We had gone out a couple times and had dinner. It was casual and there was no physical relationship and then I went to another campus and he came out there for his department. And he started staying with me. When things were moving along, I sort of stopped and said, 'You know there is something I have to tell you.' Because I didn't want to just pop the scars on him. And things were progressing to the point that he was going to find out soon anyway. So I explained the whole thing to him, and he didn't have much of a reaction. He said it just didn't matter."—Victoria

"I guess I haven't dated a whole lot, I don't know why. I guess I'm not really so interested. Sometimes I think I just prefer to be just left alone and just to enjoy everything I know I can enjoy. I don't know, I guess I'm just kind of tired of jacking around with men. It's silly sometimes. Some men just react like, 'Oh my God.' They don't know how to react to it. It scares them a lot of times. When you get enough reactions, after a while you just say, Who needs you anyway?"
—Angela

Telling someone you have had cancer is tricky. For some women the "by the way" statement takes on monumental proportions. A few women were comfortable with casual dating and not mentioning cancer until intimacy was imminent. For some the information is presented as a challenge to reject them—"By the way, I've had cancer and if that's a problem, tell me now." Remember that this kind of news may take some digestion.

Kim says she understands their reluctance, recalling that two of the three men she had dated up to the time of our interview really didn't understand what she was saying. *"They don't want to hear about cancer. I can understand. They are thinking, Why should I have a relationship with a woman who had cancer at thirty-one? Chances are that she'll have it again."*

At the time we talked, Kim was not dating anyone, but said she was feeling great about herself and having fun with the house she had bought the previous year. More than a year later, Kim met a man to whom she is now engaged. Kim, who had bilateral mastectomies and immediate reconstruction, said she didn't bring up the cancer until *after* their first sexual encounter. *"In the dark you can't tell, but I wanted him to know what he was getting, so in the light, I said, 'Look at my chest,' and I took my blouse off. He really doesn't care. What we did talk about were his concerns that since I had had cancer so young, would I get it again. I said I didn't know."*

For some, the vulnerability of opening up to a man who may reject them has led to a decision not to date at all. Chris, who divorced after her diagnosis, said she has only dated four men in seventeen years. She decided that she always wanted them to know up front. *"I did that because, if there was no relationship, I didn't have to deal with the fact that it was the cancer, if it didn't work out. If I waited until there was a relationship, then I could tell immediately if they couldn't handle it. I never got that close to anyone. Probably if I hadn't had the mastectomy, I would have dated more."*

"I worry about getting in a relationship. Before I get too involved, I have to be more sure of where I stand with a person, what kind of person he is."—Debra

"I figured sex would never happen to me again. I felt deformed. My attorney had been my lover years before and became my lover again.

He let me know it was okay to have sex. He said that the surgery wasn't me. It lasted for two years. It wasn't what I wanted, but if I had not taken the chance, I may never have again."—Sonja

"I was in a relationship at the time all that happened, and he took off, and part of it, I think, was the cancer. He says it wasn't, but part of me thinks that it was. I've not had an intimate relationship since then."—Marsha

"He handled it beautifully. He really did. He is probably the reason why I have not been reconstructed, because he just doesn't care. It doesn't bother him. He doesn't really want me to go through the surgery again, because there would be pain and discomfort involved."—Diane

PANIC ATTACKS AND FEAR— THE SHADOW KNOWS

"I have had cancer at least twenty times since the surgery. Every little thing. If I have a bowel movement that looks strange, I am sure I have bowel, rectal cancer. If I am tired, I have leukemia. I can't have a hangnail without having skin cancer."—Mary H

"The worst part now for me is her coming up with what would normally be considered little aches and pains and upset stomach or diarrhea and immediately her perception is cancer somewhere."
—Harriett's husband, Donald

"If I have a pain anywhere, it's cancer, and I am terminal within the week. I just have time to make out my last will and testament and I'm gone."—Judy D

I had my first panic attack in February 1987, after I had been diagnosed the previous October. It began with a phone call to a woman who led a Brownie troop that met at my church. I was planning an all-church event and wanted to talk with her about the Brownies taking part. We chatted for a while and agreed to get back together. I told her I would be unavailable for a while since I was having my last chemo treatment that week. She paused and said she too was taking chemo and she also had breast cancer. I asked her how she found hers and she said it was on New Year's Eve, when she sneezed and the pain in her back was so intense that she had to sit down. Pain in her back? Well, she said that by the time they had found hers, it was in her spine already. I knew what that meant and so did she.

It was the first time I had met someone for whom the disease had metastasized to another location in the body. It was the first time I talked with someone who knew she was dying from this disease.

Within twenty-four hours, my upper back was literally in spasms. I was in tremendous pain. Within forty-eight hours I was convinced that my cancer had metastasized to my back and I was dying. I convinced Tom I was dying too. We scheduled another bone scan to confirm what I already knew. I began, for the first time, planning my death. I asked specific friends to take over aspects of my daughter's upbringing.

When Becky, Dr. Mennel's nurse, breezed into the examining room the day after the bone scan, she said, "By the way the bone scan was fine and why did you have one? We just did one three months ago." She looked up to see me and Tom in tears.

"My goodness," she said. "You were worried, weren't you."

I wish I could say that was the one and only panic attack I have suffered. I can't. In fact as I write this, I know that it has been five months since my last one—and another is lurking. They are not nearly as intense as that first one, and I can usually talk myself out of them now. But I also know now that when I begin to feel a big wave of panic, the best way to get over it is to go in and have a checkup.

In the past two years, I have come to the realization that my fear of recurrence is as painful as anything I have faced in cancer. I also know enough about the disease to know that I probably won't be able to tell if the cancer is back until something is amiss in my blood work, and I get a checkup frequently enough to know that I will find it there before I feel it in my body. At least that was what my oncologist told me after I ordered yet another bone scan two years ago. It was time for one and I was having a panic attack, so I ordered my own bone scan. When I went in to see him two weeks later, he looked at my file.

"You had a bone scan?" he queried.

"Yep, I was having a panic attack," I replied defiantly, waiting for him to challenge me.

"You know that I would be able to tell from your blood work if there was any indication the cancer had metastasized," he said sweetly.

"Oh no, I didn't," I said, somewhat sheepishly, before adding. "But the reality is that I probably wouldn't have believed you." He nodded.

Luckily, I have a wonderful oncologist, who is by now used to my personality and my stubborn efforts to control my response to this disease. But he knows the pain I have suffered from fear, and he has never said I was silly or ridiculous.

In the years since that first attack, I have begun to recognize indications of an oncoming attack. They are strangely similar to those that occurred to the women I interviewed for this book. To me they seem to follow a post-traumatic-stress reaction. They are triggered by memories or events that remind us of some aspect of the cancer or diagnosis, when the feelings of death are strongest.

First, any well-publicized death from cancer sends us scurrying to the doctor in droves.

Second, unusual physical aches and pains—most of which are connected to aging, not cancer—are always thought to be cancer. I have had women tell me they panicked over elbows, moles, knees, ankles, headaches, fingers, you name it. Shoulders are a favorite since many of us hold our tension there.

Third are regular checkups. Many women begin worrying weeks before the visit and, by they time they get there, have created painful tension in their bodies that they are sure is metastasis.

I have found that the best way to deal with the panic attacks emotionally is to talk about them as soon as they hit—laugh about them with my group. "Hi, I'm Kathy and I am dying this week," and to face directly what I will do if the cancer does come back.

This last part has been the toughest part. Because the reality of this disease for all of us is that it may come back and no one knows why.

"The hard part is just thinking that it's really not gone. There are stages when the logic is just fine, and you go along, and there are points where something overtakes that, and then comes the fear."—Elizabeth T

"I gave myself the five-year mark as when I was going to stop worrying."—Debra

"It just comes crashing back when you try to go back to your old life. But you can't go back to your old life. You've changed. This is kind of backwards-sounding, but if I don't think about it all the time, if I let myself get happy and let go of it, then I'm scared it's going to sneak up on me and I'm going to get the rug pulled out from under me again. So I keep it in the back of my mind all the time. Does that make sense?—Amy

"I keep this fear inside. I don't voice it very much. I feel like the more I voice it, the more afraid I become, and when I hear the fear in other women, I get a little more afraid for myself because I know my odds and I know how bad my cancer was to begin with."—Mary-T

So what do we do with the fear? Where do we turn for reassurance when this disease offers none? It hit me in 1990—four years after my surgery—what this fear is all about. I have all my life loved the Twenty-third Psalm, but now it has a special meaning for me: *"Yea though I walk through the valley of the **shadow of death**, I will fear no evil."*

The hardest work I have done with this illness is to consciously stop trying to outrun the shadow and to turn and face him—and make peace with him. I see it as the only way to assimilate this experience into my life.

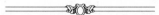

Tip—In order to fully assimilate cancer into our lives, we must face the unknown, which for many of us is the possibility of recurrence and death. Yet it is through this very painful work that we find our gifts in this disease.

I tend to personify the shadow in my life. He tends to remain behind me these days. I know he is there, and a day does not go by when his presence reminds me that life holds many uncertainties. Then he is summoned by a headline or a fear or an ache and he envelops me, distorting my view of the world and causing a dark pall over all my life. He whispers into my ear of recurrence and death; he whispers into other women's ears of loneliness, disfigurement, and uncertainty; and yet into others' of decisions already made. His screaming chorus—"what if?"

Craig and Leanne have had to struggle with a very real shadow after Leanne had five positive nodes. That fear was exacerbated by her first oncologist, who told her she had a 50 percent chance of survival after five years. Leanne had a two- and four-year-old when she was diagnosed. Her husband, Craig, and I talked three years after her diagnosis and she was still fine—but the fear is an ever-present visitor in their home. *"One of her arguments to buy a video camera is so we will have films of her for the kids to have. She makes these comments in jest, but they're not in jest all the time. She needs dental work and says she'll wait until after her test—no use doing it now if it's not going to be necessary. I'm concerned about how stressed out she is in dealing with it. I can't make her deal with it."*

Craig said Leanne's fears have worsened as she approaches the five-year mark without recurrence. They have discussed her need to get support. But the argument continues. *"There is the balance issue. How much truth does she need? You have to have it all or you don't get the benefit of any of it. But how will she do with each piece? Will she take them in balance, or will she hear the real fears for her five nodes and concentrate on that too much? It's kind of a bind—is closing your eyes and worrying about it better than finding out the truth, which may be scarier?"*

I hate the shadow and have made him the focus of my unresolved anger. "Get out. Go away." It is amazing how I can diminish his claim on my psyche through personification.

The shadow lurks in decisions: If we didn't have chemo, we begin to question that decision. If we chose lumpectomy over mastectomy, the remaining tissue gets massaged excessively. If we chose mastectomy, we are beginning to question whether we should have had a bilateral. Does my husband really love me, or does he feel sorry for me? We are scared and we must confront and make peace with the cancer that has entered our lives.

"When she has one of these attacks of whatever, there's no point in telling her everything's fine, because she's not going to believe me, whether I think it is or not, so there's not really a whole lot I can say

except that I love you and I'll be here or be there or go with you or whatever you want."—Harriett's husband, Donald

Most of us live with the shadow in some form or another. Marjorie said that for a time, she was afraid to leave the house, beset by a form of agoraphobia. *"I wasn't afraid of cancer, I was afraid of sudden death. My whole experience was transmuted into the idea that I could be walking along, not paying attention, and I could get hit by a bus, because that's what happened to me. I was walking along, not paying attention, and I got hit by cancer. I became afraid of everything. Crossing the street. I was afraid of strangers because I thought they were going to mug, rape, or kill me. That fear soon became fear of cancer in the other breast."*

I don't know if we always will be beset by irrational fear. I can only hope that time will diminish it, but at five years post-op, the shadow is still evident in my life, somewhat diminished but still popping up sometimes when I least expect him. He likes my nights, just before I go to sleep. *What if, what if, what if.*

We all learn to counter the shadow in our own way. Lynne put on her running shoes and ran, literally running until she dropped. Others have stayed busy enough to avoid him or to pretend he isn't there. Some had never truly felt his presence or were quite able to ignore him. Others have talked and talked and talked about him until his powers are diminished merely by their acknowledging his presence. This is where support groups are invaluable.

"I feel if I talk about it, it'll become a part of my life and it'll become so everyday with me that it'll be like eating and sleeping and it won't faze me. It'll be something that's okay."—Emelda

In the past year, I have learned to counter the shadow with my own vision of the second part of the statement: "Yea though I walk through the valley of the shadow of death, I will fear no evil for thou art with me."

Reared a Christian by Catholic-turned-Episcopal-turned-Methodist parents, I embraced Methodism for my own life. But I would call myself a New Age Methodist, for while believing that my gifts are from God and my life should be something that makes this world a better place, I also believe strongly in self-determination. I believe in angels, but also in meditation and the power of positive thought, which some would call prayer. I believe in the sanctity of life, but I believe in evil and its presence on earth.

One of the strongest women I know also happens to be a Methodist minister. Rev. Sue Ann Hill was leading a women's retreat in September of 1990 which I had joined, and where, during a guided meditation, I received a gift from God.

As the thirty women present lay on the floor, Sue Ann had us visualize walking by a nearby lake, where we would meet Jesus, who would have for us a gift. Never having done such a visualization before, I moved along with her words and was indeed greeted by a child's picture-book version of Jesus in flowing white robes. In his hands was a box that fairly glowed from its seams, and in the box, barely distinguishable through the bright glow, was a beating heart.

When the meditation was through, I opened my eyes and Sue Ann asked who among us had received a gift. I raised my hand, expecting that others had been equally touched. No one else raised her hand and all eyes were on me. Only then did I feel the power of my vision, and as I relayed it to the women in the room, many of whom had provided me with love and support through my cancer, I felt the tears of a truly profound experience and God's gift for me to use against the shadow— the gift of life. Since then the vision has come both at my bidding and on its own. It is the strongest when I meditate and open myself to my fears.

I have tried not to overanalyze my vision, preferring to let it be what it is in my life.

Finding your path to cope with the shadow must begin by exploring those fears the shadow holds for you.

"I made the decision to live, but I also had to deal with the decision of how to die. And I think you can make that decision, too. Of course, I can sit back and say it with a lot more confidence now than I did then. But I did go through that. I had to process that."—Diane

"My fear was that I did not want to die a terrible death. I guess I came to grips with death and I realized death might not be as bad as you think it's going to be. I just didn't want to leave right now, I was having a good time and I wanted to see my children grow."—Mary-T

DISFIGUREMENT ISSUES

"After my mastectomy, but before I was going to be reconstructed, I didn't like myself. It didn't matter whether I had on my favorite dress or my sweats. I hated the way I looked in a nightgown, and my self-esteem was terrible. After I was reconstructed, I felt so much better. It was a sense of disfigurement. I wanted to be put back together again."—Lynne

"I think it is normal to look in the mirror and say, 'Gee, I wish I were whole.' Then when I stop and think about what I would wish for if I could wish for anything, I think I'd wish for perfect teeth or eyesight. I realized I hadn't wished for a breast. I guess it isn't important to me. You would think it would be first, but it wasn't even on the list."—Kit

"I don't believe we ever accept the loss of our breast. I believe we adjust to the loss of our breast. I believe that we learn to make the most of our life and adjust to that loss. But if somebody asks me, do I want my breast back? God, I'll give you all my jewelry and all my recipes."—Teresa M

"I've had fifteen major surgeries in my life. I weighed a pound and a half when I was born. I wore a brace until I was fourteen. None of it compared to this. The reason is that you can't avoid the visual. All the other surgery, I didn't have to look at. With this, every time you take a bath, it's a reminder."—Lola

They have been called the ultimate blend of form and function. And in the breast-oriented society we live in, they receive more than their share of attention. No woman wants to lose her breasts. They are a part of our body. We were born with them and it's reasonable to want to leave the world with them intact.

Yet how badly the loss of our breasts affects us may be different for every woman, depending in part how much of our self-esteem and self-image comes from our physical self. One woman's significant loss is another's inconvenience. For Betty B who was diagnosed during pregnancy and gave birth to a healthy baby after chemotherapy, the overriding issue for her is still the loss of the breast. Body image is as unique to a woman as her personality, and there are no generalizations. I have talked to very young women who struggled with the loss of the breast more than any other issue; nothing in the experience has been as painful as the flat portion of their chest where their breast used to be. But the pain of disfigurement is not an age issue.

Mary C, who was seventy-one when diagnosed, chose a lumpectomy because she *"liked to go dancing and wear sexy clothes."* She agreed with her surgeon that if the tumor was more extensive, they would do a mastectomy. She was barely out of the anesthesia when the nurse told her they could not get clear margins and had to remove her breast. *"My friend down the hall said she could hear me screaming,"* Mary said. Over a year later, when we talked, Mary had still not resolved the issue of losing her breast. She is planning on reconstruction in 1993.

Mary-T, a striking woman, held a number of beauty titles from college and struggled with self-image after the loss of her breasts. She was reconstructed with her tummy muscle, which the surgeon divided, using half for each breast. Her husband, Leonard, said it has been a difficult adjustment for both of them. *"It is tough to deal with when you know that you are a very beautiful lady and that now you have all these scars all over you. We call it a reposition of assets. We do a lot of that in my business; we repositioned her assets."*

> *"I realized that men aren't as concerned as we thought they were. It is just that I guess I just don't feel as sexual sometimes. Well, it is something that we have to work at."*—Mary-T

Teresa M said that looking back, she may have been a little casual about the loss of her breast. *"I didn't expect my husband to say wonderful things and gush all over me. I expected him to be honest, and he was. And it was okay. And I could, from that moment on, undress in front of him. Maybe I was a little bit too casual, because I was not reconstructed for two years. My friends would come to the apartment sometimes and I'd open the door and I'd be in a nightgown and I'd have a boob on one side and nothing on the other. That was easy for me, but I didn't realize it might be difficult for them. I finally got to a point where, Hey, am I scaring them? Will I prevent them from doing what they need to do when they're fifty or sixty? I better start being sensitive to them."*

"It's been hard for me. You can't look at it and not feel that you have been maimed."—Dot

"When it is cold, I can still feel my nipples and I can feel nipple sensation against my shirt. It is like phantom pain."—Mary H

"You kind of just have to go with it and refuse to let yourself be caught up in the physicalness of our society. You have to detach yourself from it. I'm beautiful. Just stay with me. Just because I've lost a breast doesn't mean I'm not beautiful. I say these words now, but sometimes it's the hardest thing to do. But if you can at least think it and start making yourself believe it, then you get through it."—Andrea

PARENTING AFTER BREAST CANCER

Our children are, in many instances, what keep us going. They are our life's work and the thought of not rearing them can be a pain like no other. Yet they also take immeasurable emotional and physical energy, and for women trying to process the breast cancer experience, they can become yet another drain. Indeed, few professionals would argue that children can sense our fears and uncertainties as clearly as if we had said them out loud. These fears and intense feelings are often reflected by our children in their behavior—and ours.

Craig says that when Leanne is approaching her checkup dates, she often finds herself overwhelmed by their two small children. *"She called me and said, 'Come home,' and had locked herself in the bathroom. She will have fears and then the children add to it and she feels like she can't take it anymore. That seems more intense right before any tests."*

I wonder if part of this irritation is the angst of just looking at our children's faces when we must face whether or not our cancer has recurred. In my own relationship with my daughter, I am aware that I obsess about her health and something happening to her. Jo Anne has expressed the same feelings about her son.

I am now convinced that my compulsive overspending the Christmas after my diagnosis was a direct result of my fears that I might die. I wanted my daughter to remember me as a giving parent who bought her everything her little heart desired. And I almost succeeded. Christmas brings about all the strong generational and family feelings we may not have during the year. And for those of us who live with fear of recurrence there is that constant question in the back of our minds: Will I be here next year?

This realization struck me in February 1992, when I realized I had made it through January without my annual panic attack and for the first time in four years I was not struggling to pay Christmas bills. Was there a correlation? Betty B confirmed that she saw herself doing the same thing. *"I bought my son the bike he wanted, with all the bells and whistles, even though I know he will grow out of it in a year. Even he told me I didn't have to get him the one he wanted. Why did I do that?"*

I know why—it's the same reason that I let my daughter get her way more often than I should. There is a little voice that says, You might die, and is it really that big a deal if her clothes match today or she has another cookie?

One of my greatest fears is that my daughter will figure out that I look at her with awe, as a miracle, every day of my life. Can "Mom, I want a Porsche" be far behind?

MALPRACTICE

After researching this book for more than two years, I can say that there is one area about which I am totally ambivalent: the issue of malpractice for delayed diagnosis.

One the one hand, I detest that we have become a nation of people who sue. We don't want to take responsibility for our actions, preferring to threaten a lawsuit or go through with one instead of understanding that people make mistakes and doctors don't cause cancer, they just find it. Lawsuits seem too easily justified and result in additional costs to the consumer as the prices of malpractice insurance are passed on. I want women to know their bodies first and foremost and then to know how to find a good medical professional, to act responsibly as a partner with that professional, and accept that medical science is not perfect nor are those who offer it.

On the other hand, the insurance companies which must pay malpractice claims for delayed diagnosis are warning doctors not to ignore lumps in women. As long as doctors refuse to listen to their female patients and must be threatened into action, lawsuits should and must be pressed. For while it is easy to say we are responsible for our bodies, we are also placed in a position of having to trust medical professionals. All too often doctors are condescending to their patients, reassuring women and not listening to them when they could biopsy the lump or refer the woman to a surgeon. The traditional paternalistic attitude of doctors must end. It is litigation that frequently changes policy to more fully protect the consumer and the doctor.

Susan (not her real name since she still works in health care) knew years before her diagnosis that her breasts would always need special medical attention. Her mother had had breast cancer when Susan was a toddler. *"I knew it was in the genes. Mother was real honest about that. Her surgeon said, 'Make sure your daughters know that they may have multiple lumps, but never, ever let one of those lumps go, because the one they let go is going to be the lethal one.' So, this was my first lump. And my sister, who is ten years older than me, had a lump when she was twenty-four, and it was benign. And my other sister, who is eight years older than me, has never had anything."*

Because Susan was working in the health-care field at the time, she went immediately to her primary-care physician. She made it clear that she wanted to treat the lump aggressively. The doctor assured her it was nothing because the lump had come up quickly. A mammogram indicated nothing suspicious. Subsequent visits to another doctor got the same results. She was told she had traumatized her breast and that it would take six months for the swelling to reduce. Neither of the doctors she saw biopsied the lump. *"It's pretty evident in my charts that I knew there was a family history of cancer and that I wanted to be aggressive if there was the slightest problem. I went to the doctor in May, June, August, and December before anything was done. Twice in May, twice in June, once in August, and once in December."*

Eight months after the first exam, Susan went to a doctor outside her system. The breast specialist she visited did a needle biopsy in the office and drew out fluid that was suspicious and turned out to be malignant. Susan had a modified radical a week later, followed by chemotherapy and radiation. At that point she engaged an attorney out of town to pursue action against her company and the doctor.

Her case was thrown out a year later by a judge who said that since the outcome was not bad, there was no negligence. *"In other words, if I had died I would have won."*

Mary-T found a lump and visited a gynecologist who was suggested by a friend, since she was new to the city. The doctor, who she later discovered had had his privileges revoked at a local hospital but was still practicing, sent her for a mammogram in December. When he called to tell her it was clear and that the lump she felt was nothing to worry about, she was relieved. Later she would learn that the mammography equipment was malfunctioning on the day of her mammogram, a note that was on the report but not relayed to her. *"The surgeon called me the next day and said he talked to the imaging center and they said it was a cyst. It was nothing to worry about. Come back in a year."*

Because the lump was getting larger, Mary-T called the doctor in February. He told her he was sure it was nothing, but he would look at it. *"I went in and he looked at it and he said, 'Well, I am not a betting man, but if I was, I would bet it is nothing. I'm not really concerned about it, but because it is so large, it really needs to come out. There is no hurry, so just go home and find us some clear time on your calendar.' I said that in a month we are going to be going on our wonderful trip to Australia, so I would like it to be done before then. He said, 'Oh, it's not going to be any deal, you'll only be down maybe two days at the most.'"*

Finally, on March 8, Mary-T had the "cyst" removed, which turned out to be a 6-centimeter malignant tumor. She underwent six months of chemotherapy, radiation, and then three more months of chemotherapy. She and her husband filed a suit, that is still pending, against the doctor and mammography location. *"I have a lot of things that I want accomplished with this lawsuit. This mammography center, which is one of the largest in Dallas, now has a new machine and they are now accredited with the American College of Radiology. The new machine was purchased after I filed my suit. And they became accredited after the suit. I feel directly responsible for that."*

BECOMING A CANCER SURVIVOR

"I didn't stop and smell the roses before my surgery. As a matter of fact, I never saw the rose bushes, I was going so fast. And even though I'm going real fast now because of my career, I still appreciate things more. I like myself so much better now. I really do."—Kim

"You're not going to get distance from it. It's a constant part of her body. I mean, it's part of her. The best thing you're going to do is integrate it into your life, not run away from it or close your mind down about it. You can't really close the page and go on to the next one."—Marjorie's husband, Chuck

"I don't think it will ever not be a part of my life. It's there and is with us every day that goes by, and every time I go in for a checkup and they say everything is okay, that helps to put it a little more behind me. I don't think about it and worry about it and I don't let it interfere with my day-to-day living, but I'm very conscious of it."—Dot

In the mid-eighties, it became apparent that there was a new movement emerging in this country that addressed the issue of cancer survivorship. Because of increases in the number of cancer patients, advances in treatment, and earlier detection, many thousands of cancer patients were surviving—and all of a sudden they were visible and present, asking questions, attending support group meetings, and addressing the as yet unknown aspects of what it means to have had cancer.

In October 1986, twenty-two individuals from around the country who were interested in the issues of cancer survivorship gathered in Albuquerque, New Mexico, to discuss this new, emerging community. Half were cancer survivors; the other half were those whose profession or missions addressed the needs of cancer survivors.

What they first defined was survival—what did it mean? Fitzhugh Mullan, an M.D. and survivor, put into words a phrase that the group continues to use. "Survival, quite simply, begins when you are told you have cancer and continues for the rest of your life."

Since that time the original group of twenty-two has become the National Coalition for Cancer Survivorship (NCCS), its mission to explore all the aspects of survivorship, with the understanding that those of us who survive don't want to be called victims and don't want the fact that we have had cancer to be held against us economically, emotionally, or in any other way.

When we are considered cured and sent home by our physicians, we no longer want just to live, but we want to have a quality of life. Yet while we have been given physical rehabilitation, we have been given few clues about emotional rehabilitation—and what exactly it means to be a survivor.

While the survivorship movement, which has blossomed also in support groups and through many cancer centers, is relatively new, the areas that it has identified include

- Understanding that the medical treatment for most of us is a matter of endurance, with standard treatment protocols, while the emotional healing process is unique and that survivors want information and access to information about all aspects of living well, including nutrition, stress reduction, increasing joy, and finding spirituality.
- Understanding that we want to be informed medical consumers, with up-to-date information about new applications of treatment and about the long-term effects of those we have undergone.
- Understanding that we have a strong voice in policy, legislation, and legal issues pertaining to survivorship issues such as employment, discrimination, and insurance.

This is not to say that you have to join a group or become a protester, although those options are present. But there is, from those who have gone before you, the sense that at some point you will decide what kind of survivor you will be.

Someone asked me once if I referred to myself as having **had** breast cancer or as **having** breast cancer. That is a hard question that goes beyond whether I have disease in my body. I am clear of cancer, and if someone asks, I say I "had" breast cancer. Yet in a sense breast cancer still has me and always will.

At some point, it seems, we must decide what we will do with the cancer experience—how we will assimilate it into our lives from this point forward and what kind of survivor we will be. The dictionary says that to assimilate is to "absorb or incorporate into one's body or one's thinking." I suppose for us it is both.

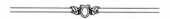

Tip—Assimilation cannot take place until the woman has progressed through the grief of the ex-

perience. Unresolved issues surrounding the cancer block assimilation.

Some women are comfortable just *being* with the fact that they had cancer. Their personal direction doesn't change significantly. Others feel that they have to *do* something with the cancer. What to *do* with the fact we have had cancer can take many forms as we get on with our lives. Breast cancer became my life for a period of time—by choice as I wrote this book. For me, writing became the process of assimilation. Others, in the arts, brought their cancer into their work.

Wendy was one of the first breast cancer patients in the state of Texas to get a bone-marrow transplant. After the 1989 transplant she became a vocal presence for young women and breast cancer. For more than a year she was asked to speak, and appeared a number of times in the local media. In 1991 she decided to move to Florida to begin a new life. Only a few close friends know her history. *"I just decided that I needed to get away from Dallas. I needed to move. I wanted to be in the sunshine and water. I got a new start. No one here knows about my health. It's not that I'm trying to hide it. It's that I don't want everybody feeling sorry for me. I just want to be a regular person."*

What we do with our cancer experiences will vary. Some of us will wear it on our sleeves, hoping for chances to talk about it—for us, talk is cure and help. Others turn to more active involvement in their churches or synagogues, where they will take a leadership role in educating women. Others move into fund-raising activities or Reach to Recovery. These women turn their breast cancer and their anger at the disease into a job or a mission. Some find a meaning in life through their cancer—an identity and a goal.

Lynne is a good example. A few years after her cancer, Lynne decided to give back what she had learned by becoming a Reach to Recovery Volunteer. She talks with women and shares her story while providing a listening ear and heart for their stories. *"It helps me as much as it does the patient. It makes me feel like I am really helping someone. I know what they are going through and there is a bond there between two women who have lost a breast. It doesn't matter who you are or what you do. We have the same fears and concerns."*

Lynne's husband, Norm, says that because of the cancer experience, Lynne is a different woman. *"She's a more resilient woman than she was nine years ago. She's a lot tougher. She's done a lot of things that she never thought that she would ever do: speak in front of large audiences of people, be on television."*

Betty B said that the cancer experience helped her find a new strength and allowed her to separate from her parents for the first time in her life. Betty, who was pregnant at the time of the diagnosis, faced chemotherapy, the birth of her daughter, and radiation—all within a few months. Her parents were pressuring her to move to a larger house. *"I was ready to move and we looked at new houses, and then I came home and finally I talked with my therapist. I suddenly realized, I don't want to do any of that right now. I just want to enjoy my children. Kelsey couldn't care less whether she has a closet in her room or not. So it's not really a bedroom. She doesn't care. It was the very first time I went against my parents. And I'm now suddenly realizing that it's okay if they don't like my husband. I do, and I'm the one that lives with him."*

Nurse Counselor Jan Pettigrew, R.N., Ph.D., has seen women at all stages of the breast cancer experience. She said that the women who come through the experience are different. *"I see them get stronger and like themselves better and find out who they really are as a woman—that they are more than a breast. They see that there is a part that is way deep down inside. At first it is exposed so radically. It seems that your whole facade is ripped off. It's distressing and you feel vulnerable and out of control, but in the end it is the vulnerability that works for you. It is a crash course in therapy. You are tossed in the ocean and told to swim to shore, but they don't tell you where shore is.*

"Relationships are strengthened and her understanding of herself as a person and a woman in all her roles have been further defined. She comes away with a more certain attitude about who she is and that there is a meaning and purpose in life. I have seen women have a spiritual experience out of this and get in touch with a relationship with God that they have never had before. The whole experience is life-changing. So they are healthier with cancer than ever before. I think that is a healthy goal to shoot for: to come out of this stronger. Maybe not healthier physically, but certainly healthier emotionally and spiritually."

FINDING CANCER GIFTS?

"I was okay just the way I was before, but I didn't know that. You see, I didn't think I was okay. Now I know I was, but it was a tough lesson to learn."—Sheila

"The good from the cancer was trusting myself and knowing I would count on myself in a crisis. I had always felt spoiled and immature and I had always counted on other people. I really counted on myself."
—Debra

At the end of each interview I conducted for this book, after the fear, pain, anger, tears, and assorted other emotions, I always looked forward to the answer to the question "Has anything positive come out of this experience?" Usually, the woman or man or both would talk about the positive aspects of what they had been through—even if it meant a painful transition from an old life to a new one or from old perceptions to new ones.

Many women *have* made positive life changes as a result of a breast cancer experience.

Dr. Michael Fitzpatrick, chief of Consultation-Liaison Psychiatry and associate professor at the University of Texas Southwestern Medical School, was instrumental in establishing the six-week program through the American Cancer Society that women can attend immediately after their surgery. He has counseled cancer patients for many years and found an adjustment that occurs in those who find the positive.

"The process of recovery is hard work, both physically and emotionally. Phenomenologically, the experience most closely resembles bereavement. Grief work involves calling a spade a spade. It means feeling rather than avoiding all the emotions evoked as new experiences bring to mind the losses incurred and their impact on day-to-day living—i.e., looking in the mirror, making love, dressing up, or watching a TV show about someone with cancer. It means actually learning to live without the breast. It means taking action. The women who do the best make positive changes in their lives by reframing their experience as recovery proceeds. They make the loss an opportunity of some sort. It may be an opportunity to become more of an independent person; it may be the opportunity of service; it may be the opportunity of a changed relationship with a spouse; it may be the opportunity of redefining one's identity. That's the process of recovery."

It really comes down to a choice: Either you can grow emotionally from this experience, or you can become bitter, angry, and hostile. You can look for the positives about what such an experience means, or you can shut down the feelings and your life. You decide. Yes, there were a few women who answered the question with a scowl, but not many. Most of the answers were like these:

"The positive thing is that life has a different meaning. I am more aware of me. I'm more comfortable with me. I seem to know who this really is."—Emelda

"Health is just so much more important than things, and if you've got that, you can enjoy everything. Simple things, like just sitting at home watching the birds chirp, watching the squirrels climb in the trees. I find those things just real pleasant."—Angela

"I think it's become a greater priority to not put things on hold, to go ahead and seize the day, and not wait to take a trip or to do whatever, which I think is very positive."—Elizabeth T's husband, Hugh

Doris said it took her years to realize that her family was emotionally out of contact, and when she was diagnosed she tried the stoic approach that had worked all her life. When she found she couldn't keep the emotions under control, she sought help from her surgeon, who suggested a support group. *"You really just finally explode, and it's not fair to other people. But if you're not getting in touch with how you feel, you don't know why you're acting this way, either."* Through group, Doris became more comfortable with hugging. She began to be more comfortable with herself and more accepting.

For Marsha the cancer was a key to learning to take a risk. She had always wanted to travel but was afraid to go places alone. A year after her surgery, she planned a trip to Palm Springs for herself. *"I went and I had the neatest time. It was really fun. And everything worked out, and I learned a lot, so the next time I go somewhere I'll do something a little differently. Before, I would have waited around."*

Joanne was running seven 18-wheelers coast to coast when she was diagnosed. *"I would never have chosen to have cancer. But I would choose to learn some of the lessons I've learned. I was a very controlling person. My family has always said that there is the right way, the wrong way, and Joanne's way. I don't think I was that bad, but I have always been a perfectionist, and I don't have to be anymore. I discovered that I am all right and I don't have to prove anything to anybody. I have a choice."*

"Early on, I'd say it was very negative. But now, eighteen months past diagnosis and staying clean, I'd say it's positive; it's more of a positive experience. Of course, I've opened up myself a lot more than I ever had before. I've met some wonderful people through the support groups. I've reached out; I haven't waited for people to come knocking at my door—I've done the opposite."—Julie

Marjorie's husband, Chuck, says that for him there have been a number of personal positives. *"You know I look back on it and I don't have a particularly great self-image about how I handle situations, but I did good. I look back at what I could have done in that small range I had to work with and I am very proud of myself. I acted the way I wanted to act. For the most part, I think I helped. It worked pretty well."*

Chapter 8

LIFE AFTER BREAST CANCER: THE PHYSICAL ISSUES

LYMPHEDEMA AND INFECTION

"I think my lymphedema is severe, but not according to the doctors. To me it's severe because my right arm is two inches larger than my left arm."—Teresa M

"I felt the lymphedema and infection issue was not stressed enough. Not that there's anything in the world I could have done about it, because I did not have an infection. I think mine was more of a scarring down. It just was closed, blocked and closed off."—Sylvia

Like everyone else, I was warned after surgery not to have blood drawn or blood pressure taken on my affected arm because of the risk of swelling—or lymphedema.

Lymphedema, quite simply, is an accumulation of lymph fluid that causes swelling. Primary lymphedema occurs in people for no apparent reason. Secondary lymphedema occurs after an infection or trauma to the lymph nodes—or their removal. For women who have undergone a mastectomy and the removal of the lymph nodes, the risk of lymphedema in the affected arm is greatly increased. But, why one woman gets lymphedema and another doesn't is still a mystery.

Untreated, lymphedema can result in an arm that is much larger than normal, resulting more in embarrassment than reduced function. But an arm affected by lymphedema is also prone to infections more often and can be painful.

380

In general I remember a warning to be careful with my mastectomy arm. I don't remember anyone looking me in the eye and saying, "Now, this is important." Yet I am one of those people who ended up in the hospital—for a longer stay than my mastectomy—because of a hangnail. And as a result of that infection, I have chronic lymphedema of the arm.

Immediately after surgery, my arm healed to its former strength very quickly. I promptly thought of the arm as healed. I was worried about cancer returning in my liver or lungs, not about my arm swelling. Then—three and a half years after my surgery—I got an infection.

I had a hangnail that wouldn't heal on my right thumb. I soaked it in hot water and tried to clear up the infection that was now under the skin. It remained sore, but I thought little about it. Then on a Saturday morning, when I was entertaining an out-of-town friend for whom I was giving a baby shower that afternoon, I noticed that my hand was sore above the thumb. I thought that strange but continued with the shower preparations. During the baby shower that afternoon, I was vaguely aware that my arm was sore to the elbow, but I still didn't realize what was happening. There was no redness, just a pain that felt like I had pulled a muscle. That evening we went to dinner and in the middle of the meal, I turned to my husband and said very simply, "Take me home; I am sick. I feel exactly the way I did during chemotherapy when my blood count would drop." I had chills and fever—AND STILL DIDN'T GET THE CONNECTION.

I went home, took two aspirin, and went to bed. Luckily, my house guest was a former nurse, because when she saw my arm the next morning, the color visibly drained from her face. There was a wide red streak from my hand up the inside of my arm and it had banded around the upper arm. The whole arm was swollen and I felt terrible. I called my surgeon immediately, and she knew by the description I had an infection—a bad one. She called in a prescription for some Cipro antibiotic and told Tom to go get it immediately, give me two, and bring me to the office in the morning.

By Monday morning the red had worsened and was moving onto my chest wall. We were at Dr. Knox's office at 9 A.M. and I was in the hospital on an IV antibiotic by 10, and there I remained for five days— longer than for my mastectomy.

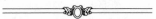

> **Tip—An infection in your arm can move quickly and become very serious in a matter of hours. Don't wait.**

Of course, I know now that by the time I got to the surgeon's office, I had a case of blood poisoning. The infection had traveled up my arm and was onto the chest wall in less than forty-eight hours.

Since then I have had two infections—one as the result of a mosquito bite, and another when I scratched my arm on a nail. Now I keep a filled prescription of Cipro at all times. At the first sign of the mottled red skin on my upper arm that indicates the beginning of infection, I call my surgeon.

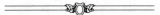

> **Tip—Women with repeated infections may want to consider long-term treatment with antibiotics as a preventative. They are usually given for one week each month.**

Quite simply, lymphedema develops when the lymphatic fluid in the arm cannot be moved by regular channels out of the arm through the lymphatic system. So the lymph fluid sits in the soft tissue and acts as a rich culture for bacteria, which cause infections, which in turn cause swelling that does not go away.

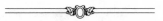

> **Tip—Lymphedema is not curable, it is only controllable. There is some evidence that early usage of a sequential pump will prevent further damage to the lymph system and may prevent infections.**

Be careful of any kind of wound, watching carefully for signs of infection. If there are any, DON'T WAIT. Call the doctor.

> *"My surgeon said if I cut the hand or burned it or scraped it—anything—not to think I can get it well myself. She said put on Neosporin or another antibiotic cream and give her a call so they can give me medication."*—Judy D

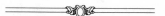

Tip—Time does not diminish the need for caution. One woman had her first infection seven years after surgery.

Many of the women who have lymphedema report that theirs began as mine did, with an infection. Others said it just appeared one day and hasn't gone away. For some, the swelling is mild and insignificant; for others it is painful, debilitating, and unsightly. While lymphedema was a significant problem for women who had the Halsted radical, it still affects around 15 percent of the women who have a modified mastectomy.

Other women, who must wear long sleeves year round to hide their swollen arm, say they are reminded more frequently about their cancer by looking at their arm than at their chest.

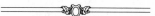

Tip—The earlier you notice lymphedema and begin treating it, the better your chance to keep it under control. Watch for signs of fluid retention in your arm—tighter rings, or cuffs that won't button as easily.

There are a number of treatments for lymphedema that vary in their effectiveness with each person. They range from simple elevation to manual lymph drainage to sequential pumps to compression sleeves. Some women have found that one system works, while others have found that it takes all methods in combination.

Elevation: Since the goal is to remove fluid stored in the arm, keeping it elevated as much as possible will help but will seldom provide an answer when used alone.

Manual lymph drainage: A physiotherapy technique in which a specially trained therapist physically massages the fluid out of the arm. Introduced in Europe some sixty years ago by Dr. Emil Vodder, this method is gaining in popularity in the United States. This technique takes special training and often it takes word of mouth to locate a therapist near you. You can also call the number here in the U.S. for the Austrian clinic where the technique is taught (1-800-642-2046) for more information, or contact the physical therapy department at various hospitals until you locate someone who can refer you locally. Do not assume that because someone is a massage therapist, he or she is trained in manual lymph drainage.

Sequential pumps: A number of sequential pumps are also available for lymphedema. The pumps work like a large blood pressure cuff that extends from the shoulder to the hand. But instead of one chamber that presses and releases, there are a number of them, which contract and expand one after the other up the arm. The pumps that are the most effective have a larger number of chambers. Once the pumps have removed the fluid, it takes constant maintenance to keep the arm reduced in size and the fluid moving. For those women with severe lymphedema, this process may take hours a day. Some women find they can "pump down" during the night. The time needed on the pump will vary for each woman, depending on her individual physiology and how closed down the channels have become and how quickly her arm swells again.

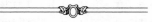

Tip—There are a number of sequential pumps on the market. Some are more effective than others. Shop around.

Compression sleeves: These sleeves are custom-fit and made out of material that puts pressure on the arm, much like a girdle. The sleeve can be quite uncomfortable, and while it keeps the swelling down, it does not keep the arm from reswelling after the sleeve is removed. The sleeve should be worn only after the arm has been pumped down or had the fluid removed manually, to keep from further compressing the channels.

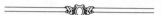

Tip—Be fitted for a sleeve only by a professional.

Complete decongestive physiotherapy: This approach, which has been used in the United States for only a few years, combines good hygiene, manual lymph drainage, and exercise with compression and bandaging of the arm.

Unfortunately, there seems to be no one source for comprehensive information about the varied techniques. Call the physical therapy department of your local hospital—or one in the next largest city, until you find a medical professional who has dealt with lymphedema. The National Lymphedema Network, (800) 541-3259, also provides information about the location of centers for the treatment of lymphedema. There aren't many in the country, but a few long-distance calls could help you find the right pump or treatment for you.

A number of the women interviewed for this book had pumps, which they used with varying success. Joan first noticed that her arm was bigger during radiation. The radiologist said it would go away after the trauma of surgery, which sometimes takes three years. But Joan noticed it kept getting worse, and two and a half years after surgery, her surgeon admitted that it wasn't going to go away. At that point Joan began looking for a pump. She liked the LymphaPress but chose the FlowPress because it was less expensive (pumps range in price from around $500 to $5,000). The FlowPress has three chambers, compared to the LymphaPress's ten. *"When I first used the FlowPress—I had it home for a weekend—and, boy, my arm really went down. My watch was off my hand. But I used it three hours on Saturday and three hours twice Sunday, and all Saturday night and Sunday night. And that's really what you've got to do, and it's just hard to find time to sit and do it."*—Joan

Joan says it varies, when she uses the pump, how long it takes her arm to swell again. *"Once you get the swelling down, then you go on a maintenance thing to keep the arm down and the time that takes on the pump varies, too, according to your body."*

I tried the LymphaPress, which, because of its number of chambers, is the pump of choice in the the Dallas medical community. The swelling in my arm did reduce for a day. But to maintain the arm's regular size requires daily use. Most insurance plans cover both the sleeves and the pump.

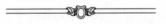

Tip—Check with your local American Cancer Society office to see if it has loaner pumps, for two months with a prescription from a doctor.

Although my lymphedema is not severe, I have bought a pump to use at those times when I am at risk of infection to help my arm battle the bacteria. My surgeon agreed that a pump may help prevent an infection. *But she warned that a pump must not be used with an existing infection.*

Tip—For information on where to find the Lympha-Press, call Camp International, at 1-800-492-1088

For Sylvia, a dentist, the lymphedema in her hand can be more than a nuisance, since it can actually interfere with her work. She first noticed at a soccer game that her hand seemed swollen. *"It was a real slow thing. We'd gone to a soccer game and I had my hands in my pockets. When I pulled my hands out, I noticed there was a crease in my right hand. I thought, My goodness. And it was sore there. And I thought, What on earth? And, of course, you immediately think, Oh my gosh, I've got bone cancer in my hand! And then I started thinking about it—well, now wait a minute. This is probably lymphedema. And then if I'd hold my arm up, I could feel like a tight band running all the way down to the back of my hand."*

Sylvia thought perhaps the tools she uses in her dentistry practice, which vibrate her hand, caused the initial swelling. Sylvia said she was religious about wearing both the compression glove and sleeve for nine months and then quit in the warm weather. She now has a pump, which she uses periodically. *"I wanted to take it off and see if the swelling gets any worse. If it gets worse, I'll put the glove and sleeve back on. If it doesn't, I'll live with this little fat hand. And so I took it off and it has not gotten any worse. I guess it goes through a period where it swells and if I start treating it like I did, I might catch it then and help some. But if this is all I have, it doesn't hurt, and I have all my feeling back—I had numbness in my fingertips for a while with it, too."*

Sylvia refused to let her surgeon remove the lymph nodes in her other arm when she had her other breast removed during reconstruction. She feels strongly that more emphasis should be placed on exercising the arm as soon after surgery as possible as a deterrent to lymphedema.

> *"If I gardened or got out in the heat, my arm would swell from the elbow down, and then it began swelling more overall. I got a mosquito bite and the next year I got a spider bite and both of those sent my fever to 105 and me to bed for a week. I started having cellulitis immediately. I would be fine and then two hours later I would be so sick. Every time you have the infection, you get scar tissue in the tiny lymph veins, so every time you get infection, it gets worse."*—Chris

There a number of things you can do to prevent and control lymphedema. This list is provided by the National Lymphedema Network.

1. Call your doctor at the first sign of infection.
2. Whenever possible, keep the arm elevated above the level of the heart. Avoid rapid circular movements that cause gravity to pull fluid centrifugally to distant parts of the limb.
3. Clean and lubricate skin of the arm daily.
4. Avoid injury and infection of the affected limb:

   - use an electric razor for shaving
   - wear gardening and cooking gloves, and thimbles for sewing
   - suntan gradually
   - avoid insect bites
   - clean breaks in skin and then use antibacterial ointment
   - use gauze instead of tape
   - prevent invasive venipuncture such as finger sticks and IV fluid
   - maintain good nail care; don't cut cuticles
   - avoid extreme hot or cold—e.g., ice packs or heating pads

5. Avoid constrictive pressure on the arm:

   - wear loose clothing and jewelry
   - carry your handbag on the opposite arm
   - no blood pressure cuffs on the vulnerable limb

6. Watch for signs of infection: redness, pain, heat, swelling, fever. Call M.D. immediately if any appear.
7. Practice drainage-promoting exercises faithfully.
8. Keep regular follow-up appointments with your doctor.
9. Return to normal use and activity gradually after healing.
10. Consciously observe all areas of the limb daily for signs of difficulty: Measure your arm width at intervals, and report any sudden increase to your doctor.
11. Sensation may be diminished. Use the unaffected arm to test temperatures of bathwater or meals you are cooking.
12. Be sure to eat a well-balanced, protein-rich diet. Consult your health professional if necessary.

Teresa M struggled with her lymphedema for a number of years before becoming frustrated. She began by visiting a lymphedema clinic in New York City, where she lives, and underwent a regimen of massages and wraps and wearing the sleeve and using the pump. *"You can get it down substantially and maybe even get it close to normal. But then it's a constant maintenance program after that. And I guess if my arm were as large as my leg, I would probably do something. But right now, I feel I can live with it."*—Teresa M

PREGNANCY AFTER BREAST CANCER

"Originally, she said wait three years. She said the conclusive studies that have been done are weak, and that from what she had been learning and following up with these cases, she didn't feel like the correlation was that strong. That getting pregnant would bring on a recurrence. So she is saying now to her patients, 'Wait one year before thinking about getting pregnant.' "—Diane

After my treatment ended, I called my obstetrician and asked what she thought about my having another child. This is the doctor who had delivered my daughter six weeks prematurely eighteen months earlier because my blood pressure had gone up significantly despite my having spent the last six weeks prior to delivery in bed.

She basically said I had one healthy child, which is more than many of her infertility patients have, and that even without the breast cancer, I was at high risk to have another premature baby, and did I have any other questions.

No, I guess that takes care of it for me. But the pain and the dreams are still there. I delayed marriage and childbearing until I was established professionally. It took two years of taking my temperature daily and a fertility drug to have my daughter and I would do it again tomorrow. But I no longer have the option. Shortly after that my husband and I agreed to do something permanent about birth control.

Many women who were interviewed for this book were unmarried, or were not yet parents, or wanted more children when they were diagnosed. For these women, the diagnosis can be a significant life loss if indicators point to a high risk for recurrence. For others there remains the difficult decision about whether to have a child after breast cancer. Asking people in the medical profession usually only complicates matters. The studies available offer little conclusive information.

In November 1991, *Oncology* magazine—a fairly readable medical journal for the lay person—included an article entitled "How Subsequent Pregnancy Affects Outcome in Women with a Prior Breast Cancer."

In the article, David N. Danforth, Jr., M.D., senior investigator, Surgery Branch National Cancer Institute, explores the existing studies on pregnancy after breast cancer to reach some conclusions that are of importance to women considering pregnancy after breast cancer. The article was followed by reviews from Richard Epstein at Harvard Medical School and J. Craig Henderson at Dana-Farber Cancer Institute in Boston and William Wood at Emory University School of Medicine.

Danforth's article offers a wealth of combined information from the studies. For example: Women *are* getting pregnant after breast cancer. Danforth says 7 percent of the premenopausal women diagnosed will become pregnant. Translated into figures for 1991, this means some 2,800 women will became pregnant after a 1991 diagnosis of breast cancer. Seventy percent of these pregnancies will occur in the first five years after treatment, Danforth says.

Based on his analysis of available studies and on his own exploration of hormonal issues, more than one pregnancy, timing of pregnancy, stage of cancer and its impact on pregnancy, and the effects of chemotherapy on subsequent pregnancy, Danforth comes to the following conclusions:

1.   Pregnancy does not appear to affect adversely the prognosis for Stage I or II breast cancer, even though it causes profound hormonal changes and many breast cancers are hormonally responsive. Most overall and five-year-survival analyses appear to remain unchanged by a pregnancy following breast cancer treatment. Similarly, no adverse effect on pregnancy has been shown in analyses of cancer patients divided by stage and axillary lymph node status. Neither the number of pregnancies nor the interval between treatment and subsequent pregnancy nor termination *vs.* term alter the outcome of the malignancy. In the absence of any evidence of recurrent disease, the pregnancy should be managed independently of the previous malignancy.

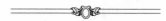

Tip—In other words, there is no evidence that a pregnancy will bring on a recurrence.

2.   The decision to conceive a child should be based not on what effect the pregnancy may have on the breast cancer but rather on the prognosis of the particular type of tumor, the time that has elapsed since the cancer was treated, the woman's ability to integrate care of a child into the psychological atmosphere of a treated malignancy.

3.   Women who have Stage IV tumors, which have a five-year survival rate of 0 to 15 percent should not consider subsequent pregnancies. If a patient with Stage III disease considers a pregnancy at all, she should defer conception for at least five years. Any Stage I or II patient whose tumor recurs should not contemplate pregnancy because of both the poor prognosis and the need for ongoing treatment.

The major prognostic variables for these types of tumors include their size and the status of axillary lymph nodes.

4.   The risk of recurrence is greatest during the first two years after treatment. Most authors caution against an immediate pregnancy. They recommend that all early-stage patients who are disease-free after primary treatment wait two to three years before conceiving.

5.   Because the prognosis for patients with positive axillary nodes may be poor, many physicians discourage pregnancy for women in this group. The fear is not of stimulating micrometastases but of the probability of tumor recurrence and the likelihood that the mother may not live long enough to rear the child. (The different doctors whose studies Danforth compiled recommended from three to five years wait before pregnancy.)

In final summary, the article reads as follows:

"The primary tumor's prognostic status is perhaps the most important factor when deciding whether a pregnancy is advisable and when conception should occur. For patients with stage I or II breast cancer and negative axillary nodes, subsequent pregnancy appears perfectly acceptable. Other prognostic factors may also help to define a particular node-negative woman's risk: nuclear grade, estrogen and progesterone receptor content, S phase, ploidy, epidermal growth factor receptor content, or cathepsin D. Although the optimal timing of a pregnancy for a patient with a good prognosis is not defined, it is reasonable to suggest that she wait 2 to 3 years. The risk of recurrence becomes less with time; in turn, if adjuvant chemotherapy was used its risk to the pregnancy, if indeed there is any, would also appear to be reduced."

It is important when reading any medical literature that you understand that studies can be interpreted many ways and that in the studies cited in Danforth's piece, the largest number of women followed was one hundred.

Indeed, in two of the reviews that follow this piece, while generally praising Danforth's article, the authors take exception to some conclusions that Danforth has reached. In one of the reviews, the doctor questions a statistic cited by Danforth that says that a review of nineteen pregnancies after adjuvant chemotherapy showed no fetal malformations. The review, by Richard Epstein, instructor in medicine at Harvard, and Craig Henderson at Dana-Farber in Boston, Mass., says that a recent publication has documented an 8 percent incidence of congenital anomalies in the offspring of 110 chemotherapy-treated patients. The exact figures, drugs, and case histories are not available in either of these articles, making clear again the confusion of information surrounding this issue.

Epstein and Henderson also question the waiting period of two to three years for patients with small, node-negative tumors.

"Our main reservation about his otherwise praiseworthy review is that the author has elected to pass sentence in an equally conclusive manner. To maintain that pregnancy appears 'perfectly acceptable for patients with node-negative disease while stage I/II patients with subsequent recurrence should not contemplate pregnancy' may be overstating the case. Early-stage patients who experience recurrence within the breast following breast conservation therapy may remain eminently curable by mastectomy, whereas 30 percent of node negative patients will die of metastatic disease within 10 years of diagnosis, irrespective of intervening pregnancies. We believe that too much weight is given to the 2 to 3 year 'waiting period' so popularly advocated by the authorities quoted. Patients with small node-negative tumors may gain nothing except lost time by waiting . . . "

I particularly like the closing of the Epstein-Henderson review. In this they present the issue I hear most from women considering pregnancy. It is not the physical act of giving birth that concerns women as much as the guarantee that they will be around for the next eighteen years in order to launch that child into adulthood. Their conclusion:

"Underlying the debate as to whether subsequent pregnancy affects breast cancer outcome is one final dilemma—a dilemma that is barely touched upon in Dr. Danforth's article, one which surely must be uppermost in the minds of those considering pregnancy in the context of a prior breast cancer. It is one thing to be able to reassure a woman that a pregnancy should not significantly influence the course of her disease; it is quite another, however, to be able to predict whether a mother with a prior breast cancer will live to see her child through to adulthood. As every clinician who treats breast cancer patients knows, the spectacle of a woman dying while still in the process of rearing young children is truly heartbreaking. No amount of prognostic or biologic information gives a physician the right to say yes or no to this most difficult decision. The best that we can do is to help the patient and her family understand the uncertainties and risks involved and to trust that the decision appropriate to priorities and circumstances will be made."

The second review of Danforth's article, by William C. Wood, M.D., chairman of the department of surgery at Emory University School of Medicine in Atlanta, distilled both pieces even further. He also was complimentary of Danforth's piece with this conclusion, entitled "What We Should Tell Women." His list of the important information to convey to a woman is as follows:

"1. *Choosing to carry a child will probably not significantly affect her prognosis.*
2. *Our best estimate of her prognosis and the ranges on either side of that estimate.*

3. *Assure her that we will support her decision.*
4. *Only if requested, state our own personal viewpoint about a woman with such a life expectancy carrying a child. Although we bring prognostic knowledge to this matter, I am not convinced that we bring any special wisdom regarding balancing prognosis and the bearing of children."*

Wood also questions the waiting time recommended by doctors. Wood points out that while extremely aggressive tumors recur within the first two years after treatment, the actual annual risk is relatively linear over the first ten to twelve years.

"Factors that perhaps are equally important to these biologic considerations are the psychosocial considerations of women who are experiencing breast cancer. The reverberations associated with this major trauma of a woman's life remain strong even 1 or 2 years later. Similarly, bearing a child and beginning its rearing are major emotional stresses. A woman might be asking too much of herself when she tries to cope with a recent breast cancer, a pregnancy, and the beginning of childrearing all in a short period of time. These psychosocial stresses contribute to the oncologist's strong belief that some delay between oncologic treatment and conception is appropriate. Dr. Danforth has combined the major available bodies of data into a single review to help us guide our patient through this murky area."

Basically, this and other medical information on the topic remains inconclusive. Getting pregnant when you are healthy and haven't had chemotherapy and radiation is a gamble. Getting pregnant when you have had breast cancer, chemo, and radiation adds to those odds. For some women the gamble is worth it. I know healthy women whose desire to bear a child is so strong they have devoted years and thousands of dollars to getting pregnant.

For others the gamble isn't worth it. If you are struggling with this issue, learn all you can, consult with enough doctors that you feel you have a balanced view, and then discuss it with your husband. To put it bluntly, he will be the primary caretaker of the child should you die.

Those of us whose diagnosis came during or immediately after a pregnancy cannot help but wonder if the hormone-rich environment created by pregnancy led to our tumors, although there is no scientific link. I have also talked to a number of women who took hormones, as I did, to get pregnant. No link has been established, but like with the pill and all other medications that influence our hormones, you have to think twice.

Debra wanted another child after her breast cancer became the catalyst for a reconciliation with her husband. Debra had chemotherapy and a year of tamoxifen for her estrogen-receptor-positive invasive tumor. She became pregnant with Ashley a year after her diagnosis, shortly after stopping the tamoxifen.

The pregnancy was normal and she had a mammogram every month on the other breast. Ashley was born in March 1987 and is healthy, as is Debra. *"My ob was unusual in that while I was going to him, he had four women who had had breast cancer and were pregnant. Three were fine and one had a recurrence."*

Debra says her oncologist approved of her decision to become pregnant, and her plastic surgeon thought she was crazy. Debra was reconstructed when Ashley was two with the TRAM procedure, in which her stomach muscle was used to reconstruct her breast.

Victoria was childless and in the process of divorce when she was diagnosed with intraductal carcinoma, which is a very early stage, and had a bilateral mastectomy. She married John two years later and their son was born in November 1990. She felt secure in her decision and was not concerned about recurrence. *"My surgeon had a specialty in oncology, and he has been very reassuring. He tells me not to give it a second thought, and I believe him."*

Ann knew immediately after her surgery for an early-stage intraductal diagnosis that many of her decisions about reconstruction (she had no adjuvant treatment) would be based on the fact that she and her husband wanted another child. Her son was sixteen months old when she was diagnosed. *"The doctor said wait until we have the second child. Then I started talking to Dr. A, and he said he didn't want me to breast-feed because of the longevity of the time with having been pregnant and not being able to have a mammogram."*

Ann and her husband visited a geneticist at Southwestern Medical School, and although he went through the library and found very little on pregnancy after breast cancer, he recommended that she wait at least three years and preferably wait five. *"He said, 'Do you want to be around here for your child, the one you have now and another you might have?' You don't know about estrogen receptors. So he put a whole different thought in my mind. I wasn't thinking in those terms. So there was a period when I thought I didn't want to go through that—being scared during the whole pregnancy."* Ann's second child was born in December 1992. She and her mother are fine.

PROPHYLACTIC REMOVAL

The prophylactic—or preventive—removal of a breast or both breasts is usually performed when a woman is at extremely high risk for a second new breast cancer, has a precancerous condition, or has already had breast cancer in one breast and, for a number of reasons, the other breast is suspect.

Women who have had breast cancer in one breast may be somewhat more likely to have it in the other breast, depending on pathology, their age, and family history. No matter the risk, the decision to remove that breast is one that should be made with deliberation and consideration.

"I said take them both, and he said, 'You need to think about that a little bit. It's kind of a shock to lose both breasts.' After losing one, I think it was even more of a shock to look down and have one stupid-looking breast! You know, I thought that was the dumbest thing I'd ever seen. Anyway, I did not have him remove both breasts at that time. I went back and had the other one removed a year and a half later."
—Sylvia

"The real reason I had the second breast removed was cosmetic. I looked like a unicorn. I never wear a bra, and I like to wear polo tops and shorts and I hated my prosthesis and without it, I looked weird. With both gone I just look flat-chested. None is better than one."
—Mary H

"To have the subcutaneous mastectomy was probably the harder decision because there was not a clear medical line of thought. She's premenopausal; she's had cancer. She's had fibrocystic disease in the other breast. We'd just gone through the hassle of going in and con-

*firming that it was a benign lump. They were going to have to do
something with that breast anyway after reconstruction, to make it
symmetrical with the reconstructed breast. So if you're going to have
to monkey with it, why the hell not eliminate the risk. She asked me
what did I think, and I said, 'No. It's a decision you have to make.' "*
—Lynne's husband, Norm

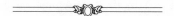

> **Tip—Unless there is clear medical evidence that it
> is needed, most surgeons will not remove your re-
> maining breast at the same time as doing your mas-
> tectomy. If you are considering this before surgery,
> you may want to delay reconstruction, to allow
> yourself time to consider having the other breast
> removed and both reconstructed at the same time.**

There were a number of women who decided at diagnosis that they
wanted the other breast removed. Either their tumor did not show on
the mammogram or there was a strong emotional reason that prompted
their decision. Factors to consider in making the decision are both emotional and medical.

1. Are you at high risk for a new breast cancer in the other breast?
2. Are your breasts hard to mammogram or examine clinically be-
    cause of dense tissue?
3. Have you consulted with at least two doctors?
4. Have you waited long enough to know that this is not a purely
    emotional decision related to the cancer diagnosis?

When my mother was diagnosed in October 1991, she chose to have
a bilateral mastectomy for a number of reasons, with comfort being
primary. She had large breasts and some women have back problems
from the lack of balance after one breast is removed. She also knew that
she would be more comfortable not having to wear a prosthesis daily,

which she didn't. She was pleased with her decision after surgery and only wore her prostheses on a few occasions.

Removing your other breast is also a very personal decision and one that you alone can make. Some women combined the decision with that about reconstruction, opting for a subcutaneous mastectomy on their other breast at the same time, to allow for better matching.

Be aware that there are different terminologies applied to surgery for prophylactic removal. A subcutaneous mastectomy may leave enough breast tissue that you will need to continue mammography of the breast.

Diana and Kim both decided on a bilateral subcutaneous mastectomy after a diagnosis of lobular carcinoma in situ—a condition that increased their risk of invasive cancer in the future. Diana's mother had died of endometrial cancer four years earlier. She was also a very good friend of mine and was my daughter's godmother and had seen first-hand what breast cancer could do. *"We researched it and found that the lobular carcinoma in situ has a higher likelihood of appearing in the other breast. I have very dense breasts and I was concerned that we wouldn't find it. Our decision was confirmed when Dr. B came out after surgery and told Bruce that he had found a small invasive tumor behind the area where the lobular carcinoma was. It had not shown on the mammogram. So I know I made the right decision."*

Diana's surgeon explained the importance of removing adequate breast tissue in a prophylactic mastectomy, describing his procedure as a total glandular mastectomy (TGM). *"The subcutaneous may leave breast tissue that could develop a tumor. And with the subcutaneous you will have mammograms to deal with in the future. He took off my nipple, scraped all the tissue off, and then X-rayed it to be sure there was nothing suspicious. Then he put it back on. He also sampled the lymph nodes to be sure they were clear. I was really glad about that because I would have had to have that done anyway, since they found an invasive tumor."*

Tip—Ask about different kinds of mastectomies and be sure that all the breast tissue is going to be removed. If it isn't, you will need to continue mammography in the future.

Despite the presence of the invasive tumor and the literature that supported the bilateral decision, Diana's insurance company refused to pay for removal of the second breast. Diana and her husband threatened to sue, and eventually the insurance company agreed to pay.

Barbara Blumberg is the director of education for the Komen Alliance Clinical Breast Center in Dallas. She is also a rare individual in that her specialty is risk analysis. Her background combines genetics, epidemiology, health education, and counseling to help a woman understand her risks of developing breast cancer in the future or, if the women is a survivor, her risk of developing cancer in the opposite breast and the risk of other female family members. Blumberg's own mother died of breast cancer in 1975. Blumberg frequently counsels with women about prophylactic removal of the other breast. She says that women considering this should move slowly.

"My goal is not to make the decision for someone but to slow them down so they can make a decision for themselves that is not based on emotion but on as much fact as possible. I would carefully analyze her personal and family medical history and gather records on the woman herself and other members of her family who had cancer histories. I'd get a second pathology opinion if the pathology had not been reviewed by someone familiar to me. There are certain factors about the first breast cancer that can tell us whether the woman is more at risk of developing a second breast cancer in the opposite breast. In addition, other factors related to her specific diagnosis need to be assessed."

Blumberg says that an emotional decision is not wrong but that a woman needs time to understand all the facts before proceeding.

"Once you take the breast off, it's off. And that's not to say you shouldn't take it off, but you should think about it as completely as possible. Take the time. If the opposite breast is totally clear, if there's no cancer there, how would you feel? How would you feel if you had that opposite breast removed and a few years down the line you were diagnosed with colon cancer? These are examples of areas a woman needs to think about. In addition, the woman should ask her doctor how easy or difficult it is to examine her remaining breast and how easy it is to view on a mammogram. A woman needs to consider the surgical options available to her as a result of early diagnosis such as lumpectomy as well."

*"My surgeon offered me the choice. I'd already had three biopsies on the other side, and he said he could make a case for either way. If I wanted to have both of them done, that was fine. But he said a lot of times after you get through with the treatment they go back and do the other side. And I just said I don't want to do this anymore. I don't want to go through this—the mammogram and the worry—because I'd done it four times now. The worst fear is that waiting to see if that's going to be it. So I really appreciated that he allowed me to make that choice."—*Harriet

Sadie said that her daughter decided on prophylactic mastectomies at forty-four, after she had undergone four biopsies, *"The doctor told her she was a prime target, because her mother and grandmother had had breast cancer. So after her fourth biopsy she said, 'I'm having them both removed and implants put in.' She was tired of worrying about it. She was waking up at night worrying about it. This was before all the stuff about implants, but she said she still thinks her chances of breast cancer were much higher than having problems with implants."*

Tip—A new test developed recently at the University of Michigan can identify women who have inherited a gene that indicates a strong possibility of breast cancer. If you have a number of first-degree relatives who have had breast or ovarian cancer and are considering a prophylactic mastectomy, ask your physician about the availability of this test.

UNDERSTANDING BREAST CANCER RISK

"I walk every day with a woman who has been a neighbor for years. She's always refused to have a mammogram. I said, 'Carrie, what the hell's the matter with you? You've got three kids.' She said, 'Well, it's not in my family.' I said, 'Sure and the car's in the street, which means you won't get hit.' " —Bridie

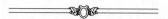

> **Tip—Remember as you read this: Your greatest risk factor is your sex, followed by your age, and 70 percent of women being diagnosed have none of the recognizable risk factors.**

A number of factors must be taken into account when discussing breast cancer risk for all women. Those that are commonly addressed and which researchers know from studies have an impact on risk:

1. family history of breast cancer
2. early onset of menstruation (before twelve) or late menopause (after fifty-five)
3. never having had a child, or becoming pregnant for the first time after thirty

In addition, researchers are accepting that there are many environmental factors that may increase risk, including diet, exposure to carcinogens, and life-style issues. These are much harder to evaluate.

While the vast majority of women being diagnosed with breast cancer have no family history, having first-degree relatives who have had the disease may play an important role in risk. Whether the relative was premenopausal or postmenopausal will indicate how high that risk can go.

For this reason, it is important that women *know* who in their family has had breast or other cancer.

While it seems inconceivable to me that a mother would keep that information from her daughters, I have talked to women who did not know that their mothers had breast cancer until they themselves were diagnosed. Rula was only nine when her mother died of breast cancer in her early thirties. *"I never knew from my dad that my mom passed away with breast cancer. I knew it from friends, but my dad would not say anything about it, because you didn't say the word cancer."* Indeed, Rula's mother had had cancer in both breasts, a fact that may have increased Rula's risk and that of any daughters she might have.

Harriett's mother died of breast cancer. *"She must have been in her fifties when she was diagnosed. She died when we were first married. Mother never really said much about hers. I knew she had had a mastectomy, but I don't even know that I ever really knew it was breast cancer until I had mine."*

Other women met similar reluctance from their mothers to talk of their own experience—a fact that was disheartening and made their own experience worse. Doris says her mother would not talk about it to her or her sister, shutting them out. *"She never showed us what it looked like. Now, she had the Halsted radical, so I thought it was a great open wound, a great sore place. It was all hush-hush. The Big C, was what one of the nurses called it."*

Betty B was pregnant with her daughter when she was diagnosed. *"My mother never talked about it. I knew that she had had it, but she never talked to me about any of her feelings about it. I guarantee that it's going to be different with Kelsey. My mother pretended it never happened. And that was what she did. She gave me no words of protection, no anything."*

While a certain degree of caution is called for by women facing a history of breast cancer, panic is not called for. Some possible suggestions that have emerged from the professionals include:

1. Beginning mammograms earlier, with some experts recommending you begin five years younger than the age at which cancer was diagnosed in your mother or aunt, taking into consideration the ineffectiveness of mammography for women in their twenties.

2. Seeing a breast specialist for annual mammography and exam. A suspicious area that changes from one year to the next may or may not be caught by a radiologist unaware of family history but would get closer attention from a breast surgeon tracking possible early breast cancer.

3. Possible inclusion in the tamoxifen trial now under way in the country for women who fulfill specific risk guideliness that become more rigid with decreasing age. Tamoxifen, the estrogen block, has

properties of reducing estrogen in the breast and is thought to reduce the possibility of developing breast cancer for those at risk. Discuss this with your breast specialist to learn where in your vicinity tamoxifen trials are under way.

A new discipline—and one that, unfortunately, is still available in only a handful of cities—will most certainly be critical in the lives of our daughters and sisters as they face this disease: **Risk analysis** is a combination of counseling, education, and genetics, during which a woman can learn her true risk of breast cancer. Andrea's story is a perfect example of how the procedure works.

After watching a talk show on breast cancer, thirty-year-old Andrea decided that because her grandmother had had breast cancer, she wanted to know what her true risk was. She contacted Barbara Blumberg, the director of education for the Komen Alliance Clinical Breast Center and one of only a few "risk analysis" specialists in the country. *"She goes over everything, all the research that she has looked at, and she also teaches you how to look at things you see in a magazine or read and try and discern what they're saying to you. You know, like you read the magazine articles or whatever, and that's fine and dandy, but look at what the research is saying. Look at what kinds of groups they surveyed and what kind of margin of error there was. Don't just take at face value what it shows you. And that helped me a lot. And she talked to me about alcohol and the risk of smoking, which I don't do, and caffeine and diet."*

Andrea met with Blumberg in six different sessions, all of which were covered by insurance. *"She told me a lot about how breast cancer starts, the theories about what makes it start, and what my personal risk was based on my family history with my grandmother having cancer. That was something they factored into it. They said that because she had it, that didn't mean that I would get it, but it was a risk factor to take into consideration."*

Midway through the counseling, when mammography was being discussed, Andrea decided to go ahead and have a baseline. It showed clustered calcifications that turned out to be malignant. She decided on a modified radical mastectomy and reconstruction. *"Barbara told me that I probably saved my own life, which helped me cope with the emotions of the cancer and the loss of the breast."*

RISK ANALYSIS PROFESSIONAL BARBARA BLUMBERG, SC.M., DIRECTOR OF EDUCATION AT THE KOMEN ALLIANCE CLINICAL BREAST CENTER, TALKS ABOUT THE REALITY OF RISK

Barbara Blumberg joined the Komen Alliance after working in patient education for the National Cancer Institute, the Fox Chase Cancer Center in Philadelphia, and the American Cancer Society in New York City. She did graduate work at the School of Public Health at Johns Hopkins. Each visit with her is one hour and costs $80; it's covered by most insurers as a service of the breast center.

Explain risk analysis.

Risk analysis is really a combination of an education and counseling program. The goals of the program are to help a woman learn what her risk is of developing breast cancer in the future or, if she has breast cancer already, to learn her risk of additional disease to the opposite breast, risk to other family members, and to help her make some kind of sense out of all the statistics and mass of information she gets.

Can you tell me the circumstances of Andrea's situation?

Andrea was about thirty when she came in. She was really concerned. She had been diagnosed as being fibrocystic and was really afraid that she wasn't going to be able to find something amiss in her breast either by self-exam or mammography. She's a take-charge woman, and she couldn't take charge of that part of her body. She was basically being told she didn't need a mammogram because she wasn't thirty-five and there were no symptoms. She had a family history of breast cancer that she knew about. Andrea and I talked, and from our conversation I learned that something was telling her she needed a mammogram. I encourage women to trust their intuition about their bodies. She had a mammogram,

(continued)

suspicious calcifications were found, and she had a choice of either waiting, because they had no other mammogram to compare them to, or to have them taken care of right away. We spoke to the radiologist together, and she came back to my office and we talked it out. I did some reflective listening with her and I told her what I heard her saying. She was saying, "I want this taken out now." Her intuition held her in good stead—resulting in a mastectomy and reconstruction as a result of a diagnosis. I went through all of this with her and served as her support and advocate. I told her I was sorry that her intuition was correct, but she should realize she probably saved her life. I still get chills when I talk about her. I'm delighted to say I went to her wedding recently. It was wonderful.

She was a real success story for what you do.

I've had a number of other people in similar situations, who are dealing with a diagnosis that needs to be verified. We get it verified by our pathologist. I teach people how to get the best possible opinions they need and how to get a second opinion. There's so much misinformation about breast cancer, even pertaining to our whole concept of risk. It's my goal to let them cut through all of the misinformation. I don't give yes or no answers. Rather, I want a woman to understand why she's hearing one day, "Don't take birth control pills," and the next day, "Take them." She hears one day, "Don't drink wine," and the next day, "Have a glass."

So you act as a sounding board?

I think that a lot of women who are diagnosed are frightened. A lot of physicians are willing to talk to a woman and a woman doesn't know it. I serve as a complement and supplement to the physician. I'm there to talk about risk and deal with it from an emotional as well as a medical perspective.

(continued)

Can they come to you before surgery?

I have people call me before surgery. I do a lot of reflective listening to see if they understand. There are videos, literature. I help a woman come up with the questions she wants answered by her doctor. In addition, if you've been told you have breast cancer, you only hear so much. A woman will come to me and say, "I didn't hear." Sometimes you just need somebody to say to you, "Tell me what you heard," someone objective, but interested and knowledgeable. Sometimes I'll go back to the doctor and ask what was said to the patient. I want to be able to reinforce medically what they've said.

If a woman is insistent that she wants the other breast removed, what do you say?

I try to get her to slow down, in order to provide her with the information necessary for her to make an informed decision. I try to steer them in the right direction and slow them down from making a decision before they're really ready to make one. But in terms of the ultimate decision, that's up to them.

What can young women do? Or what can mothers do to help their daughters?

They need to practice the best possible early detection they can. A woman needs to start self-exam at age twenty. I just started seeing a woman who's twenty-two and she's been doing self-exams since she was seventeen. There needs to be more of that. Nobody should feel that they are immune to breast cancer. We need to take some of the scare out of it. How can a lump that's just in your breast do harm to the rest of your body? It's when it has a chance to spread that it presents a problem.

Resources for risk analysis:

Dana-Farber High Risk Clinic, Boston, (617) 632-2178.

Baylor-Susan G. Komen Breast Centers Breast Cancer Risk Analysis, Dallas, (214) 820-6975

Alta Bates Comprehensive Cancer Center Cancer Risk Counseling
Services, Berkeley, (510) 204-4286.

CHECKUPS

"It's in my past and I can put it behind me. But it's not over with, and it'll never be over with for the rest of my life, because I'll always worry is it going to come back, especially every six months when I go in for tests. When I go in for tests, it's horrible. I get nervous the day before, and I stay a nervous wreck until I can get this over, and when the results are in, I'm fine for another six months. I live my life in six-month increments."—Leanne

"Every time I go for a checkup and the result is good, I tell myself it's silly to keep going. But every time I go and am waiting for the chance to be called in, I am a nervous wreck and I cannot get the results myself. My husband has to call on the phone. I cannot hear it on the phone again that something is wrong."—Lise

Except for those women who are diagnosed with metastatic disease, meaning it has already moved to another organ of the body, most of us will end treatment NED, or No Evidence of Disease. Now we wait and get on with our lives, assuming that we are well and returning to our surgeon or oncologist regularly to be sure.

After treatment has ended, the surgeon or oncologist will set up regular checkups for a specific length of time. Every three months during the first year or two is fairly standard, with the length between visits extended to six months or a year at some point down the road.

"I didn't realize how much she was worrying about going in for that annual checkup, and this was something that I made her schedule for when I was in town. After she had been through it, it was like this huge weight had been taken off her shoulders."—Dot's husband, Jack

These checkups have got to be a least favorite experience of most of the women interviewed for this book. For in the blood work and various tests and scans the doctors are, to be blunt, looking to see if the cancer has recurred.

Tip—Eighty percent of women who will have re-currence do so in the first two years. Thus the more careful follow-up during this time.

Yet they are the doctor visits we love to hate, because as much as we hate going, the oncologist's blood work becomes a lifeline, a reassurance that we are well.

Continued care after treatment includes seeing your surgeon and/or oncologist regularly, during which you will talk with him or her and discuss the results of a number of tests and scans including

1. an annual mammogram
2. blood work on a schedule suggested by your oncologist (Those women at higher risk for recurrence will be checked more often for the first two years.)
3. a chest X ray, the frequency of which will be determined by your doctor
4. follow up scans, such as a CAT scan and bone scan, to be deter-mined by your doctor

When Leanne was diagnosed at twenty-eight, she underwent a year of chemotherapy, after which her oncologist had her go to the hospital for tests every three months and then every six months after a year. She would have her blood drawn and have a CAT scan, bone scan, and a chest X ray. She would wait for the results of her tests the next day. She said at one point how much she disliked her oncologist and how glad she was that she did not have to see him. He was convinced her cancer would recur and told her there was no reason for him to see her until then. After we talked, she changed oncologists. Her new oncologist explained that she didn't need all the tests every time she came in. The blood work would give indicators if there was a need for a bone scan or liver sonogram.

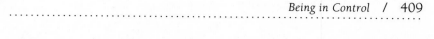

Tip—You should have a hands-on physical exam and consult with your doctor at every checkup.

Your visits to the oncologist will begin with blood work that will specifically identify chemicals in the body that may be out of balance if there is a recurrence somewhere.

Joanne says the fear of death really began for her when her doctors extended her checkups. *"The doctor says, 'We're not going to do a skeletal on you now. You can wait a year and a half.' You don't know if you are glad or sad. You think, Aha! We will wait a year and a half, but what will happen in the next six months when what he is telling you is that you're better."*

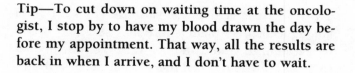

Tip—To cut down on waiting time at the oncologist, I stop by to have my blood drawn the day before my appointment. That way, all the results are back in when I arrive, and I don't have to wait.

BEING IN CONTROL

"Now it really gets me. I smell those chemicals and the same familiar smells. And every time they have to take blood one more time, I get tense—usually because I know they're going to have to try three or four times to find a vein and it hurts and I don't want to do it."
—Sherry

As time has passed since my cancer, I have learned more and more about medical procedure and how labs and doctors' offices work. I have also learned I am what is called a "hard stick." Chemotherapy leaves scars on the veins, making them unusable. Since we can only have blood drawn from the same arm used for chemotherapy because of the danger of infection and lymphedema, the good veins go fast. It takes a real pro to get blood out of my arm, and I have developed some very clear personal boundaries about who draws my blood and how it is done.

Harriett says she has also drawn some firm boundaries about being stuck. She has her own personal needle-sticker in the lab and won't go in if she is not there. *"When I had the CAT scan, I went in and the technician came in and he lays me down, and I said, 'You get two sticks and then I'm gone.' And he started laughing, and I said, 'I'm not kidding you!' And he looked at me and said, 'No you're not, are you?' And I said no. I said two sticks. So he sent for the doctor."*

Harriett says that one tech stuck her nine times—something she will not let happen again. I also learned—the hard way—to ask for the IV team when admitted to the hospital. If a tech comes around after you go into the hospital, tell him or her you are a hard stick and you will wait for the IV team and let them draw blood.

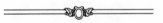

Tip—There is a definite variation in skill level among techs. Ask them before they stick you not to fish around in your arm for a vein. Tell them what to expect if they do. Tell them to get the best if they aren't. You have a right to request that a certain tech take your blood. You have a right to expect competency from those who will check you. Be polite but firm.

I have also found that I expect a certain level of interaction from residents and other medical professionals. In fact, I sent one resident packing after a checkup where I again got results back that showed I had beaten the reaper after a particularly gruesome panic attack.

I had already passed my doc in the hall and told him I was feeling feisty, since I now knew I was going to live at least four more months. He mentioned he had a new associate who was seeing patients with him. I said, "Send him in. I'm ready."

When I explained to the resident that I was there for blood work as the result of a panic attack, his body language or facial expression read CONDESCENDING.

He grabbed a paper gown and handed it to me on his way out the door, saying, "Get undressed and I will see you in a minute."

I simmered while he was out of the room. When he returned, I had indeed put on the paper shirt but had my arms tightly crossed.

"Where is Dr. Mennel?" I asked. "I want him to see me."

"He is coming, but I am going to examine you first," he said as he moved into my space. "Is that all right?"

"No, as a matter of fact, it isn't. I came in here today thinking I was dying and you don't have any idea what that feels like. I want my doctor."

He stomped out of the room, and I immediately felt both empowered and guilty. I had really taken him on, and in the frame of mind I was in, I didn't know if I had been fair.

When Dr. Mennel walked in, I began to apologize. He said, "I think he was what you needed today, and maybe you were what he needed."

Elizabeth T had the same problem with her annual mammogram. When the tech kept asking for additional views and wouldn't explain why, Elizabeth assumed she saw something. When it was finally made clear that the tech was just inefficient, soft-spoken Elizabeth became angry. *"I know which technician is going to do it, and I'm going to interview her before she does them. Because I had to end up having twelve views taken. I'm getting control of that situation."*

Judy D was unduly alarmed by a thoughtless nurse, who casually told her that her liver counts were up, an indicator on a blood test that can indicate a metastasis. *"I lost it. I went bananas and said, 'Please explain that to me.' Well, nurses will tell you nothing. So I called my surgeon and said I had to talk to her as soon as she came in. She called and I said I wanted to talk about my blood test. She said, 'What blood test?' She hadn't even seen the report yet. Well, she looked at it and called me right back and said there was nothing to worry about. I had already called my doctor about a sonogram and was primed and ready to be facing a recurrence. She said it was a minimal elevation and could be caused by anything, including the effects of chemo. She said it fluctuates and there was nothing to worry about."*

I really feel that every medical student, nurse, tech, or resident should be assigned his or her own personal cancer survivor for a few weeks.

There are certainly enough of us—1.5 million women alone have survived breast cancer as of 1993.

What would I tell my student?

I AM NOT A DISEASE. I AM A PERSON. KNOW ME AS A PERSON FIRST AND A PATIENT SECOND.

YOU ARE NOT GOD AND YOU DO NOT KNOW MY BODY BETTER THAN I DO.

I DID NOT HAVE BRAIN CANCER, I HAD BREAST CANCER. DON'T TREAT ME LIKE MY INTELLIGENCE IS IMPAIRED.

I WANT HUMANITY FROM YOU. I AM NOT A SET OF CLINICAL CLUES OVER WHICH YOU WILL BE TESTED. I WANT YOU TO CARE ABOUT ME AS A PERSON.

I WANT US TO BE A TEAM—LET ME HELP YOU—HELP ME, I'M FRIGHTENED.

GIVE ME HOPE—IT IS THE CHEMOTHERAPY OF THE SPIRIT.

GIVE ME TRUTH—I NEED IT TO DECIDE HOW TO LIVE MY LIFE.

UNLESS YOU KNOW WHAT IT FEELS LIKE TO THINK YOU ARE DYING, DON'T BE CONDESCENDING WHEN I AM AFRAID.

FEAR CAN BE MORE PAINFUL THAN SURGERY.

LISTEN TO ME AS MUCH AS YOU LISTEN TO MY BODY. MY HEARTBEAT IS CONNECTED TO MY SOUL.

CONNECT WITH ME. LOOK AT ME, TOUCH ME—IT IS A HUMAN CONNECTION. IT IS EVEN OKAY TO HUG ME.

AND FORGIVE ME IF IN MY FEAR AND ANGER I DUMP ON YOU.

WHEN CANCER RECURS

"If you have metastatic disease, the majority of physicians feel that you cannot be cured. You can be treated. You can get it under control. You can get rid of it for a period of time, but it'll come back."—Robert Mennel, medical oncologist

When breast cancer recurs it can be local or distant. A local recurrence means a new tumor has begun from stray cells left locally near the site of the original breast tumor. It can appear in the same breast or remaining breast tissue or in the underlying area of the breast—the sternum or rib. A local recurrence can be treated successfully and result in No Evidence of Disease. A metastasis occurs when the breast cancer cell, through the blood, travels to a distant organ and begins to grow again. And while there are certainly cases of cure for metastatic disease, it becomes more a battle of containment. Yet in the past few years there have been tremendous strides in the treatment of both local and metastatic breast cancer.

Elaine's recurrence in a number of spots in her bone and scalp was put into remission by tamoxifen, which had just come on the market. Today she has no evidence of disease. The spots are gone.

Tamoxifen also was effective in controlling Theresa's recurrence to her rib. The cancer is still there, but not growing.

Elizabeth P, whose cancer recurred in her sternum in 1986, was put into remission with chemo and radiation after having a portion of her sternum removed and reconstructed. Today she is fine.

Others have faced a darker picture as their cancer progressed more quickly and did not respond to further treatment.

For those who do respond, new drugs can hold the metastasis at bay, allowing precious time for even newer drugs to hit the market. Those who do not respond must come to terms with the emotional reality that this disease may, as one woman said, "have its way with us." How we choose to walk this path reflects our individual outlook and support.

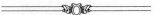

Tip—A 1990 study of women with metastatic breast cancer showed that those women who were part of a support group lived significantly longer than those who were not.

For each of you who face this journey—and this fear—I hope you will meet someone like Marilyn.

Marilyn is an angel of sorts. I have collected angels since a friend brought me one in the hospital when I had my mastectomy. Since then I have read about them and felt their presence in my life. Not in the gold, glowing, celestial-winged sense that many of us imagine, but the walk-on-earth variety. The thing about angels is that they come for a reason—to help you or give you a message. Marilyn did both for me.

I met Marilyn the night she joined my support group in mid-1990. I was immediately drawn to her incredible ear-to-ear smile and bright disposition. As was the custom of the group that when someone new came in, we each gave our sixty-second story, after which the new person could, if she chose, tell us where she was in treatment. I assumed Marilyn was facing surgery. She seemed too cheerful to have recently undergone her mastectomy.

When we were all done with our individual recitals, she introduced herself and explained that she had had a modified radical in June 1983 and nine malignant lymph nodes. In May 1987, her cancer metastasized to her liver, lung cavity, and bones. Since then she has been on a number of different drugs, each of which has worked for a time to control her illness.

I was shocked. Here was someone who, for the last three years, had been experiencing my worst nightmare. And she was smiling. In fact, Marilyn's enthusiasm for a good time soon became infectious. She found out the group always had dinner at the same restaurant after every meeting and put a stop to that immediately by insisting we try a new place every time. She came with the city dining guide and we were soon experimenting with all kinds of food. If there was a party to plan or shopping to do, Marilyn was ready.

As I learned to love Marilyn, I also began to battle my shadow by watching her battle hers. Earlier in the year, I had vetoed a suggestion by our group leader that we invite some women into the group who were coping with recurrence. At the time no one in our group fit that category. I didn't want to accept that this disease could kill. I didn't want to be a part of that struggle.

Now here in front of me was a role model for coping: someone who clearly knew she was very sick, but refused to die emotionally before her time. It's something we all fantasize about being able to do. She was doing it, and I needed to know how.

Nor was hers an unusual battle or one based on denial. Indeed, if anything, Marilyn's zest for life has come from adversity. She had polio in 1952 at age eleven in her right side, leaving her with a right leg that was somewhat smaller and weaker than the left. She lost two sons in infancy and then adopted a baby girl. She had watched her mother struggle for five years with colon cancer, which eventually took her life, and initially refused chemotherapy for her own diagnosis after watching the toll it took on her mother. *"I realized I was going to do chemo, but it took me a couple of days to accept it. I was forty-two and had to fight for my life. I don't think it really hit me what nine out of twenty-one lymph nodes meant at first, that it was really in the lymph system and I needed to fight."*

Four years passed until, during a checkup, Marilyn told her doctor that she was having trouble breathing. *"I thought it was because I was too fat. But I noticed that when I'd try to play golf, I couldn't walk up the hills without puffing. He recommended an oncologist, because we had just moved to the city. They did all the scans and took two liters of fluid out of my lung cavity. I was on tamoxifen and he switched my medicine. The scan also showed it had metastasized to my bones and liver—but after a year, when I had another liver sonogram, the doctor could hardly believe that my liver was so good."*

During this time Marilyn was using visualization techniques. *"I love Bernie Siegel's tapes and used his imaging tapes a lot. I would imagine these holes in my bones and liver and plaster them using little red raiders and they would plaster my bones and back. You know, fill in the holes. That worked for about a year, and then they drew two more liters out of my lungs and switched my medicine again."*

The next drug was the male hormone, which resulted in a rich baritone voice, thirty pounds, and facial hair, all of which Marilyn took in stride. Marilyn's coping mechanism was to draw attention to her voice and her new facial hair, laughing in her infectious, vibrant way. Life continued; her daughter left for college. Her husband, she says, felt helpless. *"My husband is an engineer, you understand. He's real quiet. But we've talked about it. For example. I don't believe in graves. I am going to be in heaven with both my parents. And I have two babies in heaven, so it's hard to be sad about dying. But I think he forgets about it. He helps me since our daughter left because he knows my limitations. I think when you have cancer, you just know what you're going to die from. Everybody is going to die. We just know we're probably going to die from cancer. That doesn't mean we can't go out and have a car accident."*

Marilyn spent her time doing the things she wanted to do: traveling to visit retired friends in warm climes, taking other friends to chemo, and enjoying life. Marilyn said it was a heart to heart with her doctor that helped her attitude. *"He took me into his office and said—you always know it's serious when they take you into their office—'Marilyn, you have a chronic disease. You respond to treatment. This just might be manageable.' He said, 'You are a tough cookie and you have a good attitude. We're just going to treat it.' And that's all I get. I have a chronic disease and it responds. But the idea of doing chemo again, I just go arghh, but I've already decided that if I have chemo again they're going to come to my house and I'm going to have it here."*

And she laughed her incredible booming laugh. For most of the time Marilyn called the cancer an inconvenience. She did begin chemo again in late 1991. She had a catheter inserted and wore a battery pack. The chemo was attached once every three weeks and infused for three days. She didn't lose her hair and still made it to group like clockwork. The chemo helped her bone pain for a while, but in summer 1992, it became clear that the chemo had stopped working. Scans showed abdominal shadows and she began having fluid buildup that made her look pregnant. Her coping mechanism, as always, was humor. *"I told Dr. Jones that if this weighed nine pounds, I was going to name it after him."*

She kept her good spirits and still dressed according to the holidays (except for St. Pat's Day, because she didn't look good in green). Marilyn and I walked in the Race for the Cure in October 1991. In October 1992, I, along with a number of group members, pushed her in a wheelchair for the race, that brought 9,000 women to Dallas. At the time, I knew as she did that I would wear a sign in her memory in 1993.

We went shopping on December 18, 1992, at a cluster of craft shops near her home. We talked about dying and Marilyn gave me a pig angel for my collection. We laughed and chatted.

On January 5, Marilyn died at home, less than twelve hours after she had been walking and talking. Her memorial service was typical Marilyn. She donated her body to the medical school, explaining that despite the fact that a few pieces were missing, someone might learn something. Instead of flowers, she filled the church with red and purple balloons.

Her eulogy brought as much laughter as tears as the pastor assured us that with her last breath, Marilyn had told him to keep it upbeat. It made me think of something she had said to me: *"There are so many other things worse than having cancer, I just refuse to die before I die."*

And she didn't.

RESOURCES

———⸙○⸙———

Tip—Although most medical journals are hard for the lay person to fathom, I found *Oncology* fairly readable. If you are interested, take out a subscription to *Oncology* or its sister publication, *Primary Care and Cancer*. Both will keep you up to date on studies about breast cancer, and other issues. Call the publisher in Huntington, New York, at (516) 424–8900 for rates.

———

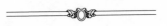

Chapter 9

WHEN LIVING WITH CANCER BECOMES DYING FROM CANCER

FACING DEATH

"I told him I wanted six months' notice so I could get my photo albums in order. He said he would try. I also told him I wanted to be able to talk until the end. He said he was sure I'd have the final word."
—Marilyn

"I said to the doctor, 'If you take me off the chemo and we try the hormones, let's come to some agreement about what our goal is. I would like to plan on as good a life as possible. I would also like to plan on as good a death as possible.' He agreed with me 100 percent and he's with me all the way."—Ida Rose

"A healthy death is one in which a patient has had the opportunity to say his or her goodbyes, to complete unfinished business, and to make peace with his or her Higher Power, whatever that term means to him or her."—Hospice philosophy

---

Tip—Breast cancer is the leading cause of death in American women ages thirty-four to fifty-five. It is the leading cancer death and second overall cause of death in women fifteen to thirty-four. In 1992,

126 women died every day from breast cancer—
46,000 in all.

Where to begin. How do we talk about dying? When I began this book, the outline did not include the word *death*. I didn't want to talk to women whose cancer had metastasized. I didn't want to face what was for me the greatest fear.

A number of events changed my mind. Indeed, I became convinced as this book progressed that this chapter was the most important in the book, for while death is our greatest fear and accepting our mortality often painful work, to do so is a gift of life. For when I was forced to accept death as a fact of my life—and perhaps one that I would face sooner rather than later—I finally had the big picture about my cancer. I could look at the past and the future and know that there were no guarantees, but that I could make the decisions about what I could control. From that came an indescribable peace.

The first significant event that began this process for me was a call from Louis. I had sent a survey to his wife, Janece, and when I hadn't heard from her, I sent a postcard to remind her. He called with the news that Janece's cancer had metastasized to her liver only fourteen months after she underwent chemo and radiation. She was dead eight weeks later—at age twenty-nine. I was shocked and felt the panic rise to my throat. I tried to end the conversation as quickly as possible. But Louis wouldn't let me. He said *he* wanted to talk to me. He had some things to say about Janece and death and their three-year-old daughter, Laura. I reluctantly agreed to talk to him.

He arrived at my office in July 1990, five months after Janece's death, with pictures of Janece and Laura. He talked about his wife and his pain from losing her and how fast it had happened.

Everyone was prepared to help Janece live, he said, but no one was prepared to help her family understand that *now* was the time to help her die in a way that would be healthy for her and hopeful for the future of those who lived after her. Indeed, Janece learned of her recurrence from the radiologist who performed the liver sonogram. Louis heard her screaming and ran to the room. *"She had read the books and she was crying, saying, 'I'm going to die. It's in my liver.' We went immediately to the oncologist's office, and she was in shock. I was trying to comfort her, but you can't say it's going to be all right. The oncologist told us up front that she wasn't going to make it, that it wasn't very treatable. He said she had three months without chemo, and probably three more months with chemo, but we could try it."*

Louis said that they returned home in a fog and called her parents. After they arrived it was total despair. He removed the guns from the house but remembers little else because of the shock of those days. *"After a week we hit a point where we felt we had to get it together. I said to her, 'You are alive now and you do feel well now and we are all going to die.' You have to keep saying these things and keep reinforcing that you have to live one day at a time. That did have an impact on her."*

Louis says that Janece went right back to work despite being eligible for disability. She wanted to stay busy. Louis saw it as her desire not to give up as she moved into denial, refusing to believe death was imminent and that they wouldn't find something to cure her. *"We could talk about it to some extent, but we basically lived day to day."*

Louis says Janece never began the process of ordering her life. She did begin chemotherapy and felt well until the week before she died. On Sunday she had cleaned house and cooked dinner for their minister. On Monday she began to feel ill; she died on Wednesday. Louis sat in my office and cried. *"I wish I had known she was dying. There were some things that she could have done. She could have sat with a tape recorder or written Laura letters. She didn't do anything for Laura. I wish there was something for me to give to her on her sixteenth birthday: Dear Laura. I wanted that for Laura. I got cheated out of saying goodbye. We never said goodbye. She worked until Friday and died on Wednesday."*

I asked Louis what he wished had been different. His answer was heartfelt. *"I wish she had told me how she was feeling and had not been so strong and felt she had to shield me from how bad she felt. She didn't want to hurt me or Laura, and her only concern was what would happen to us. She didn't let me be a part of her death. I wanted her to enjoy what she had left and to spend as much time with Laura as possible, doing the things that are memory-making. Laura was only three, so it was on the edge of where her memory was. I have memories at three, so it would have been neat to have some time with her and shoot some VCR film."*

When Laura began asking about her mother, Louis answered her questions very clearly and to the point. He made her a memory book of all the snapshots of her and her mother. It is her own book that she can keep in her room. Louis said that they spend many nights poring over the pages.

After my conversation with Louis, I knew that the thousands of men who face the death of their wives this year and next year and the year after that would benefit from his story—and the stories of others who had suffered the loss of a wife or mother to breast cancer. Theirs are the only truths when it comes to loss. And while there is no right or wrong, there is definitely better and best when facing death.

I talked to Louis again in January 1992. He was planning to remarry and had begun speaking locally to groups about the importance of early detection; he often told his and Janece's story. About a year after her mother's death, he took Laura to visit a psychologist. *"He said she was fine and very well adjusted,"* Louis said.

Louis recognizes that Janece's death was unusual in its speed, but still recommends to those he speaks with that they not wait to take the special vacation or make their wishes known. *"I just tell them not to wait. Do it now."*

While Louis spoke to the needs of those surviving such a death, the woman who had the greatest impact on my attitudes about death—and the possibility I would face it in my own life—was my friend Judy W. Diagnosed with inflammatory breast cancer that revealed fourteen malignant lymph nodes in October 1988, Judy came gradually to the realization that her prognosis was poor. We met first in our surgeon's support group, where her sincerity and humor was a major ingredient in the group's success. She had just finished chemotherapy when we met and her hair was growing back.

When the cancer recurred in her bones in March 1990, Judy began a new regimen of chemotherapy treatments, none of which worked. Soon, those of us in the group felt firsthand the power of moving with someone toward death. We didn't talk about it directly, but the acceptance was there. Judy's fondest wish occurred in May 1991, when her son graduated from high school with his mother and father and other family in attendance. Judy continued to work until mid-November 1991, when what appeared to be a minor stroke slurred her speech. By

December it appeared that something more sinister was at work. Judy's cancer had metastasized to her brain in a number of small lesions. She began radiation shortly before Christmas. When I saw her on December 26, she was tired and her speech was jumbled, but we visited and hugged. Judy died on January 14.

As I looked back on what her life had meant to me, I realized that being part of her dying process gave me more courage than anything I could name. I had always privately felt that if I had a recurrence of cancer, I would end my life before allowing my family to see me deteriorate. Judy's death changed that for me, for in it I saw all the gifts that her life and death offered those of us who loved her.

Tip—Tell your oncologist that you want to know when he or she knows that your disease will result in death. Tell him or her you want time to prepare yourself and your family.

Will I be able to apply this knowledge if I must? I believe so. But what I have come to understand is that resolution of one's death is a singular act that takes time to process and resolve. Our age and our life's desires and whether they were fulfilled will also impact this passage. But no one can even begin this process without open and honest communication among patient, doctor, and family. So it hit me that I wanted to control what I could about my death: No life support, plenty of time to put things in order, and to do that, I had to accept that the time had come.

The understanding that one's own death is approaching is a unique journey. Sorting out the feelings, keeping hope alive, and yet preparing for the inevitable make for a tricky balance.

For those who have made this journey there is a place called hopeful reality—choosing to live fully until they die. The only knowledge there is comes from those who have been there before you and from the professionals who counsel with these families.

From their words, I hope you will find the wisdom to know what is best for your own situation.

BRAD AND A'LORY

"You grow up fast. We have already talked about burial plots and things that, when you are first married, you usually don't talk about."—Brad

One of the most difficult interviews I did for this book was with A'lory and Brad. Incredibly young to be facing death, A'lory was twenty-seven and Brad twenty-nine; we talked the week of their first wedding anniversary.

A'lory found the lump initially at age twenty-one while a college student. A negative mammogram and a doctor's reassurance that it was nothing delayed her diagnosis until she was twenty-four. She had a modified radical in November 1988 that revealed thirteen positive nodes.

She met Brad at one of the many Country-Western dance bars in Fort Worth, where she broke her rule and gave him her phone number after he asked her to dance. *"I didn't date in high school and started going out some in college, and it wasn't how your mother tells you it's going to be. It was all of a sudden that we just felt really comfortable together."*

A'lory had been dating Brad for a year when she had surgery, and together the two endured her ten months of chemotherapy and radiation, feeling certain that all would be well. Brad, who had been a rodeo cowboy for twelve years, shared A'lory's desire to have a ranch somewhere where they could rear children and raise animals. A'lory had graduated with a degree in interior design in 1987 and was managing a wallpaper store when she was diagnosed.

Whether there was ever a discussion of prognosis at the time of surgery, neither could recall. They both felt that the oncologist was telling them that they would lead a normal life and be able to have children. That ended in July 1990, when A'lory felt pain in her stomach and returned to the oncologist to learn that her cancer had returned to her liver and lymph nodes in the neck and in her spine. The oncologist referred her to another oncologist, who specialized in breast cancer.

A'lory immediately had a hysterectomy and began hormone therapy and additional chemotherapy. She and Brad married in October 1990, despite the fact that A'lory was again bald. She had postponed the wedding initially to wait for her thick black hair to grow back to her shoulders—only to lose it again when the cancer recurred. Their wedding picture shows a beaming young couple with A'lory dwarfed by 6-foot-2-inch Brad in his Western-cut suit, his tanned face beaming.

When I interviewed them in October 1991, A'lory had begun receiving disability payments and had already been hospitalized once for direct chemotherapy treatments to her liver in an effort to stop the cancer growth. They lived in a tiny house in a suburb of Fort Worth, and with A'lory's parents in Illinois and Brad's in Washington State, they relied almost entirely on each other for support. Brad was working as a heavy-equipment operator for the city, and they had just bought a small house in a better neighborhood and were looking forward to moving. They clearly were very much in love, and while the issue of death was not addressed directly, both Brad and A'lory alluded to an understanding of her condition.

Brad recalled trying to pin down the oncologist while A'lory was in the hospital in July. *"I asked him what percentage was getting worse and how much liver she had left. He said that 30 to 40 percent was already gone. I asked how fast it was progressing and he hemmed and hawed around and would go off on other things."*

At the time we talked, it was clear that both Brad and A'lory knew that she was desperately ill.

> *"We aren't denying that I can die of cancer. We just live day to day and we just don't talk about it much unless something comes up and we have to. A month may go by or at least a couple of weeks and we won't have talked about it at all."*—A'lory

> *"You can't sit and dwell in it. If I sat there and dwelled on it, I wouldn't even get out of bed. I would just think, What am I going to do? What am I going to do?"*—Brad

As they talked, it was clear that both were struggling with the intense feelings such an illness elicits. But their love for one another was as readily apparent. Brad bought A'lory a dalmation puppy on the Fourth of July to help get her up and moving during the day, and the focus on the puppy had clearly helped. A'lory was eager to put her design degree to work in their new home.

> *"I love her. It wouldn't matter. I mean sometimes she says she doesn't feel like a woman. All that other stuff is beside the point besides her as a person. She is the best thing that ever happened to me in my whole life. It really is. She has really straightened me out."*—Brad

I phoned A'lory in January 1992 to see how she was feeling and to talk with her about hospice care, knowing that she and Brad would need help. Her parents were visiting from Illinois and she said she was feeling better than she had in the past few months and didn't feel that they were ready for hospice. I told her I had written a commentary about her for the campus paper at SMU. She was excited that her story may keep other young women from not acting more aggressively on lumps.

On February 20, 1992, some three weeks later, A'lory died at home in Brad's arms. One of her final comments when we talked in October was that she didn't want to end up in a nursing home, where she would have to be cared for.

I talked to Brad six weeks after A'lory died and he said he was doing okay, except in the evenings before he went to sleep. He had left the house exactly as it was when A'lory died. *"She told me two days before she died that the doctor had told her no more chemotherapy. So we knew what that meant. I just wish he had told her from the beginning that she wasn't going to get better. I always felt like she put off doing things because he kept telling her she would feel better."*

KEVIN AND BARBRA

> *"The only thing you can say to someone is that the process of grieving must be expressed. You have to let it go. You have to experience it, because you're just going to postpone it—not lick it. It'll manifest itself in other ways."*
> —Kevin

In 1987, six months before she was diagnosed with breast cancer at age thirty-seven, Barbra told her husband, Kevin, that she was going to

Antarctica to take photographs. While not that out of the ordinary for this well-known and well-traveled photographer, Kevin says that the landscape photographs she brought back possessed a stark bleakness that would foretell the next two years of Barbra's life. *"She took pictures of accomplished people for twenty years. She never took a picture without people in it. Then she went to the Antarctic for almost the entire time between Thanksgiving and Christmas in 1987. She was the kind of person who would do intuitive things, and I never questioned them."* The resulting landscapes of the forbidding terrain, Kevin says, were about death and eternity.

Barbra and Kevin could have been called a charmed couple. She photographed the country's fashion designers and newsmakers. He designed interiors and furniture for the best and brightest. And by all accounts they had already beaten death; Barbra faced and overcame cancer at age fifteen, when she lost a leg to cancer, and then underwent numerous operations to remove lung tumors. They met and began living together as college students before marrying in 1972. Their first daughter, Jersey, was born in 1982, and Addie came in 1986.

It was shortly after Barbra finished breast-feeding Addie that she noticed that her breasts seemed off-balance. A mammogram indicated no problem, and she was told to stop drinking caffeine. The doctor, who was chosen based on Barbra's history, did not biopsy the lump. Nor did he biopsy it when she returned four months later. But he sent her to a surgeon to have the mass removed. *"It was as large as an orange. He told her that she had advanced breast cancer and that she had to have a mastectomy immediately or she would die."*

Kevin and Barbra immediately turned to the oncologist who had treated Barbra's cancer during adolescence. *"We went into his office and he cried. He couldn't tell us. He loved her like his daughter, and truly, we were friends. He dropped in and we'd go out for pizza. He did what he believed in, but he did not tell us everything. He didn't tell us that the chances that the chemotherapy would do anything were really, really slim. But I think he believed that Barbra lived the first time not because of the treatment but because of an incredible and immeasurable will to live. So he put her on really extreme chemotherapy before surgery to reduce the size of the tumor."*

In September 1988, after preoperative chemo, for which she required hospitalization for an extreme emotional reaction, Barbra underwent a mastectomy that revealed more than twenty positive lymph nodes. She continued chemotherapy until December and then underwent six weeks of radiation. She resumed chemotherapy, but quit in April to begin a regimen of alternative treatments that took her to Europe. *"She went to Germany to an alternative clinic that was worthless, but he X-rayed her and found the cancer had gone to her lungs. This was only six or eight weeks after her last chemotherapy treatment."*

Kevin says that Barbra felt the chemotherapy was detrimental to her healing and that the medical profession should be more forthcoming with statistics on its ineffectiveness for advanced breast cancer. After another trip, to a clinic in Switzerland, Barbra began another treatment with a doctor in New York City that involved juices, vitamins, and coffee enemas. *"The doctor in no way tried to sell us on the program. He tried to talk us out of it. He was very careful not to take people he didn't feel he could help. He took Barbra, but promised her nothing. He said he allowed her to do it because of her tremendous spirit. And she did it up to the week before she died. He told us she would get worse before she got better. He couldn't tell us how bad it would get, so we kept waiting for a turning point and it never came. He was very supportive, as were all the doctors."*

Kevin cared for Barbra in their New York City loft with help from the family nanny and Barbra's mother. Their daughters were three and seven. Kevin says Barbra greatly simplified her life when she got sick, asking that friends communicate through notes. Kevin says she received cards, books, and books on tape as well as music and self-help books. *"We got every smile-and-you-will-live book in triplicate. I gave them all to a cancer group, except for two."*

Kevin relied on friend and writer Jill Krementz and her book *How It Feels When a Parent Dies* (Knopf, 1988) to meet his daughters' needs, with the primary focus involving the children in all that was happening. Kevin sought counseling for Jersey and himself before Barbra died.

As Barbra began to deteriorate, the family drew together. *"She was in control most of the time. Then she started having confusion in her head, and the pain-management doctors said there were tumors in her head. It went quickly after that. She was home a few weeks with delusions and then one morning she had a seizure. While I was trying to get an ambulance, the girls took care of her, so they felt that they were doing something. It was important that they were here with her and felt that they did what they could. I told them to tell their mother how much they loved her. That was the last time the girls saw her."*

At the hospital, Kevin decided against life support. *"This very won-*

derful doctor came over and said, 'We got her upstairs and unstrapped her and the nurse turned around and within three seconds Barbra had yanked all the tubes out. I can't tell you what to do, but you should think about whether she was aware of what she was doing or not, and whether you want us to support her life.' I didn't have to think about it. I just said, 'Don't put the tubes back in.' "

During the next few days, Barbra was lucid for periods of time that allowed her moments to talk with Kevin of their life together and her impending death. *"I remember the words almost exactly, 'I've had such a wonderful life. Who lives to be eighty and has seen what I have in forty years?' We kept telling each other how much we loved each other. She said, 'You know we were together for twenty years, and that's twenty years of happy marriage. Who has that much time?'*

"Her only regret was not raising her children. She said, 'Take care of yourself and the girls.'"

Within a day Barbra died. Kevin recalls it as close to Father's Day, 1990. She was buried in a cemetery near the family's country home. Kevin chose to have an open casket and encouraged the girls to see their mother before the funeral. *"The kids looked at their mother and totally freaked out. Jersey sobbed for four hours straight. My parents felt I had done the most horrible thing in the world to my child. In fact, it turns out it was the best thing I could have done. Children just want the truth. They can handle it better than anyone. If you tell them a lie or hide something, they obsess and they leave this horrible thing around it."*

Kevin encourages the girls to talk about their mother and pictures abound in the family's apartment. *"Barbra's work is still published, and two weeks ago we opened up* The New York Times *and there was a picture she did of Ralph Lauren. And Jersey took it to school the next day for show-and-tell. We had a birthday party for Barbra and got an inflatable cake and helium balloons and put notes on them and sent it to heaven."*

Kevin says the most important area of recovery for him has been assisting his daughters' emotional adjustment. Barbra's mother remains a weekly presence for Kevin and his daughters. Barbra's father died three weeks after his daughter; Kevin says he died of grief. Kevin has begun dating again but concedes that his own healing process is ongoing. *"Barbra and I were so close, and we were sort of inseparable in many ways. I just had to relearn who I was, and grievance counseling wasn't going to be enough. I went to therapy twice a week. I am lucky because I have a therapist who is really good. It's been almost two years and I'm still not done. What lingers for me is the sense of still trying to find who I am and still the tremendous sense of loss. I am just starting to think that maybe there will be some things in the next part of my life that will be wonderful."*

RAY AND ANN

"You really do need to get on with your life with the best quality possible and live it day by day, not letting your life be dominated by death but by the present."—Ray

In February 1980, Ray's wife, Ann, died of breast cancer at age forty-two. She had been diagnosed initially in 1973, at age thirty-five and was in the process of rearing their two sons, David, eight, and Mike, five.

Ray, an orthopedic surgeon, recalls the evening that Ann found the lump. He was late returning home to prepare for an evening out. *"She was sitting at the dressing table and I came in and looked at her and knew something was wrong, but didn't know what it was. I thought it was because I was late. After we got home that night, she told me she had felt something. That was the beginning."*

Ray recalls that from the beginning Ann struggled mostly with the disfigurement of a Halsted radical, which was the common procedure at the time. Ray said that Ann had always felt that her breasts were her most attractive asset. *"She felt she was hit in her most vulnerable area. She felt she had a lot of things physically that were not particularly attractive, and she was worried about not being very attractive. She came to believe that that's what she needed as time went on. It was a spiritual issue."*

After a Halsted radical that revealed four positive nodes, Ann had chemotherapy and radiation. Ray and Ann, both Christians, had begun their spiritual journey when their first child was stillborn, and from the time of the diagnosis, the couple sought spiritual answers for coping with cancer.

Ann remained cancer-free for five years. Ray recalled the day she first felt the pain in her back. *"The dog has just puddled on the floor and she bent over right behind me where the dog was and I heard something pop. She hollered. That was her first spine fracture. It didn't hurt; it was like a sore back. But I think as far as I was concerned, I knew what it was."*

The tests revealed mestastases to the bone in a number of places in Ann's back. She began radiation treatments, which Ray said were very effective in helping reduce the pain.

Emotionally, Ray said, the next two years were a roller coaster as they coped with the spreading cancer and the creeping reality. "*There were two years of metastases—two years from the first metastasis until she died—and the first year she was pretty up that she was not going to die, that she was going to lick it. And well, even longer than that, because she was a fighter and she never gave up on the hope that something would come along to control it. So it was only in the last six months that it was just a little bit more than she could handle, but she was very upbeat about it.*"

Ann was surrounded by many friends who assisted her in her search for answers, both medical and spiritual. Ray said his commitment from the beginning was to do anything that she wanted, including trips to Mexico and trying Laetrile. "*She also did a lot with diet. She did macrobiotics and high-dose vitamins. She had read about it and was absolutely inundated with people that wanted to do for her. She let anyone offbeat do what they could for her.*"

About eight months before she died, Ann began indirectly addressing the reality of her death. "*I came in one night and she said, 'Ray, I want to talk to you.' I felt like I knew what she wanted to talk about. But she said, 'Remember when we first married, and I always told you that I would never want you to marry again if I died?' She said, 'Well, I've changed my mind.' I said, 'Oh good, now you're going to plan my life from the grave.' I was just joking with her, but I asked her why she felt that way.*

"*She said, 'If you never married again, it would be such a reflection on me that everybody would say, "Well, marrying her was so bad that he would never marry again."' She said, 'I do want you to marry again. I am serious about it.' And that was the beginning of really sort of talking about the end.*"

Ray said there were many talks after that night, time that he now looks on as Ann winding up her life and saying goodbye to the people close to her. There were even times when they could laugh. "*One humorous thing was that she wanted to see four or five of her old boyfriends. There was always one person that she had gone with who I'd heard about through the years. He was a big jock football player at the University of Texas. I guess they were crazy about each other for a period of time. So through our marriage I had heard about him, and it had always been kind of a family joke about this guy. We talked about it and laughed about it. She*

*would talk very easily about dying. She was able to tell people what they
had meant to her and vice versa. She also had some unresolved conflicts that
she took care of—misunderstandings that had occurred in childhood. She
had a real ministry."*

Ray said his two sons handled their mother's illness very differently.
The oldest son, David, who was thirteen, was able to talk openly with
Ann about her death. *"I talked to Ann about David, and six months before
she died we started David in counseling and stayed with it six months after
she died. He was certainly overwhelmed by her death, but he was pretty well
prepared for it. As much as you can be."*

Ray described Mike, eleven, the younger of the two boys, as very
outgoing and very much into being with friends. It was his way of
denying what was happening around him, Ray said. He spent the night
with friends frequently and was unwilling to go to counseling. *"Even
after Ann died, we kept trying to get Mike to go, and David talked to him
and explained why it would be a good idea. But he didn't want to and he
just wouldn't talk about it. When Ann died it was some time before he would
look at her casket. He made three trips to see in before he ever looked. And
then he cried, but he wouldn't say anything. In the year after, David and I
would talk; Mike would listen and cry but wouldn't enter in. He would never
verbalize anything. So it took about five years for it to manifest itself and
have to be dealt with."*

As the end neared, Ann began to talk to people about her life. She
and Ray had been in Bible study and Ann had been a frequent speaker.
She encouraged friends to talk with her. She also began asking to see
old friends to say goodbye. Ann made peace with her death in a way
that Ray describes as 'Why me?' becoming 'Why not me?' *"The big thing
was she really felt cheated about having taken care of the boys as babies and
she wasn't going to see them grow up and what she considered the fun time.
She didn't consider diaper changing very much fun. But she did like older
kids and did very well with them. She really felt that and was really grateful
for the seven years that she lived. Because there was a lot that took place
with the boys growing up. They were eleven and thirteen when she died, and
I was amazed at the quality time that there really was during that time."*

Two months before her death in February 1980, Ann attended a
dance with Ray. For the last two months of her life she was on pain
management and was cared for at home. She and Ray talked about
where she would die. Her concern about dying at home, Ray said, was

that the room would become a sad place in the house. At one point she had complications from the many medications she was taking and was facing death if the situation was not reversed medically. She and Ray brought the oncologist to the house and discussed whether to reverse the situation. *"We talked about it. She talked with her oncologist about what it would be like to die from uremic poisoning. She asked, 'Will I be unconscious? Will it be painful? Will it be peaceful?' It's so unbelievable that the three of us sat there and discussed it—dying now or dying later. Anyway, she decided that she didn't want to die then."*

Ann lived for six more months, ultimately suffering from metastases in the brain. Ray was with her in the hospital when she died.

Ray said the years following Ann's death were difficult. David went away to school for the last year of high school, and Ray spent considerable time with Mike, who still seemed not to have dealt with his mother's death. That came to an end when Ray's father died, and it soon became clear that Mike was depressed. *"So that led to counseling. We went together for most all the visits and the assessment was that there had been a series of losses to Mike that he had never dealt with personally. And in this process, after about six months in counseling, Mike told me he couldn't remember anything about Ann, couldn't remember what she looked like, couldn't remember anything about his mother."*

Ray said that the counseling resulted in the two finally talking about Ann and her death. Ray said that a particular issue was the day Ann died. *"Mike had plans to spend the night with somebody. I went by and told Mike and told the family he was staying with that Ann was very critical and didn't he want to go to the hospital with me to see her. And he didn't. The family knew what was going to happen. Unfortunately, they were the ones that told Mike later that night that his mother died. I arrived right after that. It came up in our counseling that he thought I 'dumped' him at this kid's house. We talked about it for several sessions, clarifying the details about what had really occurred, but his memory was that I wouldn't take him to the hospital—not that he wouldn't go."*

Ray said that real resolution occurred for both of them in counseling. *"It was such a relief when I quit crying. Ann's been dead ten years, and for five or six years, I was still driving down the road and all of a sudden I'd burst into tears. A couple of years ago David was crying and I said, 'You know, I just want to tell you that I understand this, because this is the first time you've cried and I haven't.' "* Ray has not remarried. *"I think that Ann had as healthy a death as it could be, and certainly she got a lot of things done. That was one of the biggest things that I learned. I used to say that if you have cancer and got accidentally killed tomorrow, it's almost a blessing because you'd die anyway—I don't feel that way at all about it now. I feel like there's so many benefits that can come from life being prolonged if that person wants it. And I am totally convinced that I don't think there is a single one of us that knows what he or she would do until faced with it."*

Tip—Cancer pain can often be controlled to allow a somewhat normal life. If your oncologist is not controlling the pain to your satisfaction, ask for a consultation with a pain-management specialist.

MY MOM AND ME

As I wrote the above stories in early 1992, I knew that I too would face a breast cancer death within the next few years. My seventy-two-year-old mother, Mary Josette Stevenson LaTour, was diagnosed with breast cancer on Halloween 1991. Because the tumor was against the chest wall, it did not show up on her annual mammograms. By the time it was large enough to feel, there were ten lymph nodes involved. Further tests at the time of surgery indicated that mother already had three small tumors in her right lung. After I read the pathology report, I knew that breast cancer would take my mother's life. It would also be sooner than any of us had planned or suspected.

Mother began chemotherapy immediately after her diagnosis, but a CAT scan in early 1992 revealed that her cancer was not responding. Mother began a regimen with a study drug that had been shown to be effective in metastatic breast cancer. After two treatments that left her in great pain, she decided to stop all treatment and let the disease take its course.

We talked about dying during this time. At seventy-two, my mother saw her life's work as complete. She had reared four children, burying her first born son, my brother Edward (Skeeter), in 1972. Skeeter, a naval aviator, died a week before his twenty-fifth birthday when the helicopter he was piloting crashed. During the next decade she was active in helping other bereaved parents survive the loss of their children and was a founder of the Dallas chapter of the Compassionate Friends. She had cared for my father, who suffers from Parkinson's disease, at home, finally telling my sister and me on the day of her biopsy that she was too tired to do so anymore. She had seen the births of seven grandchildren and opened her heart to four stepgrandchildren.

In early May, six months after her diagnosis, she began experiencing pain that initially was thought to be from the chemotherapy or scar tissue under her arm, since a bone scan only six weeks before had shown her to be clear of any bone metastases. But when mild pain medication failed to help, and a lung X ray showed more lung tumors, a second scan was ordered. This showed that her cancer had moved to a number of spots on her spine and rib. Until this time, my mother had lived alone in the family home, with frequent visits from children and friends. We had found nursing-home care for our father earlier in the year. When it became clear her cancer had metastasized to the bone, my sister took my mother to her home and she was scheduled to begin radiation therapy to help the pain.

I had already called the local hospice chapter, recognizing that we were moving into a constant-care situation more quickly than any of us suspected. We had scheduled an intake interview for the week of May 18.

When my sister, Marylee, called me on Monday the eighteenth, she was crying. Mother's pain has become unbearable, she said. We had to do something. By that afternoon we had admitted Mom to the hospital for pain management. I had called in a pain-management specialist and my mother was clearly relieved on the morphine she was receiving. She was scheduled to begin radiation on Tuesday. When our oncologist visited, he suggested we move her to the hospice floor at the hospital since Medicare would pay 100 percent.

When I returned to the hospital on Wednesday afternoon to spend the night, it was clear that my mother's breathing was much more labored. I told my brother, Larry, that she seemed much worse. He agreed. When we arrived at the hospice room an hour later, we were met by Barbara, the nurse on duty and someone I have added to my list of angels. She helped us arrange my mother and get her comfortable.

I explained to Barbara that we wanted to begin talking with home health nurses. She listened carefully. When I finished, she motioned for us to come to the hall, where she gently explained that Mother would not need home health care. She said Mother was dying. She explained that Mom's breathing was clearly labored and her lungs were filling with fluid. She also told us that she could not respond and had her eyes closed, but she could hear us.

When Larry and I recovered from the shock, we cried. Barbara cried with us. We spent that Wednesday night on either side of her bed, telling her that we loved her. She opened her eyes and spoke a few times. I told her that Skeeter would be coming for her soon, and her eyes widened in delight, and she said, "Really?" Larry asked her if she was afraid. She shook her head strongly, no. We called her brother in Los Angeles and told him that his planned trip next week would be too late. Come now. He made reservations for Friday. We called the others who we knew would want to say goodbye. They came on Thursday, as did her grandchildren. The room was abuzz with small children telling Grammy about their day.

As she slipped further under from the increased morphine, her responses diminished. She opened her eyes and responded clearly to my sister, Marylee, on Thursday afternoon. Because her blood pressure was still strong, I went home to sleep Thursday night to be ready to return Friday morning. That night, some people from Larry's church came with an electronic keyboard and sang her all her favorite hymns. Larry called me at home so I could be a part of one of their hymns. He also called her brother in Los Angeles and put the phone to Mother's ear, sensing that Friday would be too late for this last goodbye. The hospital floor resounded with song.

We had been told that a severe drop in blood pressure would precede her death by two to three hours. It never happened. Larry called at 3:30 A.M. When the phone rang, I was sitting on the side of the bed. I was not aware of being awakened, but I was awake. Larry said that Mother was taking her final breaths. I rushed to the hospital. Larry had held her as she died peacefully, after which he felt a force rise from her body. I crawled up on the bed and held my mother, cradling her in my arms and kissing her goodbye one last time. My sister arrived shortly thereafter and also had time to say goodbye.

I felt a new pain for those people who don't know death is approaching and don't have those precious last few hours to say all that is on their heart. If it had not been for Barbara, who clearly told us Mother was dying, we would have been cheated out of those final moments that are so precious to us now.

We celebrated Mother's life as we built her casket together the next day. Larry, an expert woodworker, explained as we stood in the casket room of the funeral home that he wanted to build Mother's casket himself. That evening my husband, Tom, stepson Brad, and brother-in-law, John, joined Larry and a number of the men of his church in his workshop. As the women prepared the meal and the grandchildren ran in and out, a beautiful ash casket took shape. I bought a white satin comforter, and Marylee and my sister-in-law, Cindy, and I cut, glued, and sewed it to line the casket and cover the interior of the lid. We delivered it the next morning, to the total amazement of the funeral home director. My only regret is that Mother didn't see it. She would have loved it.

HELP FOR DYING

"Hospice provides support and care for persons in the last phases of incurable disease so that they may live as fully and as comfortably as possible. Hospice recognizes dying as part of the normal process of living and focuses on maintaining the quality of remaining life. Hospice affirms life and neither hastens nor postpones death. Hospice exists in the hope and belief that through appropriate care, and the promotion of a caring community sensitive to their needs, patients and their families may be free to attain a degree of mental and spiritual preparation for death that is satisfactory to them. Hospice, to the maximum extent possible, accepts patients regardless of ability to pay."—Texas Hospice Organization Guidelines

"Although it may be a literal place, Hospice is actually a concept of care. It focuses on the quality of life remaining for the person in respect to her personal dignity during that time."—Joanne Pryor-Carter, grief counselor with Hospice

There was a time in this country when every family was familiar with grief. Before the availability of antibiotics and the level of medical care available today, most families cared for sick relatives who ultimately died at home. The community served as a grief-support system to aid with sick family members and to be there when they died. Food, funeral arrangements, and the funeral itself were often living room arrangements, with family and friends there to offer their personal perspectives. We grieved together more readily.

Today, many of us are isolated. Families move in and out of neighborhoods with the seasons. Churches may provide community, and they may not. People may reach adulthood and never have suffered the loss of a close friend or relative, making them uncomfortable with an acceptance of death. Medical technology has made such advances that often people expect they will be cured when really they won't. Doctors, who have committed to keeping their patients alive, are reluctant to stop treatment, which would allow them to begin thinking of death. If a patient does finally face the fact that treatment must stop, the decision is frequently made without the social support that will help families know what to do next. These factors make it more difficult for a family facing such a crisis, for they must seek out the help that used to be readily available.

Tip—Doctors can only follow their patients in providing information. You must tell the oncologist directly that you want to know best-case and worse-case scenario. Remember, their reluctance may come from the fact that they just don't know how cancer will act.

When there is some acceptance on the part of family or the woman that treatment options have ended or that they are no longer effective, it is time to find someone who can help with the process of healthy dying, which means, quite simply, a death that is resolved and has as much closure for the dying as possible. For the living it means goodbyes and practicalities of plans for after the death. Sources and resources for this process are numerous in most metropolitan areas if the family has adequate time to look for them.

The hospital chaplain's office is a good place to start. There are usually social workers and grief counselors available. Your local American Cancer Society should have a list of grief counselors, those therapists specializing in grief. Depending on where you live and the network available in your city, you may have a local Hospice chapter.

Hospice, a nationwide network, offers those who have been identified as within six months of death a wide range of services and support, both for the dying woman and her family.

FAMILY HOSPICE COUNSELOR JOANNE PRYOR-CARTER, ED.D., TALKS ABOUT HEALTHY DEATH

Joanne Pryor-Carter, Ed.D., is a grief counselor with Family Hospice in Dallas. She says that while the concept of Hospice is nationwide, services may vary from city to city. Hospice costs are usually covered by insurance, but most Hospice organizations have funds to assist the uninsured. Medicare covers Hospice for anyone eligible for Medicare Part A. Medicaid also covers Hospice services.

What is the procedure if a family is considering Hospice?

Hospice is really based on the concept of holism. That means that a person is not just composed of physical parts but spiritual and emotional and psychosocial parts as well. So we have an interdisciplinary team, composed of doctors, nurses, social workers, counselors, volunteers, chaplains, and home health aides, who address the varying needs of the whole person. Usually, a visit from the nurse, chaplain, and social worker could be expected within a week after admission to the program. Follow-up visits would occur as family needs arise.

(continued)

How do you get the doctors to tell them they're dying?

That's a pertinent question, and I wish I had the answer for that. So many times we see families at the very end. Doctors feel they've failed their patients when they haven't cured them. They believe if they refer them to Hospice, they've given up hope. We tell people that we don't want them to give up hope. But hope changes as the disease progresses. It might be hope for a good day without pain. Or hope for a good morning. It might be hope for a reconciliation with an estranged family member. We help to continue to keep hope alive.

A key factor in Hospice care is expert control of pain and other distressful symptoms. As these symptoms are controlled, the patient has energy to say her goodbyes, complete unfinished business, and deal with emotional and psychosocial issues involved in the dying process. Hospice is the only health care organization that treats the family and the patient as a unit. The emotional well-being of the family is as important to us as the physical condition of the patient. As each member of the care team makes visits, he or she addresses whatever needs are presented at that time—whether they are the needs of the spouse, family, or children. The goal of the care team is a blessed and peaceful death for the patient and ample emotional support for the family.

Is there a plan for helping them accept death?

There's a process you need to go through. What we try to do is meet people where they are. They may be in the denial stage because they've just heard the information and they can't believe it. Surely there's something else they can do, they think. So we try to meet them wherever their emotions are. We don't try to talk them out of their denial or fear or their anger. We gently confront them. "Well, you've said your doctor said this. What else did he tell you?" And then maybe they've gotten some other test results. Maybe that's what has precipitated the move to hospice. Because they've done the treatments and they thought they were working

(continued)

and now they find out there's been a recurrence. So slowly, with the new test results, the reality is beginning to dawn on them. They really aren't going to be cured. We try to provide knowledge and education about the process, because this helps to reduce the fear of the unknown.

Denial is the first stage, then what happens?

Elisabeth Kübler-Ross talked about five different stages she felt that patients went through: Denial is first, and there are some positive aspects to denial, because it protects a person from having to absorb all the information at one time—the unacceptable truth she has to face. It allows people to maintain control. Our efforts to help the patient during this time would be to respect that need and allow her to be there—not try to talk her out of it, but just allow her to be there, just listen nonjudgmentally. Recognize that during this stage families may refuse to follow the recommendations that the nurse gives them. They may not comply with the medication regimen. This is just evidence of their denial. We have families right up to the very end that just can't believe they're going to die. During this stage, we try to reassure and listen to her feelings.

What comes next?

Anger. Again, there are some positive aspects to the anger stage. It might provide some energy to complete unfinished business that she hasn't been able to do. In this way, anger may function as a positive force for change. We also find it can be negatively directed toward family members or doctors or nurses. Why didn't she find out ahead of time? Why didn't this treatment work? It may be also directed toward God. It's just so important for us to listen and allow her to express these emotions. We all get the message that it's not acceptable to talk about anger; it's not nice to have that feeling. As members of the Hospice team, we can be that outside, objective, nonjudgmental listener who can allow the

(continued)

patient to express those feelings of anger and know that it's okay. If she can express it verbally, she can work through it.

What comes after anger?

Bargaining. God, if you'll just let me live for another month for the wedding or whatever, then I'll promise to be a better person. Again, it can be a positive stage. It might explore a new source of energy. Maybe the patient didn't care about living at first. She was so depressed. These stages don't always go in a particular order and people jump back and forth, even within a morning or a few minutes. The patient may be in shock and denial and then experience anger or depression and then go back to shock. These are just kind of a guideline that families can expect. Perhaps the patient may experience this time to complete a bargain she made with a significant other.

Is there a certain intuition about knowing when you're going to die?

Yes, our patients know much more than we do about when they're going to die. Dying patients have an intuition about their death and that may influence when they die. They may wait for a family member to get in from out of town to see them one last time. Or there's something really important happening and they hang on for that. In contrast, they may die before certain family members get there. This is a common occurrence in grief counseling. "I wasn't able to see them. I couldn't get there before they died." We reassure survivors that, "Maybe she felt like that was just too hard for you, that it would be too painful for you, so she just died before you got there."

What do you do when you've got children involved?

We try to visit with them if the family member feels it's important for us to do that. We will meet with them and try to find out what they know about the illness, the death. "Do you know

(continued)

that your mother is very sick?" We try to find out what they know. Children are very perceptive. A lot of times parents postpone trying to talk to them because they're afraid that they're not going to know how to answer their questions. Children don't want real involved answers, usually. They just want to know simple things. When they want to know more, they'll come back to ask for more details. It's important when dealing with children not to talk with euphemisms, like describing death as "going to sleep" or say that the person who died is "on a long trip." Children will not want to go to sleep and they might have nightmares. The most important advice regarding children is to just answer their questions openly and honestly. Remember that what you don't tell children, they often make up with their imaginations. Often what they imagine is much worse than the actual event itself.

What about children and funerals?

It's important for families to use their own judgment about whether or not the child attends the funeral. Recognize that it's better if the child goes for just ten or fifteen minutes than if he or she doesn't attend at all. It's important not to *force* children to go but to allow them to go if they want to, explaining ahead of time what's going to happen. We think that it's going to be upsetting to children, but we often worry needlessly about that. I think, again, we should take cues from the child, answering his or her questions openly and honestly, letting the child know what's going to happen at a funeral, and giving each child the option of whether to go. Funeral-home personnel are too often overlooked as a valuable source of information. They usually have numerous videos that are excellent resources for parents during this time. The videos are often donated to interested persons. Literature may be provided as well.

Hospice assists with the stages and listens to the patients; what else?

Part of what the Hospice team does is to provide education and information about what the death process is going to be like. They

(continued)

provide information about the signs and symptoms of approaching death. What people often fear is the unknown. If we can help provide information about what's going to be expected and what's normal, that will be more reassuring for families. We do have a Hospice presence at death if the family needs or wants it. The nurse facilitates all the legal details of a death at home. In Texas, Hospice registered nurses are certified to do death pronouncements. Hospice nurses assist with making all the necessary calls and assist the families with details.

What does Hospice do for the family after the death?

We provide ongoing bereavement support for the family and friends for approximately thirteen months following the patient's death. The follow-up includes calls, letters, and visits. A memorial service is held twice a year to celebrate the memory of our patients.

We had a lady who died several months ago and she left four little girls—six, eight, ten, fifteen—so we've visited with them and taken one of them a birthday cake for her birthday. The husband had forgotten the candles and the ice cream. He said he'd never had to do that before. His wife always took care of all those things. He was going through those adjustments.

What about Medicare patients?

Some of our patients are on Medicare Part A and do not realize that they have a Medicare Hospice benefit. The benefit pays for all Hospice services, team visits, and all the equipment and supplies, such as wheelchairs and hospital beds. It also covers all the medicines related to the terminal illness. Our services are financed through Medicare or Medicaid or private insurance. We try not to let anybody fall through the cracks. We do have a memorial fund through the Heart of Texas Foundation. Last year approximately 10 percent of the care given by our Hospice was nonfunded care.

CHILDREN AND DEATH AND GRIEF

"I'll never forget the morning my sister died. Her daughter said, 'Daddy, how could Mommy die and not say goodbye to me?' And I thought to myself, how could you not say goodbye to your child?"
—Patrick

I know that I speak for every mother I interviewed when I say our greatest fear is dying before our children are old enough to know us. How, then, do we face this? What are the gifts we want to give our children through life and how can we do that in death?

First is to not deny that we are dying, but to talk about it with even your very young children in terms they can understand. Denying the issue seems to provide protection from emotions, but it is a selfish and irresponsible act on the part of parents—and Dad will almost certainly have to cope with these unresolved issues at some point in the child's life.

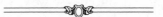

Tip for Dads—For some women accepting death is impossible. In these cases you must take emotional care of yourself and your children.

Patrick spoke of the day his sister died and returning home, where his three nieces, ages six, nine, and eleven, waited. *"My sister had a terrible time dealing with this emotionally and psychologically. As a matter of fact, they never, ever sat their children down and discussed what was going on, and I was there the morning she died. I was with her when she died and I drove home with her husband so he could tell the children. They were just in utter disbelief that their mother had died. It never crossed their minds that this was coming. It was like—what? I sat there and watched him tell those girls, who were as unprepared for that moment as you could ever imagine. Because they had done no groundwork and no preparation whatsoever."*

Patrick recalled his sister's struggle to say goodbye and her denial that cancer would take her life. She would not allow the word *cancer* mentioned in front of her children. Patrick, who lived in another state, had contacted his sister's doctor about visiting at Thanksgiving or Christmas. The doctor recommended Thanksgiving. "*We were at her house, and I'd watch her. My brother was there the same weekend. And she just—she was trying like hell to say goodbye to everybody, but she didn't know how to do it. I'd be standing over by the refrigerator and she would just walk over—she wouldn't say anything, she wouldn't look at me, she wouldn't make eye contact. But she'd just lay her head down on my chest for a second and walk away. And I watched her do it to my brother a couple of times. Her kids knew that she was sick, but they were doing what kids do. They were running around the house. Every once in a while one of them would come over for something, and I'd watch her. She would put her arm around them and then they'd walk away. I'd watch her and I knew what she was thinking. I mean, I knew what she was doing. But no one ever said anything. No one talked about it. It was just so weird. Everybody was trying to say goodbye, but nobody could do it or knew how to do it.*"

As I have coped with my own fears of death, I have allowed, as the issue has presented itself, my daughter to explore the idea of death. I had a very good friend die of AIDS when Kirtley was just six. She knew he was sick and she asked if he would die. I told her he would and she wanted to know about that. I explained that when his body was too sick, his spirit would leave, kind of like letting the air out of a balloon. His body would then be honored at a gathering for friends that is called a funeral. This was a way to thank the body for its good work when his spirit lived there. I said the hard part about this was that we can't see his spirit and we still want the body we knew. But we have to remember his spirit is free.

This explanation worked well, and despite the brevity of the conversation, she has repeated it to friends. Think about death and what you think it is. How would you tell a six-year-old? What do you want her to believe?

When my friend Judy died, I was crying and Kirtley wanted to know why. I explained, and in the purity of a child's wisdom, which we should listen to more frequently, she said, "And you are missing her body, aren't you, Mom." I said yes and that it was okay to miss her body and be sad. Then she said, "But remember, her spirit is free."

While I have never heard the words *you are dying*, I can honestly say that during my first panic attack, when Kirtley was sixteen months old, I truly thought I was dying. It was then that I thought about what I would want for her in my absence. I needed closure on this more than any other aspect of my life. I knew my husband would probably remarry and that he would be a good, kind, loving father for her. I knew that my brother and sister would give her strong family support and that her stepbrothers and -sisters would provide a great extended family as she grew. But strong women role models have always been important for me, and I knew I wanted the same for my daughter. Besides, Tom would need help. I recall making a list of the things that were important to me and eliciting a promise from my close women friends that they would be in charge of these areas. Diana, Kirtley's godmother, is an excellent cook and master of many domestic areas such as sewing and handwork. I asked her to teach Kirtley these things were I to die. Because I always battled the bulge as an adolescent and never felt like I looked right in clothes (and because I know that my color-blind husband would put shopping at the bottom of his list), I asked Dianne to take Kirtley shopping and be sure that she felt good about how she looked. I knew Dianne's daughter, who is my goddaughter, would be a great friend also. Terry was drafted as the education consultant, and since then I have asked SueAnn to take care of Kirtley's spiritual growth.

I have also gathered some ideas from women and men and children about how a mother can specifically leave a legacy that will help her child or children deal with her death. The first realization in planning this is to understand that children's needs will vary at different ages. The loss of a mother when you are a child is a life-changing event. Young children may seem to understand on one level what is happening, but as they grow and become teenagers, children will have an entirely new set of issues as they begin to examine who they are and begin to grieve as if their mother had died yesterday. When they become young adults, another set of questions will develop, and when they are adults, with children of their own, a different issues will come up. One of the angriest women I ever met was denied the opportunity to tell her mother goodbye because her father refused to believe she was dying.

From the beginning, the greatest gifts a parent can give a child are information and participation in the death process. Let them be a part of the death. Even the smallest child can fetch things for Mom and feel that he or she is helping. Adult children need all the information in order to make their own decision about how they want to express their grief.

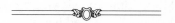

Tip—You may want to begin counseling for your children and yourself when you can determine the end is a few months away.

All children need to be prepared as much as they can be for what will happen when the end comes. Will Mom die at home or will she die in the hospital? Then what will happen?

Other ideas come from a variety of places:

1. Videotape the funeral. This may sound macabre, and I don't mean to have bright lights and close-ups. Do it discreetly. Very young children may at some point in their life ask what it was like and wish they had been there. If the funeral is a celebration, this may be even more important.

2. Create a memory book of letters to the child from his or her mother's close friends. Ask at the funeral that all those who knew her write of specific instances that will give the child an insight into her personality. Ask that they recall times when the child and mother were together.

3. Let the children be involved in the funeral or memorial service. Ask if they want to place something in the coffin with their mother—a toy or stuffed animal. Older children may want to chose a favorite piece of clothing for her to wear. Whether the child should see his or her mother after she has died is a very personal decision. The child shouldn't ever be forced to do anything. Yet a parent should encourage older children by explaining what they will see. For a reluctant child, a picture may work in the future. Unfortunately, funerals are one-time events; a child cannot choose to regain that experience once it has happened.

When my mother died, my twelve-year-old niece, Kendra, went with me and my sister to the funeral home to see Mother's body before they began the viewing. We allowed her to move at her own pace, reassuring her that there was no right or wrong way to feel during this experience.

When they brought Mother into the viewing room, my sister and I did not like the way she looked. We added her glasses and the earrings she had asked to wear. They had not applied any eye makeup, and the lipstick was all wrong. We began redoing her makeup when we noticed Kendra had moved from the other side of the room and was standing at our side. She looked at her Grammy and cried. Then she said, "Grammy's wig looks terrible. I always fixed it for her." She asked for a comb and began fixing Mother's wig to her satisfaction. When we finished, the three of us knew Mother would be pleased. She looked like herself at last. For Kendra it was a special moment.

When my six-and-a-half-year-old daughter arrived at the viewing a few hours later, she came slowly into the room and stood a number of feet back from the coffin. No one suggested that the children do anything they did not want to. Kirtley slowly approached the coffin and eventually began stroking Mother's arm. I watched as she began stroking her face. She then came across the room to where I was sitting. "Mom, Grammy is cold and hard," she said. "That's because her spirit is gone," I replied. "A person's spirit is the warm part that makes them laugh and talk and walk and hug." She accepted this and returned to my mother, where she again gently stroked her face for a number of minutes before returning to me. "Mom," she said excitedly. "I think she's warming up." I smothered a laugh and gently explained to her that once a spirit has left a body, it can't come back. She accepted this news and began to ask her cousins specific questions about crying at the funeral. My nephew asked me to take a picture of my mother in the coffin for him. I did.

4. Ask the children if they would like to be included in the funeral, and don't forget to be sure that their friends are also present. Children need their support system also.

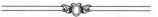

Tip—Dads should be aware of the grief process and the stages: shock and denial, anger, acceptance. A few visits to a child therapist may help understand how these stages will appear, depending on the child's age.

A most valuable source of what should be done comes from those who have been there. Barbara was four when her mother died of breast cancer at age thirty-three. Barbara, who was thirty-seven at the time of our interview, is the director of the YWCA breast-screening project. Barbara says that she has discovered that the pain of the loss of her mother is more acute now than when she was a child. *"When I had my son, my only child, at thirty, that made a difference in understanding the loss, and then when I turned thirty-three, I was the same age she was and my son was close to the age I had been. That brought it all up. It was time to deal with some of those feelings that I had not dealt with before."*

What Barbara had to face was the magnitude of the loss. She felt that as a child she just coped, as most children do, not facing the issues until later. *"The funny thing is that the older I get, the more I miss her, the more I wish I had a mother, and then having my son, I really understood the great love you have for your children."*

Barbara says she only has vague memories of her mother and that the family did not handle the loss openly or well—leaving her now with a *"great hunger to understand who she was and what happened."* Barbara and her sister, who was four years older, were separated and went to live with various relatives after their mother's death. Barbara eventually settled with her mother's mother and always felt that talking about her mother was taboo because her grandmother had been so hurt by her daughter's death. She says that message has remained with her into adulthood, leaving a subtle barrier even now when she wants to talk about her mother with relatives. Barbara says her sister has always been curious why their mother did not make plans for who would care for them after her death.

Mostly, Barbara wishes for a gift—something personal from her mother for both her sister and herself—a letter. *"Both my sister and I have said that we are sometimes angry at my mother for not having done that. We don't know if it was denial or she wouldn't accept that she was dying. We both have some of her things, but nothing personally from her to each of us. We long for some message."*

Just before we talked, Barbara had begun the process to get her mother's medical records. *"The main thing I need to say is that she wasn't real to me, and that's what I long for—something that makes her real—and that's part of why I asked for the medical records even though some people might think that is morbid. That makes her real to me."*

GRIEF COUNSELOR REVEREND JUDY KANE-SMITH TALKS ABOUT DEATH AND DYING

The Reverend Judy Kane-Smith has a master's degree in marriage and family counseling and a divinity degree in the Church of Religious Science. She counsels individuals and families in the vicinity of her California home.

When did you begin grief counseling?

When I was in high school, I worked in a geriatric center, where I was at the bedsides of people when they died. But I became the most aware of the grief process when my own father died suddenly at age fifty-five of a heart attack. I was a member of a church in Kentucky at the time and my minister said a number of things that helped, particularly, "People are only a thought away, no matter where they are. In your mind you can talk to them." So I became aware that while time eases the pain, there are specific things to do such as writing my father a letter to say goodbye. In my ministry I dealt with families in other churches who faced death and it became clear to me that we do not know how to grieve in this society. We minimize the pain. I have heard people say to others who are grieving, "Aren't you over that yet?"

How did you cope with your father's death?

I cried. It was a deep-grief kind of sobbing. Someone, to bring me back to my senses, slapped me because he thought that was the thing to do. Something inside me said strongly, NO. It's important to emote. I think we should have padded rooms for people to be, places where they can hit the wall, hit a pillow, get the physical energy out.

But ironically, we get a lot of support in the community for being "tough." Showing emotion is weak.

We do a Jackie Kennedy, which gets us a lot of respect. I always wanted to believe that in private someone held her while she

(continued)

sobbed. I had an uncle who at my grandfather's death gathered us before the service and said, "Let's show respect for Grandfather by not crying tomorrow at the service." This included my brother, who was a teenager, and this was his Gramps and he was supposed to go up and say goodbye and not cry? The result of this attitude is that people stuff the emotion inside and get nauseated and sick. There is a tremendous need for physical release.

What needs to be done to face death?

There are the tangible things you want to do, to put your estate in order so that it's left in a good place for the family. Then there's dealing with the grief, communicating with each significant person in your life to the extent that they want to and are physically able to.

People need to share what they feel before someone dies. Think about what you would miss and what would you regret not having done or said. Individually, everyone who is close to the person needs to see if there are any issues they are still angry about or family relationships that need clarifying so that's not a barrier to closeness. Wouldn't it feel good to get letters from people who love you before you go, about the value you are to them.

How does a friend talk about death? Where do you start?

Ask what they want to talk about, what they have been thinking about lately, because it doesn't matter where you start. But as you talk, when the tears start to well, you know you're starting to get to what is really saddest as well as anything about which they are hurting. Then they may pass through sad to some anger. You have no idea what emotion is going to pop out. You do a lot of listening and just looking into people's eyes and letting them know you are not going to interrupt but keep silent because there is a process that they're going through.

Friends can assist with this then?

I encourage people to find others to talk to. Start thinking. Who do you know who's gentle? They don't even have to know how

(continued)

to talk to you. It is best if they are a gentle and comforting presence around you. They won't judge how you are, and you can feel safe.

What about children and grief?

Parents need to make themselves available to each child individually. If a father doesn't know his children, this is the time to learn what their personalities are like. I do not accept when a parent says two weeks after the mother's death, "Oh, she [the child] seems to be doing fine." I don't accept that when the child's pet dies after two weeks. "He is doing fine and never talking about it." That's a warning sign that all is *not* well. But it doesn't mean you confront the child and say, we've got to talk about this right now, but you let yourself be around the child enough and even do other things. Sit and fish; go places. This gives them the opening to say something about Mom or anyone who has died or is dying, and you can say, 'What do you think about Mom?'

Remember, children emulate adults and if the adults are keeping a stiff upper lip and not talking about their mother, then that's what they will do. If they are in an environment where people are remembering and laughing about what she did and then crying because she won't ever do that again, then it's part of the conversation. This was a significant living person in this child's life, and in a fantasy life this mother is still there. If you have a child who isn't a talker, you can suggest writing. If the children are at the age where they can use crayons or write, give them a book and just say, "This is your book and nobody's going to look at it. You can write anything you want."

What kinds of things can women do with their children for remembrance?

A journal, tapes, a personal letter about what I dream for your happiness, a letter for the day you get married and for the day

(continued)

you have a baby—make it special and tangible. Take the child to a favorite store and buy a favorite something in the price range you can afford. Make it a lifetime object, some token you can take with you forever. And say, "Whenever you hold it, I'll be there, because I am always there."

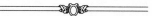

Tip—One woman approaching death wrote out birthday cards for her daughter for each year until she was eighteen, then one for each decade. She wrapped small items like a piece of family jewelry or a keepsake to be opened at Christmas.

RESOURCES

Check with your local Hospice for their reading list, or the local library should have resources to investigate.

There are a number of good books for children that deal with death. Check with the local children's librarian. Another good source of information is from the Centering Corporation, a group that has a catalog of books that deal with death. Call (409) 764-7289 for a catalog.

BOOKS FOR CHILDREN:

Lifetimes—The Beautiful Way to Explain Death to Children, by Bryan Mellonie and Robert Ingpen (Bantam Books, 1983)

Explaining Death to Children, by Earl Grollman (Beacon Press, 1967)

Books for Adults:

Who Dies, by Stephen Levine (Anchor Books, 1982)

Healing into Life and Death, by Stephen Levine (Anchor Books, 1987)

Final Gifts, by Maggie Callanan and Patricia Kelly (Poseidon Press, 1992)

Gentle Closings: How to Say Goodbye to Someone You Love, by Ted Menten (Pennsylvania Running Press, 1991)

EPILOGUE
GET INVOLVED: A LETTER
FROM THE AUTHOR

You are now one of the more than 1.5 million women who have had this disease. And my hope for you is that you will recover both physically and emotionally and be able to go on with your life.

I also hope you will not put this experience away—but join those of us in the fight for the women who will come next year and the year after with the ultimate goal being the eradication of this disease by the year 2000. I want you to get involved.

Sometime in 1991, I got politicized about breast cancer. Perhaps it was meeting so many other women in Washington in the fall of 1991 who had traveled as I had from across the country to testify about the importance of silicone implants for women who had experienced breast cancer. Most of us go through breast cancer isolated from all but a few other women who have had this disease. In Washington, I realized that my experiences with this disease were shared by women from around the country. It intensified my anger that the implant issue, in general, was pitting survivor against survivor. Whether the women were for or against implants, we had all had breast cancer. We should have been standing together to demand more research dollars instead of arguing among ourselves.

There was a bond that I saw and have since experienced with other women. When I returned to Dallas, I felt energized. I was finishing this book, but I wanted other outlets to share in areas where I was feeling a new commitment. And most important, I had done my emotional healing. I had dealt with the big questions—during two and a half years of support group meetings twice a week—and was ready emotionally to venture outside my own experience.

I was already a member of NABCO, the National Alliance of Breast

Cancer Organizations, which sends out a quarterly newsletter focusing on the latest announcements about breast cancer. I joined the Susan G. Komen Breast Cancer Foundation in Dallas and served on its grants-review committee. Komen, which was founded by Nancy Brinker, whose sister Susan Goodman Komen died of breast cancer at age thirty-six, is the nation's third-largest funding source for breast cancer research dollars.

With my surgeon and a small group of women, we formed The Bridge Breast Center, to link uninsured women with diagnostic and treatment services. This unique coalition of private physicians and breast cancer survivors provides the only private alternative for women in the Dallas area. We created the *Link,* a quarterly newsletter for the survivor audience in Dallas, which focuses on survivorship issues, such as treatment options and emotional issues. All proceeds from the newsletter support the Bridge Clinic.

So what is the message here? Get involved. Do your personal emotional work surrounding this disease and then turn power from those emotions to some aspect of this disease. You don't have to be an orator or highly educated to make a difference. It took one angry mother, whose daughter was killed by a drunk driver, to begin a movement in this country to stop drinking and driving. Whether you live in a metropolitan or a rural area, your voice can make a difference. Find a cause and work at it. Each of us has a role to play:

- Offer emotional support for those newly diagnosed by being vocal about your diagnosis. Volunteer through your hospital or as a Reach to Recovery volunteer. Join a support group—not because you need it, but because your experience might help someone else.
- Help raise awareness of this disease in your community. Fight for education about early detection. Work toward regulation for mammography. Be sure your community offers treatment options that are up-to-date. Teach doctors about care.
- Work on the state level to ensure that mammography is paid for by insurance companies. And work for insurance regulations that will benefit women with breast cancer.
- Help raise funds for research. Below are specifics about national organizations and coalitions. Start a local chapter in your city.

- Get political. There will be 10 million cancer survivors in 2000— that's 10 million votes.
- Keep up with breast cancer research issues. Join some communication network that will keep you informed.

Remember that psychologists' recommendations for beating this disease include reaching out in the community. Get involved. Do it for yourself. Do it for your sister. Do it for your daughter. Do it for your granddaughter. Do it for the 46,000 women who will die in 1993 from breast cancer. Do it for those not yet diagnosed. It can make a difference.

I'm doing it for my daughter. She will be fifteen in 2000. In January 1992, a fifteen-year-old was diagnosed in Dallas.

WHAT YOU CAN DO IN THE FIGHT AGAINST BREAST CANCER

"I have said that if this was testicular cancer, even though it has a big rate, if it was killing men in the same numbers that breast cancer is killing women, they'd find a cure in fifteen minutes."—Bridie

Across the country, women are getting organized. Learn what is being done in your community. There are also a number of national organizations that are working for political action, research dollars, and education.

NATIONAL COALITION FOR CANCER SURVIVORSHIP

In October 1992, I attended the annual Assembly of the National Coalition for Cancer Survivorship in Charlotte, North Carolina. This grassroots organization has a board composed of cancer survivors and, with a move to Washington, D.C, in 1992, promises to become a vocal advocate for cancer survivors.

Indeed, in January 1993, the NCCS took the lead in forming a Leadership Council comprising the largest, most vocal cancer support organizations from across the country. Together, these organizations drafted a policy statement on health care reform that specifically addressed the issues of cancer care and survivorship, including access to health care for all persons, preexisting conditions in health insurance, and access to clinical trials.

At the NCCS assembly, I met cancer survivors from across the country. In addition to learning that the politicism I was sensing in Dallas was nationwide, I also joined the board of this organization, which will be speaking for cancer survivors about health care reform and a range of other issues in the nineties.

There are some 8 million cancer survivors in the United States. That is a strong constituency. Workshops at the three-day assembly focused on a variety of issues geared toward the spiritual, physical, emotional, and political health of cancer survivors. The information to join NCCS is in the Resources for Chapter 1. You will receive a quarterly newsletter and be given updates on political actions of interest to cancer survivors.

The Breast Cancer Coalition

In 1991 the National Breast Cancer Coalition (NBCC), a national non-profit information and resource center based in New York, and seven other groups formed the National Breast Cancer Coalition. The coalition is a national grass-roots effort that focuses on cancer public policy with three goals: increased research funding; improved access to screening treatment and care for all women, particularly the underserved and uninsured; and increased influence and involvement of women living with breast cancer in decision-making bodies, including policymaking and clinical-trial designs.

Women can join the coalition by joining one of the member organizations. To locate those, call the coalition at (202) 296-7477.

The power of such a coalition was seen in 1992 as the combined voices of the coalition and other breast cancer groups such as NABCO, the Susan G. Komen Foundation, and the American Cancer Society combined to bring a three-fold increase in federal spending for breast cancer research—from $93 million in 1991 to more than $400 million in 1993. The tactics and lobbying that brought about this increase were a direct result of women watching for a number of years as funds for AIDS research rose proportionately to the vocal and visible presence of those afflicted by the disease. AIDS has been allocated more than $1.7 billion in 1993, a figure that some say is still disproportionate to the numbers dying of breast cancer compared to AIDS. According to U.S.

Centers For Disease Control figures, breast cancer deaths from 1982 to 1991 totaled 404,300 while AIDS deaths during the same period were 133,232.

Amy Langer, the executive director of NABCO and a breast cancer survivor, says that she does not like to compare disease dollars, since other forms of cancer are also of concern. "A lot of people ask for comparisons with AIDS just as a way to show how quickly very large government dollars can be amassed if there is sufficient urgency. But those of us in the coalition don't feel AIDS is overfunded, but rather that health is underfunded, that we need a bigger health pie and perhaps a smaller defense pie."

Women who are part of member organizations of the coalition receive updates on the process and are encouraged to contact our government officials to press for more dollars.

Amy Langer says, "What's important is that women understand that as women concerned with breast cancer progress, they are voters and they need to act like voters. They need to hold their elected officials accountable for breast cancer policy change. They need to let officials know that *that* is how women are measuring their performance. So if they don't perform, they won't be reelected. And women can do that with the coalition or alone. Make a list of your elected representatives. Sit down and write each of them a letter and tell them the following: I am concerned about breast cancer. Here's why it is important to me. I would like to know what your record is on this issue. What have you done? What do you intend to do? How quickly? Please report back to me by letter."

THE SUSAN G. KOMEN BREAST CANCER FOUNDATION

Susan Goodman Komen was thirty-six when she died of breast cancer in 1980. If there is proof that one person can make a difference, it is apparent in the foundation that bears Susan Komen's name. The foundation was started in 1982 by her sister, Nancy Brinker, who in 1984 waged her own battle with breast cancer. Brinker, who tells her story in *The Race Is One Step at a Time* (Simon & Schuster, 1990), is a survivor today. In one decade, a sister's vow has grown to be the third-largest source of funds in the country for breast cancer research. The foundation raised more than $10 million in its first decade, funds that went to 111 grants for research, education, and screening projects across the country.

The stated mission of the foundation is to "achieve higher recovery rates for breast cancer victims by advancing education, treatment and research." And the funds for those grants are raised primarily through the Race for the Cure, a series of 10K races now held in more than thirty-five sites around the country.

Nancy Brinker, who still works full-time at the foundation, is a member of the President's cancer panel, three presidential appointees who advise the President on cancer issues. She is also the chairman of a subpanel of the President's cancer panel, a committee that will investigate the progress over the past ten years of breast cancer research and where the next decade should focus in terms of funding and research.

The Race for the Cure, the foundation's primary funding source for national research, contributes 75 percent of the funds raised to the local community that sponsored the race to be used for screening or education programs, with the remaining 25 percent going to the foundation, to be distributed nationally for grants. Every year, the foundation adds new races, assisting the local organizers with planning and execution.

In spring 1991, the Komen Foundation opened an education center in Dallas, where the national help-line operates (800) I'M–AWARE, which is staffed primarily by breast cancer survivors. There are now fourteen chapters of the Komen Foundation that are actively involved in education, fund-raising, and legislation. To find if one is in your city, call the help-line. If you are interested in starting a chapter, tell the volunteer when you call that you would like to be contacted.

RESOURCES

NABCO (National Alliance of Breast Cancer Organizations) Second Floor, 1180 Avenue of the Americas, New York, NY, 10036; (212) 719–0154

Susan G. Komen Foundation in Dallas. Call 1-800-I'M AWARE. Or call the foundation headquarters in Dallas, Texas, at (214) 450-1777. Ask about chapters in your area—or about starting one!

Let me know if this book helped you in your journey. What would you like to see addressed? Send your questions and comments to Kathy LaTour, P.O. Box 141182, Dallas, TX 75214.

Thanks.

BIOGRAPHIES: THE WOMEN AND MEN OF *THE BREAST CANCER COMPANION*

=======✲◯✲=======

AMY

Diagnosed in May 1989 at age twenty-five, she chose a modified radical for intraductal carcinoma. No positive nodes and no follow-up treatment. Amy had immediate reconstruction with an expander. Married at the time of the diagnosis, Amy and her husband divorced in 1990. Amy attributed the breakup to the cancer. She has since returned full-time to college. *"My husband's maturity level was just not where it should have been to sustain what happened. It made him look at some things he didn't want to look at. The whole idea of the possibility of death was too frightening for him and he had to get away from it. He was never turned off physically. He was just terrified."*

ANDREA

Diagnosed in September 1990 at age thirty, she chose a modified radical and immediate reconstruction for intraductal carcinoma. There were no positive nodes and no follow-up treatment. Andrea, a software marketing executive, was divorced and had been dating John, a computer engineer, for two years when she was diagnosed. They were married in December 1991. *"From the very moment after the mastectomy, I just refused to be an invalid. I would get up every day, get dressed, wash my hair if I could or get a nurse to do it, walk around. I refused to wear the damn hospital gown. I wore sweat pants and a long sweater and tennis shoes."* John: *"When I saw the scar it was very scary. It was scary-intimate. My first reaction was, Well, it's not as bad as I thought. I really pictured just grotesque disfigurement, and it wasn't that at all."*

ANGELA

Diagnosed in 1983 at age twenty-three with invasive carcinoma, she had part of the tumor removed for a biopsy, followed by chemotherapy and radiation, which eliminated the remaining tumor. Angela refused a mastectomy, due to having no insurance, and no nodes were removed. Single at time of diagnosis, Angela has remained single, attributing her reluctance to get involved to her lack of confidence that a man would be supportive. *"I think when I hit the five-year mark, that's when I think I started to let go of it. I'd had this fear. I went to a psychologist afterwards because I was just scared. What do I do now? I have been fighting for my life, but I don't know how to act."*

ANN

Diagnosed in February 1990 at age thirty-six, she chose a modified radical for intraductal carcinoma with no nodes, and no follow-up treatment, followed by immediate reconstruction with an expander. A housewife and mother of an eighteen-month-old son, Ann had her second child in December 1992. *"I figured the pregnancy was worth the little bit of risk, and when it gets right down to it, Dr. K said to go ahead. I'll be a little worried during pregnancy, especially since I can't have a mammogram."*

ANNE

Diagnosed in August 1991 at age thirty-three, she chose a lumpectomy for her 2-centimeter invasive tumor with no positive nodes. She then had chemotherapy and radiation. Anne, a computer consultant, is single. Her mother had breast cancer at forty-four, a recurrence in the other breast at fifty-four, and is currently living with metastasis to the bone. *"There is just a lot we don't know about Mom. She doesn't share. Her whole relationship with her doctors is different. I want to know everything. She just lets them tell her what she needs to do and that's what she does. I wanted our doctors to talk and she wouldn't permit it."*

BETTY B

Diagnosed in October 1990, at age thirty-nine, while pregnant with her second child, she chose a modified radical mastectomy for the 2.5-centimeter invasive tumor with three positive nodes. She began chemotherapy by slow infusion through a catheter until her daughter's birth, followed by radiation and more chemotherapy. Betty, an elementary-school teacher, is married and had one son age six at the time of her diagnosis. Her mother and both grandmothers had breast cancer. Her daughter was born in February 1991. *"I just wanted the baby to be healthy. We had had testing and knew she was a girl and she was healthy before the cancer. That was reassuring. I was bonding to a sick infant. I was sure she would be sick, because I had had five treatments before she was born. But she was fine, even though she was a week early. The placenta started to disintegrate and that was why she came early. But she even had a full head of hair."*

BETTY L

Diagnosed in January 1991 at age sixty-two, she chose a modified radical for her intraductal diagnosis that presented as a large flat mass. There were no nodes involved and she had no follow-up treatment. She decided against reconstruction. Betty was married and had one son, age thirty-four, at her diagnosis. *"Immediately after surgery, I was sort of on a high. I felt wonderful and everybody was so wonderful to me, and I just felt like everything was going to be fine. Then after a month or so, I began to get depressed. I suffered depression for several months before my family decided that I needed help."*

BRIDIE

Diagnosed in September 1991 at age fifty-four, she chose a lumpectomy for her intraductal diagnosis with no positive nodes, and no follow-up treatment. When pathology detected additional malignant areas close to the margins, she had a modified radical and immediate reconstruction with an expander. Bridie, a publishing executive, was divorced and had three children ages eighteen to twenty-two at the time of her diagnosis. Bridie's mother died of breast cancer at age eighty-four. *"The ongoing pump it up for expander reconstruction is boring. I believe, in the long run, the reconstruction will be emotionally beneficial, but I am still of the opinion to just stick a sock in it."*

CHRIS

Diagnosed in April 1974 at age thirty-three, she chose a radical mastectomy for the 3-centimeter invasive tumor with one positive node. She had radiation and chemotherapy. An interior designer and mother of three- and five-year-old sons at the time of her diagnosis, she began chemo the same month her husband filed for divorce. In 1979, Chris was reconstructed using her back muscle. She has had ongoing problems with lymphedema or swelling of her arm. Today she is a representative for an arm pump that reduces lymphedema. *"I really changed after the reconstruction. People would come up to me and ask what I had done to myself and tell me how good I looked. I know that I didn't feel so old anymore. I didn't realize it had such an effect on me."*

CINDY

Diagnosed in June 1989 at age thirty-three, she chose preoperative chemotherapy and a modified radical mastectomy for four invasive tumors that totaled 6 centimeters, with no positive nodes. She had chemotherapy, followed by radiation. She underwent prophylactic removal of the other breast and bilateral reconstruction, using back muscles, in June 1992. A public relations and marketing executive when diagnosed, Cindy had been living with Larry for five years. They were engaged in spring 1990 and plan to marry in fall 1993. *"We got engaged after I finished chemo. Neither of us had wanted to make the commitment before, but this got us off dead center."* Larry: *"I really think that what helped her the most was my being strong and convinced that she was doing fine and going to be fine throughout the process. I tried to treat it like an appendectomy. Then I would go to my office and close the door and cry for hours."*

DANA

Diagnosed in March 1988 at age thirty-eight, she chose a modified radical for a 2.2-centimeter invasive tumor with three positive nodes.

She then chose chemotherapy, radiation, and hormone therapy and is planning reconstruction for the future. A physical therapist with a large suburban hospital when she was diagnosed, Dana was single at the time of diagnosis and sought counseling a year after her surgery. *"I ran out of emotional and physical strength during chemo and began to wonder why this wasn't bothering me as much as it should be. I knew I was at home drinking—alone—two or three glasses of wine a day. And it hit me that something wasn't quite right. I should be crying or mad or going out and learning to hang glide or something. That's when I contacted a psychologist through work."*

DEBRA

Diagnosed in January 1985 at age twenty-eight, she chose a modified radical mastectomy for the 3-centimeter invasive tumor. There were no positive nodes. Debra then underwent chemotherapy, radiation, and a year of hormone therapy, followed by reconstruction with the TRAM flap in 1987. Separated from her husband at the time of diagnosis and mother of a two-year-old, Debra and her husband reconciled. Their second child was born in March 1987. They are now divorced. *"I was a really insecure person before. I didn't know how I would deal with adversity. I always thought that I would fall apart. I found out I had inner strength."*

DIANA

Diagnosed in May 1991, at age thirty-eight, she chose a bilateral total glandular mastectomy and immediate reconstruction for her lobular carcinoma in situ. A 1-centimeter invasive tumor was found behind the in situ location, but there were no positive nodes and no follow-up treatment. Diana, a free-lance technical writer and desktop publisher, was married and had no children at diagnosis. *"This was considered a precancerous condition at first because I didn't know about the invasive tumor. And at first it was easy to decide because I have very dense breasts and the constant screening would be hard. Then three weeks before the surgery I started having doubts about my decision to go ahead with surgery. I think that's when I consulted a psychologist. I think it was denial. I wanted to believe the pathologist made a mistake."*

DIANE

Diagnosed in March 1987 at age thirty-two, she chose preoperative chemotherapy for the 12-centimeter invasive tumor, followed by a modified radical mastectomy. There were no positive nodes. Diane had postoperative chemotherapy, followed by radiation; she is still unsure about reconstruction. Single at diagnosis, Diane is now engaged and planning to start a family. *"Dr. H wouldn't let me leave her office until I called a friend. She said, 'Go call a friend and tell them you've gotten some bad news and you want them to be there when you get home. Go get a drink. Go work out or whatever.' So that cued me to get the support group together."*

DORIS

Diagnosed in January 1988 at age fifty-three, she chose a modified radical for the 1.5-centimeter invasive tumor with no positive nodes. She then chose radiation, followed by reconstruction using the back flap in March 1990. Doris's mother died of breast cancer. Married and the mother of one son, twenty-nine, Doris was a word processor for an insurance company at diagnosis. She is married to Maurice, who is retired from the oil business. *"It's important to tell people where you are and how you feel about it, not to hold it in yourself, because it acts like a poison. It poisons your relationships with your husband and friends. It poisons your outlook on going to work and makes it hard to get through any kind of situation, because you haven't worked out the feelings."* Maurice: *"Doris had a lot of hostility. She would go into screaming and crying and rages. But it was very vocal, which was good for her to get rid of it and get it out in the open. You don't know how it affects women. I was surprised."*

DOT

Diagnosed in August 1990 at age forty-nine, she chose a modified radical mastectomy for several small invasive tumors with one positive node, followed by chemotherapy and radiation. She is planning future reconstruction. Dot, a school librarian, was the mother of two sons, ages twenty and twenty-two, at the time of diagnosis and was married to Jack, a salesman. *"I think most insurance companies are now covering mammograms, but if they aren't, they are making a costly financial and* *human mistake. When my cancer was discovered, it was the first mammo-gram I had ever had. I had put it off because it was expensive and I had no symptoms. My attitude was, why pay them $150 to tell me I'm healthy."* Jack: *"At night after we went to bed, we both cried ourselves to sleep. We did that a lot at night. The one thing I probably resent was that she thought I was going to love her less because she only had one breast and I don't give a damn if she doesn't have any. That's not what I married her for."*

DOTTEE

Diagnosed in June 1988 at age forty-nine, she chose a lumpectomy for the 3-centimeter invasive tumor with no positive nodes. She refused chemotherapy and chose radiation. Married and the mother of seven children, Dottee, a professional colorist, used a number of complemen-tary healing therapies and began seeing a therapist. *"They were after me to do chemotherapy, but I have been in holistic medicine for twenty-five years and I did not want the toxicity that goes with chemotherapy. So I did a natural detoxification with liquid diet for two days, followed by vegetables and fruit for the next ten days."*

ELAINE

Diagnosed in February 1985 at age thirty-seven, she chose a modified radical mastectomy for the 2-centimeter invasive tumor with no positive nodes, and no follow-up treatment. After a recurrence two months later on her scalp and spine, she chose to have her ovaries removed to stop estrogen and began taking hormone therapy. She is in remission today, with no evidence of disease. Elaine, in information security, is married to Ray, a policeman, and had two children, ages eighteen and eleven, at the time of diagnosis. *"There were a lot of nights that I would lie in bed and I couldn't go to sleep and I'd just tell Ray to talk to me—talk me to sleep. I would say, 'Tell me about a vacation we're going on. Tell me about what we're going to do when we retire. Tell me about a dream you had.' Things like that. He would start telling me about something and talk me to sleep."* Ray: *"We really turned to each other for support. We started doing some things together. You learn to appreciate each other a little more when you start thinking of the possibility that she may not be around long."*

ELIZABETH P

Diagnosed in June 1984 at age forty-two, she chose a modified radical mastectomy for a 1.5-centimeter tumor with no positive nodes, and no follow-up treatment. She was reconstructed with an implant in June 1985. After a recurrence in the lymph gland under her sternum in May 1986, she had chemotherapy and radiation, and began hormone therapy. There is no evidence of disease today. Elizabeth was a fashion consultant, married, and the mother of two children, ages sixteen and ten, at diagnosis. *"This has given me an insight into who I really am and how unimportant it is to worry about all the things I was thinking I had to be. We no longer have intercourse because of the changes in the vagina due to the hormone therapy, but it is a better relationship. Now it isn't just sex, it's the real thing."*

ELIZABETH T

Diagnosed in August 1990 at age forty-one, she chose a lumpectomy for a 1.7-centimeter invasive tumor with no positive nodes. She then chose radiation and hormone therapy. The mother of an eight-year-old daughter, Elizabeth, a hospital administrator, was married to Hugh, a psychologist. *"In my case the doctor said it was up to a 25 percent chance of local recurrence, but that statistically he would catch it so soon that the numbers didn't show it would increase my mortality rate."* Hugh: *"I think there should be a caveat to be ready for this changing every aspect of your life, possibly in a big way, a significant way. It's not something that you can sweep under the rug or try to ignore."*

EMELDA

Diagnosed in August 1988 at age forty-six, she chose a lumpectomy for the 5-centimeter invasive tumor because she was uninsured and could not afford reconstruction. There were no positive nodes and she refused chemotherapy, choosing radiation. She also saw a Chinese herbalist. Emelda, a librarian, was a divorced African-American mother of two children ages twenty-two and seventeen when she was diagnosed. Her cancer recurred in her bones in late 1992. *"When I worked for the insurance company we would have to look up drugs. I looked up things for my own information. Every drug for breast cancer had a side effect. I asked if there was nothing they could take that doesn't have a side effect. I thought, well, any drug would, and with everything God has given us, surely he has given us a way to cure ourselves without having to mix and mingle all these drugs. A friend told me about Dr. X in Houston. He is from China and mixed these bags of herbs for me to take."*

EVELYN

Diagnosed in November 1990 at age seventy-two, she chose a modified radical for her intraductal diagnosis with no positive nodes, and no follow-up treatment. She decided against reconstruction. Evelyn, a housewife, had been married to Ray, a retire army colonel, for fifty-two years when she was diagnosed. They had three grown children. *"It was just the thought of death rather than any sense of loss. The feeling of, How much longer do I have?"* Ray: *"We've been through some pretty tough times. The army wasn't exactly the best-paying profession in the world back in the forties and early fifties, so she just put up with it and me. There has to be a lot of give and take. Some of our present-day men and women are unable to make that commitment."*

GALE

Diagnosed in December 1982 at age forty-six, she chose a modified radical mastectomy for the 1.5-centimeter invasive tumor with four positive nodes. She chose chemotherapy with slow infusion. She had back-flap reconstruction in 1984. Married and the mother of two grown sons, Gale, who was fired from her job the day after her last chemotherapy treatment, now owns her own business. *"There weren't any support groups in 1982. We didn't talk about this out loud. Now we are on the cover of* Time *magazine. We have to arm ourselves. We have to be aware, and we have to do something about it. I think one of the things we've got to do is make young women aware that they're not immune."*

HARRIETT

Diagnosed in April 1988 at age forty-eight, she chose bilateral modified mastectomies for a 6-centimeter invasive tumor with two positive nodes, followed by chemotherapy and hormone therapy. She has decided against reconstruction. Harriett's mother had had breast cancer more than forty years ago. Harriett, a church secretary, and her husband, Donald, a computer software designer, had been married thirty years and had five children, ages seventeen to twenty-nine, when she was diagnosed. *"Being a Reach to Recovery volunteer has been really good for me. Some people feel that they don't want to go and see people. They don't want to deal with it on a regular basis. It's better for me if I do."* Donald: *"The older son who was in college came over first thing for the surgery and was very casual about it. He was very nonchalant. I think it was from absolute fear."*

IDA ROSE

Diagnosed in April 1986 at age seventy-one, she chose a modified radical, with no follow-up treatment, for the small invasive tumor with no positive nodes. She had breast reduction on the remaining breast and wears a prosthesis. After a recurrence in 1989 in the lung lining, she chose chemotherapy and hormone therapy. She decided to stop all treatment in fall of 1991 and died in September 1992. *"In spite of cancer in the family, we have a tremendously healthy constitution and we all get through things quickly, healthily, and easily. I was out of bed the day after the mastectomy, walking all over the hospital. I was in excellent condition at the time. I recovered so fast, I forgot it ever happened."*

JOAN

Diagnosed in January 1987 at age forty-seven, she chose a lumpectomy, followed by radiation, for the intraductal diagnosis. There were no positive nodes. After a local recurrence in the same breast in May 1990, she chose a modified radical and chemotherapy for the multiple pinhead-size points. In spring 1991, she had a subcutaneous on her other breast and bilateral reconstruction, using TRAM procedure. Joan was married and had two daughters, ages eighteen and sixteen, at the time of diagnosis. Joan's mother died at age thirty-four of breast cancer, when Joan was five. *"Chemo gave me a burning feeling right here in the ribcage, and finally I found that hot sauce—salsa—helped it. I guess the acid in the tomato or something."*

JO ANNE

Diagnosed in January 1988 at age thirty-one, she chose a modified radical mastectomy for her intraductal diagnosis, and a simple mastectomy on the other breast. There were no positive nodes and no follow-up treatment. She has decided against reconstruction. Jo Anne, a social worker, was married and the mother of a six-month-old son when diagnosed. *"During the time between the biopsy and surgery I decided that I had had enough of this shit and I didn't want to go through this fear again. When I looked at the film of the other breast, I realized that we could biopsy it, but where? It looked like it had the measles. Dr. O said the problem was that we could biopsy part and it would be free and clear and miss another area that wasn't. I just felt that I was walking around with a time bomb and I wanted to live. I wanted them off. In the big picture, it was clear that I wanted them both off."*

JOANNE

Diagnosed in September 1988 at age fifty, she chose a modified radical for the 2-centimeter invasive tumor with one positive node, followed by chemotherapy, radiation, and hormone therapy. She has decided against reconstruction. Joanne was married and the mother of two daughters, ages thirty-two and thirty, and ran her own trucking business at the time of diagnosis. *"I had the lump for two and a half years, with everyone telling me it was nothing. Then after the surgery, I went back to where I had the mammograms. They tried to tell me I had had a sonogram that also showed nothing. I told them that I didn't, but their records said I did. The nurse said, 'Honey, let me take you down to the room where they do sonograms and jog your memory.' I almost turned her on her head. I said, 'Let me tell you something, honey. I did not have a brain tumor. I had breast cancer. My mind is just fine. You don't have to jog my memory. I would remember if I had had a sonogram.' "*

JOYCE

Diagnosed in January 1989 at age forty-eight, she chose bilateral modified radical mastectomies, followed by immediate reconstruction, for her .5-centimeter invasive diagnosis with no positive nodes, and no follow-up treatment. She had immediate reconstruction with expanders. Joyce, married and the mother of four teenage sons at diagnosis, is a full-time volunteer with a breast cancer foundation. *"I suppose if I were to say what my mission is in twenty-five words, it is to preach empowerment. To help women who say, 'I have a lump, but the doctor says it's all right,' and she is now on death row. It's important to get to people who turn over their life to another human being. They give their power away. Women have done it historically, and it's time it stopped."*

JUDY D

Diagnosed in April 1991 at age fifty, she chose a lumpectomy, followed by chemotherapy and radiation, for her 1.8-centimeter invasive tumor with one positive node. Judy, who is single, is a manager for a health care organization. *"The surgeon called me and said she had taken nineteen nodes and only one was malignant and she was ecstatic because she thought that was a wonderful report. I was like, 'Are you kidding?' A wonderful report to me would be zero. She said that I would understand after I met other people. And I did."*

JUDY W

Diagnosed in October 1988 at age forty-six, she chose preoperative chemotherapy, followed by a bilateral modified radical, for the 13-centimeter invasive inflammatory tumor with fourteen positive nodes. She had additional chemotherapy, radiation, and hormone therapy after surgery. Her cancer recurred in March 1990 in the spinal column and she began additional chemotherapy. On January 14, 1992, Judy died, three weeks after learning that the cancer had metastasized to her brain. Judy, a bank manager, was married and the mother of a fifteen-year-old son at diagnosis. *"What brings me down is just messing with it all. It's not on my list of things to do. There's lots of things I want to do. Like going shopping. I can go shopping all day long and be sick as a dog and feel great. It's just the hassle."*

JULIE

Diagnosed in April 1989 at age forty-two, she chose a lumpectomy, followed by chemotherapy and radiation, for the 1.5-centimeter invasive tumor. There were no positive nodes. Julie's mother had died of breast cancer fifteen years earlier. Julie, a former nurse, was married and had three children, ages twenty, seventeen, and seven, at the time of diagnosis. A year later she decided to return to school. *"I always thought that if I ever got breast cancer, I would never have a lumpectomy. How stupid of those women. Just take the breast off. Just get it over with. That's how I thought. Then, of course, I was faced with it and I decided I didn't want that. I felt I was educated and that if I had that option, I would take it since survival rates were the same."*

KAREN

Diagnosed in October 1989 at age forty, she chose a mastectomy and chemotherapy for the 1-centimeter invasive tumor with no positive nodes. Karen was reconstructed, using the TRAM procedure, in May 1990. A self-employed financial consultant, Karen was single when diagnosed. *"I could have had a lumpectomy, but I had heard of too many recurrences. I knew there was reconstruction, and I just didn't want to take the chance. Anyway, mine was near the nipple and I have small breasts, so a lump out of it would have made a big difference."*

KIM

Diagnosed in March 1987 at age thirty-one, she chose bilateral total glandular mastectomies and immediate reconstruction with implants for a lobular carcinoma in situ diagnosis. There were no positive nodes and no follow-up treatment. Kim was single at diagnosis and is now the director of a mobile breast screening unit and has become involved in a group that visits women before surgery. *"I didn't go to the support group until more than a year later. I really didn't share much with the group because I kept thinking, 'I'm in a room of women who had breast cancer, who have had lymph node involvement and it spread.' Somebody else was waiting on a bone marrow transplant. I felt like I shouldn't even talk because I couldn't hold a candle to any of these people. I didn't feel worthy. And I always called mine precancerous. Then one time I broke down and cried and cried. I finally realized that I had to face what I had been through, too."*

KIT

Diagnosed in November 1987 at age forty-four, she chose a modified radical mastectomy for the 4-centimeter invasive tumor with six positive nodes. She then chose chemotherapy. A special-education instructor and divorced mother of three children, ages eight, ten, and twelve, when she was diagnosed, Kit married in 1989. *"It was important for me to have my children see me dealing with it. You can't crawl in a corner. You have to deal with it so if they do ever have it, they can deal with it."*

KITTY

Diagnosed in January 1987 at age sixty-three, she chose a modified radical with no follow-up treatment for her 1-centimeter intraductal tumor with no positive nodes. In July 1987 Kitty had reconstruction with an implant and had the other side reduced. Kitty, a high school counselor, was married and had three grown children when she was diagnosed. *"I had lived very happily all this time, knowing there was no breast cancer in my family. My mother was one of eight daughters and a number of them lived to be quite old and no breast cancer. I had nursed my babies and I had them young and all that. This wasn't supposed to happen to me, and it did".*

LAURA MAE

Diagnosed in 1981 at age sixty-two, she chose a modified radical for her intraductal diagnosis with no positive nodes. Laura Mae, who was a widow with one grown son, was a school librarian at the time she was diagnosed. She chose not to have reconstruction. *"I could have just lost part of the breast and have radiation or do the mastectomy with no follow-up. I just didn't want to do radiation. That's how I decided."*

LEANNE

Diagnosed in November 1988 at age twenty-eight, she chose a modified radical mastectomy for the 6-centimeter invasive tumor with five positive nodes. She then had chemotherapy, radiation, and hormone therapy, followed by reconstruction in 1990 with TRAM flap. Leanne, a preschool teacher, was married to Craig, a computer programmer, and they had a two- and four-year old at the time of her diagnosis. *"I think everybody deep down knows when there's something wrong. I was never a hypochondriac. I hardly ever get sick. But I knew something was wrong, and everybody kept telling me, 'You're fine, you're fine,' and eventually I let them convince me of that. I trust myself and my instincts better now than I did before."* Craig: *"With each series of tests her emotional state seems to be getting worse. It starts earlier. I guess it's because she is close to the magical five years. The closer you get, the more you are afraid of not making it."*

LINDA H

Diagnosed in July 1989 at age thirty-nine, she chose a modified radical mastectomy for the 1-centimeter invasive tumor with one positive node. She chose chemotherapy, radiation, and hormone therapy, followed by reconstruction with an expander in March 1990. Linda, a manager with a computer company, was divorced and the mother of three daughters, ages twenty-one, nineteen, and fourteen, at diagnosis. *"It's a very lonely thing to go through and not have someone. My parents were here, but it's not the same as having a husband who can comfort you in his arms or give you a little kiss on the cheek."*

LISE

Diagnosed in December 1988 at age forty-two, she chose a lumpectomy, chemotherapy, and radiation for the 1.5-centimeter invasive tumor with no positive nodes. Lise, a medical secretary, was married to Bill, a professor at a local medical school. They had two sons, ages eleven and four, when Lise was diagnosed. *"I don't know of one woman who would not want to preserve her breast, but also I had a young child and I want to live forever. My husband said it was my decision, and since the tumor was not that big, I decided on lumpectomy."* Bill: *"Chemotherapy was the worst experience, really. It's awfully hard to sit there and watch your wife being poisoned. I mean, in effect that's what it is."*

LOLA

Diagnosed in December 1987 at age fifty-six, she chose a modified radical mastectomy for her invasive diagnosis with no positive nodes.

She had immediate reconstruction with an expander. Lola, a humor therapist, was married and the mother of four grown sons at the time of her diagnosis. *"Before I got the nipple I bought a pastie nipple at a medical supply store and it looked really good. And my husband said, You have been through so much surgery and this looks great, so why get the nipple? But I wanted to, and about a week after that I woke up in the night and told him that there was a big bug on my back. He jumps up and turns on the light and pushed this thing off the bed and ran over and stomped up and down on it and said, 'I've got it, I've got it.' And he picked up what was left, and it was my nipple. I have a good time telling that one."*

LONA

Diagnosed in May 1986 at age forty-four, she chose a modified radical for the 7-centimeter invasive tumor with eleven positive nodes. She had chemotherapy, radiation, and hormone therapy. Due to her high risk for recurrence, she had her bone marrow harvested in June 1990, in the event she would need a bone-marrow transplant in the future. She had reconstruction in 1987 with an expander. Lona, a geriatric social worker, was married and had no children. *"Most of my family had had cancer, and in a way I always felt that I gave myself permission to have it. But as soon as I realized that in counseling after the therapy, I gave my body permission not to have it again. Since then I have given myself permission to do lots of things. Like get angry and quit a job I hated."*

LYNNE

Diagnosed in November 1982 at age thirty-four, she chose a modified radical mastectomy for a 1-centimeter intraductal tumor with no positive nodes and had no follow-up treatment. Lynne, a housewife and mother of three sons, ages two, nine, and twelve, when diagnosed, chose to have the other breast removed and underwent reconstruction using the back flap in early 1984. She now volunteers with breast cancer patients at a Dallas hospital. Lynne's husband, Norm, is an attorney. *"A month after the mastectomy I had everyone convinced I was doing great. I had my doctor convinced; I had my husband convinced. I went to church Christmas Eve with a smile on my face, and everyone said, 'Look how great she's doing.' I was a mess inside and fell apart six months later."* Norm:

"When your wife has cancer, it's something you can't control. Here is something bad coming to attack your wife and you're the protector. How do you protect? And the answer is, you're helpless. There's not a blessed thing that you can do. You can't punch it in the nose. You can't sue it. You can't kill it. You've got to rely on other people to take care of this thing for you."

MADELINE

Diagnosed in November 1988 at age thirty-one, she chose a modified radical mastectomy for the 4-centimeter intraductal tumor with microscopic invasion, with immediate reconstruction with an implant. There were no positive nodes. She chose chemotherapy and hormone therapy. Madeline, a nursing student, was married and had two children, ages five and two. *"The radiologist informed me there were extensive calcifications and sent me back to my doctor. I was so naive—I remember thinking, Well, I'll just cut down on milk and cheese. However, when I returned to my doctor's office, I was ushered into his private office and he closed the door and told me the mammogram was highly suggestive of intraductal carcinoma. I went cold, but still refused to think it was cancer. After all, I had just turned thirty-one, had just decided to return to nursing school, had two great kids and one wonderful husband. Everything was too perfect. Nothing could go wrong. Wrong."*

MARILYN

Diagnosed in June 1983 at age forty-two. Chose modified radical mastectomy for a 5-centimeter invasive tumor with nine positive nodes. She then had chemotherapy, radiation, and hormone therapy. When her cancer recurred in May 1987 in liver, lungs, and bones she resumed chemotherapy, using a variety of drugs that arrested the disease for six years. Marilyn, an elementary-school teacher, was married, with one daughter age thirteen, when she was diagnosed. She died on January 5, 1993. *"I think when you have cancer, you just know what you're going to die from. Everybody is gonna die. We just know we're probably going to die from cancer. And that doesn't say we can't go out and have a car accident."*

MARJORIE B

Diagnosed in March 1987 at age thirty-three, she chose a lumpectomy and radiation for her intraductal diagnosis. After a local recurrence in the same breast in 1989, she chose a modified radical mastectomy and immediate reconstruction, using a hip flap and no implants. Marjorie, a book editor, was in the process of divorce during her first diagnosis and became engaged to Chuck, also in publishing, after her second diagnosis. They were married in 1991. *"After the second diagnosis, before my mastectomy, Chuck said let's go on vacation. We go to what we call 'space,' in the U.S. Virgin Islands. I knew what Chuck was going to do. He said, 'I really think we ought to get married.' I said, 'I can't believe you are asking me this now. I've got so much to think about. How can you possibly ask me this now.' He said he thought I might want to know that he loved me no matter what. For the two weeks we were there he kept saying, 'I can't believe you turned me down.' I said, 'I didn't turn you down. I just didn't say yes. I can't even think of marriage now.'"* Chuck: *"The proposal turned out really good, because it gives me something that I can yell at her about for the rest of our lives. How she spurned me. How lucky she is that she's got me, and all of that. But I knew I wanted to find whatever it was that I could do to say, Look, worry about all the stuff you really have to worry about, but don't worry about if I'll still find you attractive."*

MARJORIE S

Diagnosed in 1989 at age 60, she chose a modified radical for her intraductal diagnosis with no positive nodes, and no follow-up treatment. A retired widow at the time of her diagnosis, Marjorie chose not to have reconstruction. *"The surgeon told me on the phone that they would take out the suspicious place and that I would need to give consent to have a mastectomy if it was cancerous. Then he handed the phone to his receptionist, who said, 'Well, what have you decided.' He didn't do my surgery."*

MARSHA

Diagnosed in August 1989 at age forty-six, she chose a lumpectomy, chemotherapy, and radiation for the 3-centimeter invasive tumor with no positive nodes. Marsha, a library administrator, was divorced and had no children. *"I was always that person who spent more time worrying about what I should have done than living for the day. And this really made me realize that it could all be over next year. And boy, I'm going to do the stuff I want to do as much as I can."*

MARY C

Diagnosed in February 1991 at age seventy-one, she chose a modified radical for her intraductal diagnosis with no positive nodes, followed by hormone therapy. Mary, a widow with both a son and daughter over forty, is planning reconstruction. *"I'm just never going to get old, and nobody believes how old I am when I tell them. The doctor said with my body image he thought I should consider reconstruction, but I wanted to wait a year and get more information."*

MARY H

Diagnosed in December 1987 at age forty-four, she chose a modified radical mastectomy for the intraductal diagnosis with no positive nodes, and no follow-up treatment. She decided to have a simple mastectomy on the other breast in August 1988. Mary, a single corporate health care executive, does not wear prostheses and does not want reconstruction. *"The volunteer came into my room and showed me this stuffed tit that was made out of satin. She said I could make one myself and pin it on the inside of my gown when I left the hospital so my husband would feel comfortable. My immediate reaction was, 'You are an ass, lady.' First, you should have come in here with the knowledge that I am not married before telling me that I should be concerned about what someone else thinks."*

MARY-T

Diagnosed in March 1989 at age forty-two, she chose preoperative chemotherapy, followed by a modified radical, for the 6-centimeter invasive tumor with no positive nodes. She had additional chemotherapy and radiation after surgery. Mary-T was married and the mother of two sons, ages eighteen and fourteen. She had reconstruction with the TRAM flap in June 1990. Her husband, Len, was in insurance. *"I think it is so important for a man or a friend or whoever is close to let you know that they care and to give constant reinforcement of 'I love you, I care about you, I'm so sorry you had to do this.'* " Len: *"I felt helpless and inadequate and I felt like there should be more that I could be giving her. I didn't have the answers and it was a tough time. Always before, I could figure out what to do."*

MAUREEN

Diagnosed in March 1973 at age thirty-two, she chose a bilateral mastectomy for an intraductal diagnosis with no positive nodes. In 1975 she began two years of chemotherapy for a local recurrence on the skin near her scar. At the time of diagnosis, Maureen was married and had a severely retarded one-year-old daughter. She divorced in 1987 and now teaches elementary school. She chose not to have reconstruction. *"One of the good things about having a bilateral is you can go in and be whatever size you want to be. Or you can be several sizes. I have a variety of different types of prostheses. I have a gardening type and the one I wear regularly. I have no desire to be reconstructed—in part because of the tiny things that have recurred on my chest wall. I just don't want them to cover anything up that could mask anything. And I don't want to go through the pain."*

MELISSA

Diagnosed in January 1990 at age thirty-three, she chose a modified radical mastectomy for the 10-centimeter invasive tumor with no positive nodes, followed by immediate reconstruction with the TRAM flap. She then had chemotherapy, radiation, and hormone therapy. Melissa, a health care insurance administrator who was single at diagnosis, had been very careful of her breasts because her mother had had breast cancer at age forty-two. *"I immediately went back to my psychologist after the surgery because I knew that there was going to be anger there."*

MICKEY

Diagnosed in April 1987 at age forty-one, she chose a modified radical for the 3-centimeter invasive tumor with three positive nodes. Mickey chose chemotherapy and hormone therapy. In July 1988 she had a subcutaneous mastectomy on the other breast before having a bilateral back-flap reconstruction. A former school teacher and currently a customer rep with the phone company, Mickey was a divorced mother of a twenty-year-old son when she was diagnosed. She married her boyfriend of three years while undergoing chemo in September 1987 and was hospitalized for depression two months later. *"I always blamed myself for things. I think I blamed myself for the cancer, too. I was depressed and it got worse and then all of a sudden I was thinking about killing myself and starting to plan it. When I started talking about it, my husband took me to a hospital. They helped me see I was co-dependent on taking care of everyone else instead of myself."*

NANCY S

Diagnosed in September 1990 at age forty-five, she chose a lumpectomy, chemotherapy, and radiation for her 1.5-centimeter invasive tumor with no positive nodes. Nancy, who is African-American, was single and worked as a medical-supply representative at the time of her diagnosis. Nancy's cancer recurred in March 1992 in her lungs, liver, and bones. She chose chemotherapy. Nancy died in October 1992. *"I realize that the little things I worried about, like traffic and work and other people's problems and things like that, compare nothing to having cancer. I think I have a stronger faith now."*

NANCY W

Diagnosed in June 1989 at age thirty-six, she chose preoperative chemotherapy and a lumpectomy for the 4-centimeter invasive tumor with two positive nodes. She had additional chemotherapy after surgery, followed by radiation, but refused hormone therapy. Nancy, who had just begun nursing school when she was diagnosed, was married and had three children, ages six months, two, and four. *"I told the surgeon I wanted him to talk to me while I was under the anesthesia. I wanted him to tell me the process of healing, how I was going to get better. And this surgeon is really brusque but really wonderful and willing to listen. He took a deep breath and said, 'All right.' The first thing he said to me in recovery was, 'I talked to you.'"*

PAT F

Diagnosed in August 1986 at age fifty-seven, she chose a modified radical and no follow-up treatment for her intraductal diagnosis with no positive nodes. In April 1991 Pat discovered a lump in the other breast and had a second modified radical for a second primary tumor, with one positive node, followed by chemotherapy. She chose not to be reconstructed. Pat's mother had breast cancer at forty-four. The mother of three grown sons when she was diagnosed, Pat is a former school nurse and is married to John, who is retired from the oil business. *"I went to group for about a year and then was out a year because my energy was so low and I just used that as an excuse to not go. And then with my depression, I thought, well, I need to be with people."* John: *"I kept urging her to get back in the group because of the depression."*

PAT G

Diagnosed in January 1990 at age fifty-seven, she chose a lumpectomy, with chemotherapy, radiation, and hormone therapy, for the 2-centimeter invasive tumor and two positive nodes. Pat, an artist, was married and the mother of two grown daughters. *"If you live in a rural area, find the best doctor possible. I didn't stop in southeast New Mexico or west Texas. I went to Dallas and Houston to check out the possibilities and eventually went to Baylor in Dallas."*

PAT H

Diagnosed in April 1989 at age fifty-three, she chose a modified radical for her intraductal diagnosis with no positive nodes, followed by hormone therapy. Nine months later she had the other breast removed after a benign mass was removed. Married and the mother of five sons, ages nineteen to twenty-nine, Pat chose not to have reconstruction. *"You know, if someone said with reconstruction I would have the feeling back, I would go through the whole operation. But for decoration, no."*

RULA

Diagnosed in March 1990 at age twenty-eight, she chose a modified radical for the 10-centimeter invasive tumor with twelve positive nodes.

She then underwent chemotherapy and radiation before her oncologist recommended bone-marrow transplant due to small lesions in the lung. She completed the bone-marrow procedure in October 1990. Rula, a nurse, learned after her diagnosis that her mother had died of breast cancer at age thirty-two. Rula is engaged and plans to have reconstruction in the future. *"I always tell my patients with cancer that we are gifted people."*

SADIE

Diagnosed in January 1987 at the age of sixty, she chose a modified radical and radiation for two small tumors totaling 3 centimeters with no positive nodes. In May 1989, she discovered a second primary in her other breast and chose modified radical, with twelve positive nodes, followed by chemotherapy. Sadie was married and the mother of three grown children. Her mother had breast cancer at age seventy-seven. *"If I had known then what I know now, I would have had both of them off. It's no more of a problem having them both off. Even as far as how you look in clothes, it's easier with two off."*

SANDY

Diagnosed in March 1990 at age forty-seven, she chose a modified radical for the 2.5-centimeter invasive tumor, with one positive node, followed by immediate reconstruction with an expander. She then had chemotherapy. Married and the mother of five children, ages eighteen to twenty-five, Sandy has since become a Reach to Recovery volunteer. *"I went upstairs one day without my scarf and my son looked at me, shocked. I said, 'I'm so sorry, I forgot my scarf.' He is the one in the family who can't handle a cut finger."*

SHEILA

Diagnosed in February 1988 at age thirty-one, she chose a modified radical mastectomy for the 7-centimeter invasive tumor with no positive nodes. Sheila had chemotherapy, followed by reconstruction with the TRAM flap in March 1989. Sheila was single and worked in property management at diagnosis. *"I had the tummy reconstruction on March 11 and I didn't go back to work full-time until the first of May. It took ten weeks. People were complaining about the mastectomy. It was a cake walk compared to reconstruction. But don't get me wrong. I love it."*

SHERI

Diagnosed in 1985 at age twenty-nine, she chose a lumpectomy, followed by radiation, for a 2.5-centimeter invasive tumor. There were no positive nodes. Since 1985 she has had numerous other suspicious lumps removed from both her breasts. Her right breast is now much smaller than her left, but she does not want reconstruction. Six months after her diagnosis, she left her husband and two teenage children and quit her job to pursue an art career. Today she is a free-lance artist. In 1989 she married Todd, who was sixteen at the time. *"I left home young, married young, had my kids young, and went to work young. It overpowered me before I knew it. I had spent all my life doing for everyone else. Today, I am happy."* Todd: *"I am trying to help her get away from it all and kick back and have some fun."*

SHERRY

Diagnosed in October 1989 at age thirty-eight, she chose a modified radical mastectomy, with immediate expander reconstruction, for the 2.5-centimeter invasive tumor with four positive nodes, followed by chemotherapy and hormone therapy. Sherry, an administrative aid for a major corporation, and her husband, Kerry, who managed a retail fabric store, had two children, ages six and nine, at the time. *"I was going through a very bad time emotionally. I was not really wanting to live. I felt very ignored and like a piece of furniture. When Kerry found out how bad off I was, he let me know that he did care and he did love me and I got counseling and started getting better. So after the diagnosis, I began taking much better care of me. I believe the immune system was suppressed, and while I had a good diet before, now I have a great diet. I am not going to have a recurrence."* Kerry: *"When the doctor told us about the life expectancy and this and that, he asked if she had any questions or if he could do anything more for her, and she said no. I spoke up and said, 'What are you going to do for me?' and I was quite serious about it. He gave me some medication to take care of the anxiety and just take the edge off. It was quite a help for me."*

SONJA

Diagnosed in March 1985 at age thirty-eight, she chose a lumpectomy and radiation for the 3-centimeter invasive tumor with no positive nodes. She then had reconstruction to fill out her breast with an implant and had the other breast lifted. Sonja, a secretary, was divorced and rearing her children, three, eight, and seventeen, when diagnosed. *"It has definitely gone through stages. I do not have night terrors anymore, and I finally cut my hair. I expected to lose it all when I had chemo. My attitude used to be 'when it comes back' since I had decided against the mastectomy."*

SYLVIA

Diagnosed in May 1990 at age thirty-nine, she chose a modified radical for the lobular and ductal in situ diagnosis (with one small area of invasive). She had no positive nodes. Sylvia chose chemotherapy, followed by reconstruction with an expander in July 1991. She had the other breast removed at the same time. Sylvia, a dentist, was married and had a son, nine, and five-year-old twin sons. *"I've done an MRI on my neck because leaning over patients and looking in their mouths causes my neck to give me fits. I've had that in the past, but in the past it was just occupational. Now it's cancer."*

TERESA C

Diagnosed initially with bone cancer in 1972 at age twelve, Teresa lost her right leg above the knee. At fourteen, her cancer recurred in her lungs. The tumors were removed surgically, and she had radiation to both lungs and chemotherapy for two years, after which another tumor showed up in her left lung. She had more surgery, chemo, and pinpoint radiation, which was later connected to her breast tumor. Teresa, an attorney, was diagnosed with breast cancer in April 1988 at age twenty-eight, when she was six months pregnant. She chose a modified radical and chemotherapy while pregnant for the 4-centimeter tumor and two positive nodes. She had radiation and hormone therapy after the birth of her son on July 4, 1988. In 1990 Teresa had a prophylactic mastectomy on her other breast and bilateral reconstruction with expanders. Teresa's cancer recurred in her liver, lungs, and bones in August 1992. She had her ovaries removed and began hormone therapy. *"The surgeon told me that the lump was probably a clogged duct. She said at my age there was an 85 percent chance it was benign. Of course, after what I had gone through my whole life, I'm thinking, Not me. This is going to be cancer. I am always that small percentage."*

TERESA M

Diagnosed in May 1980 at age thirty-six, she chose a modified radical and radiation for the 5-centimeter invasive tumor with no positive nodes. She had reconstruction with an implant in 1982. Teresa was married and had a six-year-old son when diagnosed. In the late eighties she began working for Reach to Recovery and is now the supervisor of eighty volunteers in her metropolitan area. *"About a year after my surgery, my son began having a really bad time. He was a very bright child and all of a sudden he wasn't learning. He ended up in therapy for a year and having nightmares that his mommy was going to die and wondering if his daddy could take care of him and then having guilt feelings. He didn't know how to sort that out at seven. I asked him when he was older about it and told him how hard it was to put him into therapy. I worried about what his friends would say and whether he would ask me why when he was older. He said, 'Mom, it's one of the best things you've ever done for me.' That was wonderful to hear."*

THERESA

Diagnosed in July 1988 at age twenty-seven, she chose a modified radical for the 3-centimeter invasive tumor. There were no positive nodes. Theresa had chemotherapy, radiation, and hormone therapy, followed by an expander reconstruction in July 1989. Theresa, a restaurant manager, had been living with Scott, a mechanic, for six years at the time of diagnosis. Theresa had a recurrence on a rib in the fall of 1991 and is on hormone therapy. *"After the surgery I was more worried about him than I was about me. I was really worried that he was going to want to stay with me more out of sympathy than out of true love."* Scott: *"Seeing a counselor did her a whole lot of good; it really did. I could come home and walk in the door. Before it was better to stick your arm in the door and see if it would come back with a nub."*

VICTORIA

Diagnosed in January 1987 at age thirty-seven, she chose a bilateral modified radical for intraductal carcinoma in one breast and calcifications in the other. There were no positive nodes and no follow-up treatment. A college professor in the process of a divorce when diagnosed, Victoria had expander reconstruction ten months later. Victoria married John, also a college professor, in 1989. Their son was born in November 1990. *"When things were moving along with John, I sort of stopped and said, 'You know there is something I have to tell you.' I didn't want to just pop the scars on him, but things were progressing to the point that he was going to find out soon anyway. So I explained the whole thing to him and he really didn't have much reaction. He said it just didn't matter."*

WENDY

Diagnosed in May 1989 at age twenty-six, she chose preoperative chemotherapy and a modified radical for the 13-centimeter invasive tumor and four positive nodes. Because of the aggressiveness of her tumor and the fact that preoperative chemotherapy failed to shrink it, she was recommended for an immediate bone marrow transplant, which she underwent in October 1989. In December 1991, Wendy had reconstruction with the TRAM flap. Wendy, a paralegal, now lives in Florida with her fiancé. *"I was only the eighth breast cancer patient they had treated with bone marrow transplantation in Texas and the doc said all the others were doing fine, but it had only been two years—so he could assure me two years. I thought, Well, that's nothing. My life is just starting. But if I didn't do it, I would have died for sure."*

INDEX

489